LANGUAGE AND COMMUNICATION DISORDERS IN CHILDREN

Deena K. Bernstein
City University of New York
and
Ellenmorris Tiegerman
Adelphi University

Charles E. Merrill Publishing Company
A Bell & Howell Company
Columbus Toronto London Sydney

Photo credits: Strix Pix, pp. 1, 31; Ben Chandler, p. 20; Lavisa Wilson, p. 46; Robert Collins, p. 64; © Harvey R. Phillips/Phillips Photo Illustrators, p. 108; © Randall D. Williams. Reproduced by permission of the Licking County, Ohio, Board of Mental Retardation, p. 153; Jeff Bates, p. 172; Rohn Engh, pp. 233, 298; Jan Smyth, p. 268; Neil G. Rankin, p. 330.

Published by
Charles E. Merrill Publishing Co.
A Bell & Howell Company
Columbus, Ohio 43216

This book was set in Souvenir.
Cover Design Coordination: Cathy Watterson
Production Coordination: Jeffrey Putnam

Library of Congress Catalog Card Number: 84-43164
International Standard Book Number: 0-675-20267-1
Printed in the United States of America
1 2 3 4 5 6 7 8 9 10—89 88 87 86 85

Contents

Preface

The goal of this book is to introduce you to the dynamic areas of speech-language pathology and special education. These areas are concerned with the heart of human experience—the investigation of how children learn language and what can be done about those children who do not. The study of children's language and communication disorders requires you to apply *theories* of child development, speech and hearing sciences, and language development and disorders to the *real world* of providing language intervention to communicatively disordered children. You will be challenged and rewarded.

We have organized this book to provide you with the most up-to-date information in this rapidly changing field. We have included clinical examples in the disorder chapters to demonstrate how to apply concepts to actual evaluation and remediation.

The fundamentals of communication and language development are presented in Chapters 1 through 5. We define language, describe language acquisition, and present an overall framework. Chapters 6 and 7 provide a bridge to clinical application. Chapter 6 covers the principles of language assessment, emphasizing concepts, methods, and diagnostic techniques. Chapter 7 provides a model for designing appropriate language intervention programs. Chapters 8 through 11 focus on four language disordered populations: the mentally retarded, autistic, hearing impaired and language learning disabled. Chapter 12 concludes with a discussion of language intervention in the school setting.

We believe this book provides an introduction to the exciting area of communicative disorders. We sincerely hope it will motivate you to keep abreast of new research results and clinical procedures.

ACKNOWLEDGEMENTS

Acknowledging those who help make a text a reality is a risky venture. There is the risk that a person deserving thanks may be omitted, and there is the risk that those who have contributed to the book during its gestation may be forgotten at its birth.

Thanks to Vicki Knight, Administrative Editor, who shepherded this manuscript from beginning to end. Her experience, advice, and gentle prodding were invaluable. Marianne Taflinger was a most valuable resource person. She started us on this project and oversaw its early drafts. Jeff Putnam was equally important in the final phases of publication.

The essence of educational writing is the critique of peers. First among equals is Richard Schiefelbusch, who foresaw the need for an introductory text about language and communication disorders in children, and helped us satisfy the need he identified. We thank our reviewers: Sharon James of Syracuse University, Kenneth Gavin of Marquette University, Linda Swisher of the University of Arizona, and Bobbie Lubker of the University of North Carolina. We offer special thanks to Judith Page, University of Kentucky, Alan Kamhi, Memphis State University, Philip Prinz, Pennsylvania State University, and John Schmitt of the University of Alabama, whose suggestions and comments substantially improved the book. Our colleagues, the contributors to this text, deserve thanks for their flexibility and patience during the reworking of the manuscript.

We thank Lynn Maniscalo, who labored tirelessly, often late into the night and under the pressure of short deadlines, to type parts of the manuscript.

Last, but not least, I express my gratitude to my family. To them I owe a debt of time taken. I hope to be able to repay my debt with time, as weekends might now belong to them. My thanks to my husband and friend Josh, whose critical eye helped shape many of the chapters. Thanks also to my children, Ariella Y. and Chaim Z., for their patience and understanding.

Although my gratitude is to others, the responsibility for the text, including all errors, is indeed my own.

D.B.

I thank my sons Jeremy and Jonathan, from whom I learned more than any course or text could teach. To my husband, Solomon—now that this book is finished, start your wish-list.

To Dr. Howard Grob, Vice Provost for Academic Research, I express my deepest appreciation for all your professional support.

To Mrs. Joan McCarthy, Assistant Director of the Preschool Language Stimulation Program and my closest friend—I owe you unlimited understanding when you write your first book.

Finally, my thanks to the professionals in the Preschool Language Stimulation Program, Lizabeth Dooley, Maryann Horan, Debbie Schneider, Patricia Sanders, Diane Metzendorf, Rosemarie Cartuscielli, Lisa Pappas, Susan Ellenis and James Grossane, who provided the stimulation for this book and who represent the spirit and the future of our profession.

E.T.

To
Jeremy and Jonathan Tiegerman,
the Preschool Language Stimulation Program,
and
my students

Ellenmorris Tiegerman

To the memory
of two of my dearest friends,
my parents,
Julius and Pearl Kahan
for whom
the love and understanding of children
were overriding values

Deena Kahan Bernstein

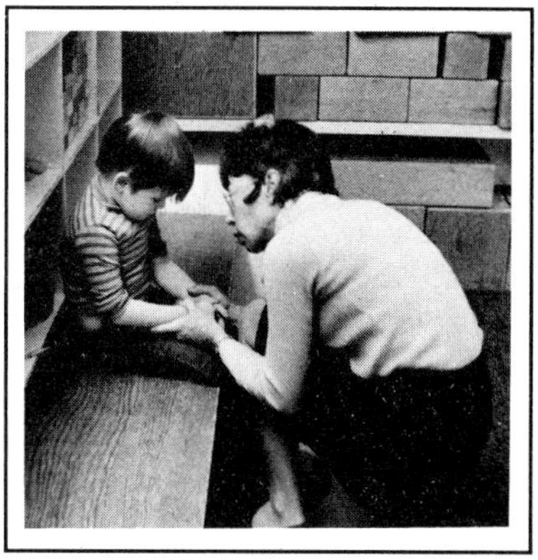

1

The Nature of Language and Its Disorders

Normal children acquire language naturally and, for the most part, without any formal instruction. Some children, however, experience serious difficulties in their acquisition of language. These children are language disordered. To overcome their disorders, such children require the assistance of various professionals, including speech and language pathologists, psychologists, and, in the school setting, special educators and resource room teachers.

The multidisciplinary nature of the study of language disorders is one of the reasons for the complexity of the discipline. Speech and language pathology, special education, sociolinguistics, linguistics, psycholinguistics and psychology, the disciplines that study language, have their own respective inventories of terms and methods. Diversity of terms, constructs, and even attitudes and biases pervades the study of language and its disorders. A cursory perusal of the writings in this field is enough to convince the student of this diversity.

A second reason for the complexity in studying language disorders relates to the complexity of language itself. Although in this decade of the 1980s we program computers to process information so that they can control a factory, cook a meal, and even fly a plane, we have not yet succeeded in programming a computer to simulate the generative nature of human language. This may happen someday, but, for the present, language remains too complex for reduction to a simpler format by programming. Comprehending language, theoretically, is a formidable task. Applying theories pragmatically to assess and to provide remediation to individuals who are language disordered is even more complex.

This chapter was written by Dr. Deena K. Bernstein, City University of New York.

The centrality of language in the human experience is a third factor that complicates the study of language disorders. Language is crucial to all social and educational functioning. Parents are most concerned that their children acquire language because they recognize that any deficiency here may have a serious effect on future educational, social, and vocational opportunities. "Language," it has been said, "may be the most distinctive attribute of human beings; its acquisition is an integral part of human development. It is not surprising that how language is learned and taught are major issues in education and other human service fields" (McCormick & Schiefelbusch, 1984, p. 2).

In this first chapter, we begin with fundamental information on three interrelated subjects relevant to language: the components or elements of language, perspectives on language acquisition, and approaches to language disorders in children. After completing this chapter, you should be able to answer the following questions:

1. What is language?
2. What components constitute language?
3. What approaches have been proposed regarding how children acquire language?
4. How can we define a language disorder?

THE NATURE OF LANGUAGE

Language is a very complex system. At the outset, it can best be understood by dividing it into various elements or components. Bloom & Lahey (1978) divide language into three major components: form, content, and use.

Form includes those elements that connect sounds or symbols with meaning. Included are three kinds of rules: rules that govern sounds and their combination; rules that govern the internal organization of words; and rules that specify how words are ordered to produce a variety of sentence types.

Content of language maps knowledge about objects and the relationships among objects, events, and people. Included are the rules governing the meanings of words and their combinations.

Use encompasses rules relating to the use of language for social communication. It assumes that the speaker has a reason for talking, a concern for his listener, the ability to use linguistic contextual information in formulating messages, and an understanding of the dynamics of discourse.

Bloom & Lahey (1978) combine these elements to define language as "the knowledge of a code for representing ideas about the world through a convention of arbitrary signals for communication" (p. 4).

The American Speech-Language-Hearing Association (ASHA), in a similar vein, defines language as a "dynamic system of conventional symbols . . . used in various modes for thought and communication" (June, 1983). According to ASHA, language is a rule–governed system composed of the five components described in the next section. It is important for the student to understand the terms for describing these linguistic components as they are the key to understanding normal language development as well as child language disorders.

Chapter 1

THE COMPONENTS OF LANGUAGE

Phonology

Every language incorporates a variety of speech sounds or phonemes. English has approximately 43 phonemes. A phoneme is the smallest linguistic unit of speech that signals a difference in meaning. The words *bat* and *pat* differ from each other in only one way—their initial sound. Because this initial sound difference produces two different words, the difference is a meaningful one. Therefore, /b/ and /p/ are, by definition, two different phonemes.

Phonemes are classified by their acoustic properties (the pattern of their sound waves), their articulatory properties (where in the oral cavity they are produced or place of articulation), and their production properties (manner of articulation).

The use of phonemes is governed by two sets of rules. One set describes how sounds can be used in various word positions. These are called distributional rules. In English, for example, the *ng* sound as in the word *long* is considered to be a single phoneme, never appearing at the beginning of a word. The second set of rules determines which sounds may be combined. They are called sequencing rules. In English, for example, the sound sequence *rs* may not appear in the same syllable. In sum, phonological rules govern the distribution and sequencing of sounds within a language.

Morphology

The second component of language—morphology—governs word formation. Morphological rules are concerned with the internal structure of words and how they are constructed from morphemes. Morphemes are the smallest linguistic unit with meaning. They may be roots, prefixes, or suffixes.

Morphemes are of two types: free morphemes and bound morphemes. Free morphemes can stand alone while bound morphemes cannot. Examples of free morphemes are *boy, tall,* and *play.* Bound morphemes, while possessing meaning, must be attached to free morphemes. Examples of bound morphemes are *s, est,* and *ed.* When these bound morphemes are attached to the three free morphemes named above, they create the words *boys, tallest,* and *played.* The bound morphemes *s, est,* and *ed* express, respectively, the meaning of "plurality," "the most," and "past tense."

Syntax

Syntax is the rule system that governs the structure of a sentence. It specifies the order words must take and the organization of different sentence types. Syntax specifies which word combinations are acceptable and which are not. "The boy hit the ball" is a syntactically correct sentence, but "Ball the boy the hit" is not. Because the words of the second sentence are out of order, it lacks meaning. Syntactic rules have two additional functions. They describe parts of speech (nouns, verbs, adjectives) and sentence constituents (noun phrase, verb phrase, etc.).

Semantics

Semantics is the component of language that governs the meaning of words and word combinations. It encompasses the meaning conveyed by individual words and the speaker's or listener's mental dictionary (called a lexicon). Words may be classified according to the knowledge they represent. For example, words that represent objects are called substantive words (e.g. *cookie, baby,* and *Mommy*). Words that map knowledge about the relationships among objects, events, and people are called relational words. *More, all gone,* and *drink,* for example, code the semantic relationships of recurrence, nonexistence, and action, respectively.

Pragmatics

Pragmatics concerns the use of language in social contexts, including rules that govern language functions (the reason for communicating) and rules that govern the choice of codes to be used when communicating (Bloom & Lahey, 1978).

The functions of language relate to the speaker's intention or goal. Greetings, asking questions, answering questions, and requesting clarification are examples of language functions.

In addition to coding communicative intentions, a speaker must use information regarding the listener and the nonlinguistic context to achieve his communicative intention. He must choose among alternative forms of a message the one which will best serve his communicative intention. The speaker must take into account what the listener already knows and does not know about a topic, as well as information about the context. The selection of the words and sentences to use to formulate a message depends upon this information. For example, knowing the age and occupation of different listeners influences the choice of words to greet them. It is appropriate to say "hi ya" to a 3-year-old, and "how do you do" to a school principal. The form of the message is also influenced by whether the topics of the message are present in the situation in which the utterance is used. For example, whether a speaker says "The doll is on the floor," or "It's over there," depends on whether the doll and the floor are in the immediate situation.

Lastly, pragmatics encompasses rules of conversation or discourse. Speakers must learn to organize their conversations to make them coherent. They must learn how to enter and initiate conversations, take turns, maintain a conversation, and close it. It is necessary to know the dynamics of discourse to be an effective communicator.

The Components of Language: Correspondence and Integration

We began this introductory chapter with a discussion of two language models: the components model of Bloom and Lahey (1978) and the functional elements model, culminating in the ASHA formulation (1983). Having reviewed both, our conclusion is that the models do not significantly differ; the functional elements may be grouped within the components. Table 1–1 depicts the correspondence. This way we make the models interchangeable and avoid confusion and misunderstanding in later discussions.

Although the components of language appear as distinct entities, Bloom and Lahey (1978) point out that they are indeed interrelated. (See Figure 1–1)

How a child integrates linguistic components is best exemplified by the $2\frac{1}{2}$–year–old child who looks through a window into the yard while his mother sits in the same room reading a book. As the child sees a kitten in the yard, he says to his mother, "Look, baby cat." As a result of this statement, the child has accomplished three things. One, he has coded two communicative intentions linguistically (*getting*

TABLE 1–1
Language Is

Components	Functional Elements
FORM	*Phonology* Rules that govern speech sounds and their combination. *Morphology* Rules that govern the internal organization of words. *Syntax* Rules that govern word order, sentence structure, and organization.
CONTENT	*Semantics* Rules that govern the meaning of words and their combinations.
USE	*Pragmatics* Rules relating to the use of language in social contexts.

attention and *describing*) by saying "look" and by describing what he sees. Next, he has linguistically coded knowledge about the animal he sees. Finally, he has expressed an utterance containing an acceptable word order. In sum, the child has successfully communicated by integrating pragmatic, syntactic, and semantic rules.

Figure 1–1. Bloom and Lahey's Model of Language

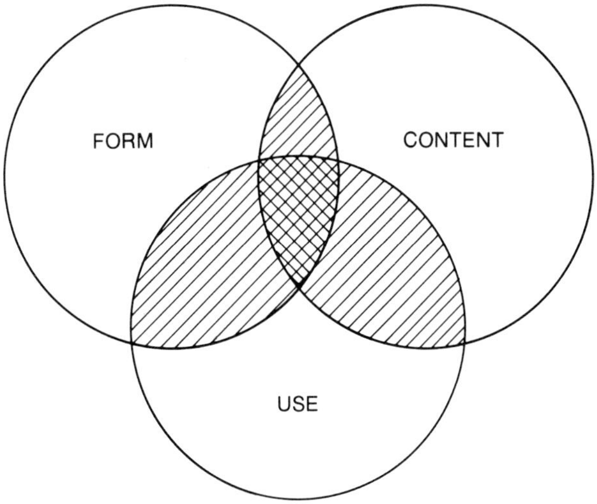

/// = overlap in components

Note. From *Language Development and Language Disorders* by L. Bloom and M. Lahey. Copyright © 1978 by John Wiley & Sons. Reprinted by permission of John Wiley & Sons, Inc.

By taking the example a step further to a 3–year–old, we are able to demonstrate the child's integration of phonology and morphology with pragmatic, syntactic, and semantic rules. Both mother and her 3–year–old child are gazing through a window as two puppies are playing in the yard.

Mother: What do you see?
Child: Two puppies.

As in the previous case, the utterance codes knowledge about the animals and contains appropriate word order. In addition, the latter utterance contains the morphological ending that codes plurality. Using phonological rules, the child "knows" that the *s* in *puppies* is pronounced as a *z* because it follows a vowel in contrast to the *s* in *cats,* which is pronounced as *s.*

Having defined language, we are now able to distinguish three very complex and often misused terms: speech, language, and communication.

SPEECH, LANGUAGE, AND COMMUNICATION

Speech

Speech is verbal communication. It involves the precise coordination of oral neuromuscular actions to form linguistic units. In addition to speech sounds, rate of speech and rhythm and intensity of sound also contribute to the speech process.

While humans primarily use speech for communicating, it is not the only means available to them. Writing and manual signing are two other formal modes of communicating.

Language

Language is the system of rules governing sounds, words, meaning, and use (see previous sections). These rules underlie both linguistic comprehension (the understanding of language) and linguistic production (the formulation of language). While children give evidence of "knowing" many of the rules of language at quite an early age, precisely how this "rule learning" occurs is still being researched by investigators.

McCormick and Schiefelbusch (1984) state that "the most important points to remember about language rules are that:

1. they are socially acquired;
2. they are not directly observable; and
3. they specify how to arrange symbols to express ideas." (p. 4)

We would like to add two other points to those of McCormick & Schiefelbusch:

4. Language is described by five parameters: phonology, morphology, syntax, semantics, and pragmatics.

5. Language learning and use are determined by the interaction of biological, cognitive, social, and environmental factors. (ASHA, 1983)

The development of the five linguistic parameters and the biological, cognitive, social, and environmental factors influencing language development are discussed more fully in chapters 2–5.

Communication

According to Muma (1978), communication is the primary function of language. It is an active process requiring a sender who encodes or formulates a message and transmits it to a receiver. The receiver decodes or comprehends the message. Each partner must be alert to the needs of the other to ensure that the messages are effectively conveyed and understood. Partners may choose to communicate in speech, in writing, or in a combination of the two.

While speech and language are crucial to the communication process, they are not the entire process. There are other aspects of communication that may enhance or distort the linguistic code. These include speech intonation patterns, stress, and the rate of speech. Nonlinguistic cues such as gestures, facial expressions, and eye contact can also add to or detract from the linguistic message.

The terms and concepts just outlined are basic to the study of language and its disorders. Definitions alone, however, are inadequate to understand language development and use. In the next section, therefore, four general perspectives on language development are presented. As this review is merely introductory, the beginning student is strongly urged to supplement it with the references noted in the text.

PERSPECTIVES ON LANGUAGE ACQUISITION

Four multidisciplinary approaches to the study of language acquisition have predominated the literature in the past two decades: the behavioral, the psycholinguistic/syntactic, the cognitive/semantic, and the pragmatic. Each approach is summarized in terms of essential elements, emphasizing background, limitations and contributions. Owens (1984) provides a more detailed description of these approaches for interested readers.

Behavioral Approach

Background. The behavioral approach to language development was first presented by B.F. Skinner (1957) in *Verbal Behavior.* Language learning, according to this approach, depends on environmental variables, which are mastered by imitation, practice, and selective reinforcement. The result is the acquisition of language through the gradual accumulation of vocal symbols and sequences of symbols. Within the process, parents and significant others are crucial because they model the appropriate utterances which children imitate and practice. By rewarding children's correct productions, parents shape children's utterances until they are grammatical and acceptable. In short, children learn language because their verbal behavior is selectively rewarded by others in the environment (Skinner, 1957). Variations on this theme are provided by Osgood (1963), Mowrer (1954), and Staats (1963).

Limitations. Chomsky (1959) faults Skinner on four counts, the first being that Skinner attempted to explain the process of language acquisition while ignoring the content being learned. Chomsky says, "There is little point in speculating about the process of acquisition without a much better understanding of *what* is acquired" (p. 55).

Second, Chomsky points out that children seem to acquire a verbal repertoire far too quickly to depend on environmental conditioning mechanisms alone. Third, Chomsky argues that children produce utterances they never heard adults use—utterances such as "I goed," and "mouses." A fourth criticism of the behaviorist model has come from research which has shown that parents rarely, if ever, correct or punish children's grammatical errors (Brown & Hanlon, 1970). Hence the role of parental reinforcement is, at best, limited and not crucial to language acquisition as described by Skinner. A further discussion of the role of imitation and reinforcement is provided in Chapter 5.

Contributions. Although in the early 1960s criticism was leveled at the behavioral school for overemphasizing parental input, recent researchers have revised their thinking to acknowledge its importance in language development. Studies by Snow (1972), Newport (1976), and others have clearly shown the positive effects of parental linguistic input to children's language development. Another contribution made by the behaviorists to the field of speech and language pathology has been to delineate "systematic training designs and their applications to nonspeaking individuals" (McCormick & Schiefelbusch, 1984; Schiefelbusch & Bricker, 1981). Structured behavioral techniques are commonly used in speech and language therapy and provide a basis for many intervention programs used with language disordered children.

Psycholinguistic/Syntactic Approach

Background. In the late 1950s and early 1960s, linguists, particularly Noam Chomsky, hypothesized that the human brain contains a mental plan to understand and generate sentences (Chomsky, 1957, 1965). This mental plan incorporates the necessary "electronic circuitry" for children to internalize the knowledge necessary for deriving sentences.

The key to Chomsky is that children have an innate predisposition to apply linguistic rules, and that the human infant is "prewired" for language acquisition. According to Chomsky, a baby is born with an innate linguistic mechanism (called Language Acquisition Device [LAD]) which is activated by exposure to linguistic input. The LAD contains two parts: a set of rules or general principles for forming sentences, and procedures for discovering how these principles are to be applied to the child's particular language.

The child's LAD processes information from the linguistic environment and generates hypotheses about the rules of his language. Through the preprogrammed LAD, Chomsky was able to explain the seemingly miraculous ability of very young children to acquire language easily and rapidly and to produce an infinite number of novel but grammatical utterances.

Limitations. Child development specialists (Schlesinger, 1977; Sinclair-deZwart, 1973) argue that Chomsky treats language learning as if it occurred independently of cognitive development. Citing Piaget's work, Sinclair-deZwart (1973) says that language development is dependent on cognitive development. Schlesinger (1977) points out that it is very difficult to ascertain from Chomsky's model precisely what children are born "knowing" as opposed to what they "come to know" and how this knowledge eventually gets linked to words and phrases.

Semanticists (Fillmore, 1968) fault Chomsky and argue that language depends more on underlying semantic representation than on syntactic rules. Sociolinguists challenge Chomsky's assertion that linguistic input is too fragmented, confused, and unsystematic to facilitate children's acquisition of language. Their data (Nelson, 1973a; Newport, 1976; Phillips, 1973; Snow, 1972), show that parental input enhances language learning. In Chapter 3 we detail the nature of parental input and its facilitating effect on language development.

Contributions. Although the psycholinguistic/syntactic approach is currently viewed as being inadequate to explain language development, Chomsky's work provided the impetus for much in-depth research on the language acquisition process. Investigators began to search for developmental patterns that crossed cultural boundaries. More important, they began to realize the value of naturalistic observations (McCormick & Schiefelbusch, 1984). A host of studies on both normal and disordered language were published in the 1960s (Menyuk, 1964; Braine, 1963; Brown & Fraser, 1963; Brown & Bellugi, 1964). Last, an alternative view of language learning evolved in contrast to the behaviorists, with the result that we currently view the child as being active and creative, rather than passive, in the language acquisition process.

Semantic/Cognitive Approach

Background. With the publication of Bloom's *Language Development: Form and Function of Emerging Grammars* (1970), there appeared a new focus in the study of language development: the meanings conveyed by children's utterances, rather than their syntax.

In her study of children's language at the early multiword stage, Bloom (1970) found that one of her subjects used "Mommy sock" on two different occasions. She used it once while she was picking up her mother's sock, and once while her mother was putting a sock on her (the child's) foot. Although the form of the child's utterance was the same in both contexts, the *meanings* the child conveyed were clearly different. On the first occasion, she conveyed possession. The sock she was holding belonged to her mother. On the second occasion, the child's utterance conveyed a meaning found between an actor (Mommy) who was doing an action, and an object (sock). Bloom concluded that children's language maps meanings. Bloom called the meaning categories that children use to code relationships among entities found in the world, semantic relations.

Bloom further postulated that children express meanings long before they know anything about syntax, and that the meanings they convey are based on prior cognitive knowledge.

Following Bloom, the cognitive prerequisites for language acquisition became the subject matter of much research. The works of Jean Piaget (1952, 1954, 1964) were reexplored and the search began for linkages between the concepts attained in early cognitive development and early linguistic constructions (Sinclair-deZwart, 1973).

The evidence (Nelson, 1973b) tends to show that children begin to use language expressively to talk about what they know, and that this knowledge is related to their sensorimotor experiences. A fuller account of the cognitive prerequisite for language acquisition is found in Chapter 3. Rees (1980) best captured the essence of the semantic/cognitive approach when she said that "children say only what they know how to mean" (p. 21).

Limitations. The semantic/cognitive approach to language development highlights the importance of meaning and cognition. However, it does not explain why some children, in spite of seemingly normal cognitive abilities, lag in their linguistic development (Cromer, 1974). It would seem that not only conceptual abilities are important to the language learning process and these abilities are not accounted for in the semantic/cognitive approach.

Three other criticisms of the semantic/cognitive view have been offered. Bowerman (1978) points out that the semantic/cognitive approach does not answer the question of *how* children acquire language, nor does it explain the relationship between later developing cognitive abilities and corresponding linguistic attainments. Schlesinger (1977) observes that the semantic/cognitive approach ignores the role of linguistic input to the language acquisition process. How could language be learned if the child is not exposed to it? Last, McLean and Snyder-McLean (1978) argue that an adequate description of language acquisition must include formulations about the nature and purposes of children's social communicative interactions. They maintain that the social environment of the child is crucial to language development.

Contributions. The semantic/cognitive approach to language development is set against a background of overall development; hence it gave impetus to multifaceted research on (a) the cognitive prerequisites of language (Sinclair-deZwart, 1973; Bowerman, 1974); (b) the universality of children's cognitive experiences resulting in a universality in their coding of meaning; and (c) the relationship between language and thought (Cromer, 1974; Miller, 1981; Rice, 1983). The role of imitation and play was reexamined (Bates, et al., 1979; Sinclair-deZwart, 1973; Westby, 1980) because scholars believed it was rooted in children's symbolic functioning. Last, the importance of contextual support (that is, the nonlinguistic context) was highlighted as being important to understanding the meanings children convey.

The Pragmatic Approach

Background. Because communicative intentions are expressed in social contexts, the pragmatic approach views language development within the framework of social development. According to Bruner (1974/1975), children learn language in order to socialize and to direct the behavior of others. Social interaction and relationships are deemed crucial for they provide the child with the framework for understanding and formulating linguistic content and form.

Within the pragmatic model, caretaker/child interactions are considered to be the originating force for language learning (Rees, 1978). As caretakers respond to infants' early reflexive behaviors and their gestures, the infant learns to communicate intentions. Infants refine these communication skills through repeated communicative interactions with caretakers.

McLean and Snyder-McLean (1978) summarize the pragmatic model in four major statements:

1. Language is acquired if and only if the child has a reason to talk. Herein it is assumed that the child has learned that he can influence his environment through communication;
2. Language is acquired as a means of acknowledging already existing communication functions;
3. Language is learned in dynamic social interactions involving the child and the mature language user in his environment. The mature language user facilitates this process;
4. The child is an active participant in this transactional process and must contribute to it by behaving in a way which allows him to benefit from the adult's facilitating behavior. (p. 28)

The pragmatic model spawned a range of new research efforts. Expanding on the work of Searle (1965), Dore (1975), and Halliday (1975), Bates (1976) formulated a classification system for categorizing children's communicative intentions, while Bruner (1974/1975), Bates (1976), and others examined the role of parents and caretakers in the language acquisition process.

Limitations. The explanation of language acquisition by the pragmatic approach leaves two major questions unanswered:

1. How do communicative intentions get linked to linguistic structures? and
2. How do children acquire symbols for referents?

Two further limitations relate to the newness of the pragmatic view. One, present researchers cannot agree on a common system for classifying communicative intentions, and two, a system for assigning a specific intention to children's utterances has not yet emerged.

Contributions. The pragmatic view highlights the social aspect of language and places language use in center stage. "It is beginning to answer many of the questions raised by other perspectives: the role of linguistic input; the continuity between gestures and words; and the ways children learn the complex social devices through which people make their intentions known" (McCormick & Schiefelbusch, 1984, p. 21).

The pragmatic approach has stimulated research on the conditions and contexts in which communication develops (Bruner, 1974/1975; Bates, 1976) and has identified the social prerequisites of language acquisition. These are discussed more fully in Chapter 2.

The four approaches to language acquisition—behavioral, psycholinguistic/syntactic, semantic/cognitive, and pragmatic—contribute to our understanding of language development and enable us to appreciate the complexity of language in the absence of a full-blown model. The need for a complete model of language acquisition, however, remains. Future research may indeed provide it, pending the successful integration of constructs developed in the four approaches reviewed here. This need for integration is best summarized by McLean and Snyder-McLean (1978):

> By nature of its content, language carries within it the products of the cognitive developmental domain; by nature of its function, language carries within it the products of social development; by nature of its form, language carries within it the complex products of all the inputs identified . . . plus the effect of the nature and functions of human physiological and neurological systems. (p. 43)

For the present, without a full model of language, we may view each approach as best describing one or more of the phases in development. As the normal child passes through these phases, different aspects of language acquisition may be emphasized. In the earliest stage of development (infancy), emphasis may be on pragmatic development. In the early preschool years, emphasis may be on syntactic development. Understanding the process of normal language acquisition provides the reader with a firm basis for understanding language disorders.

APPROACHES TO LANGUAGE DISORDERS

There are two major approaches to the study of language disorders in children: the etiological-categorical and the descriptive-developmental. In this section, we define each approach and identify the respective strengths and limitations of each. In conclusion, we present a working definition of language disorders as proposed by the American Speech-Language-Hearing Association.

Etiological-Categorical Approach

The traditional approach to child language disorders involves the classification of disorders by their causes, or etiology. Each etiological category summarizes a cluster of behaviors that differentiates the language-disordered child from his normally developing peers. McCormick and Schiefelbusch (1984) classify language disorders into five etiological categories:

1. Language and communication disorders associated with motor disorders. Included in this category are children who possess motor deficits, as well as language disorders due to brain pathology (e.g., cerebral palsy) or damage to the nervous system (e.g., spina bifida). Children in this category possess motor difficulties and may be mentally retarded, visually– and hearing–impaired, and in possession of seizure disorders. Because of the simultaneous multiple handicaps of these children and the space constraints of this text, we will not discuss this category. Instead, the reader is referred to Cruickshank (1976), McDonald and Chance (1964), and Mysack (1971) for a fuller account of this group.
2. Language and communication disorders associated with sensory deficits. Included in this category are children who possess hearing and visual impairments. Because the data on the language deficits of the blind are very scanty (Bernstein, 1978), we will discuss only hearing impairments as they relate to language disorders. (See Chapter 10.)
3. Language and communication disorders associated with central nervous system damage. Damage may be either mild or severe. Children are generally classified as learning disabled when the damage to the central nervous system is mild. When the damage to the central nervous system is severe, however, they are classified as developmental aphasics. Differentiating the aphasic from other severely language disordered children is both difficult and complex (McCormick & Schiefelbusch, 1984). Hence, we limit our discussion to the language disorders associated with learning disabilities. (See Chapter 11.)

4. Language and communication disorders associated with severe emotional-social dysfunctions. Included in this category are children who are classified as psychotic, schizophrenic, and/or autistic. These children experience a profound disruption in the development of their verbal and nonverbal interaction skills. Considerable research on this disruption has been carried out in the area of autism and is reported in Chapter 9.
5. Language and communication problems associated with cognitive disorders. Included in this category are children who are classified as mentally retarded. The cognitive disabilities of children in this group vary according to the level of retardation. Chapter 8 discusses mental retardation and the language deficits associated with it.

Strengths of the Etiological-Categorical Approach. Etiology is a convenient way of comparing and distinguishing autistic, learning disabled, mentally retarded, and hearing impaired children. Each classification is like a label that summarizes how a child is similar to, or different from, other children both within and across the disability categories.

A second and practical advantage of the etiological-categorical classification is that often a diagnostic label is needed for a child to receive appropriate services in schools. In many states today, children are placed in special education programs for speech, language, and resource services based on their diagnostic label. Furthermore, special education programs often are tailored to the etiology of a language disorder. Thus, one finds programs for the autistic, hearing–impaired, or the mentally retarded child. In this context, it is understandable that a child must be so labeled in order to be admitted to the most appropriate program.

Some advocacy groups have argued vociferously for the continuance of a categorical classification because they believe that it is better to be labeled and to receive attention and services than to be ignored. This has been especially true of advocacy groups for the severely developmentally delayed: the autistic and the mentally retarded.

A third advantage of the etiological-categorical approach is that it provides speech and language pathologists with clues as to what type of remediation might be indicated and the modalities to be used during intervention. For example, knowing that a child possesses cognitive deficits, as in mental retardation, suggests remediation that focuses on teaching the concepts that language codes and on providing the child with redundant and repetitive cues to support the language being taught. Knowing that a child is hearing–impaired may lead the speech and language pathologist to search for alternative or augmentative systems to teach language. This may involve teaching some form of manual communication (e.g., sign language) or combining manual and spoken language (e.g., total communication).

Because much of the research concerned with language and communication disorders has focused on groups of children within etiological categories, four chapters, 8, 9, 10, and 11, are devoted to explaining their findings. This information should be helpful to the speech-language pathologists working in educational or clinical settings in which diagnostic labels are used. Caution, however, is called for, as overlap among the categories exists.

Limitations of the Etiological-Categorical Approach. Drawbacks of the etiological-categorical approach are highlighted by Bloom and Lahey (1978), who point out that a particular diagnostic label does not tell the speech and language pathologist what the child really knows about language and what he needs to learn. Moreover, they state, it is rare to find a child who neatly fits into one diagnostic category. For example, it is not uncommon to find a child who is both mentally retarded and hearing–impaired or a child who is mentally retarded and also possesses autistic characteristics. In a similar vein, they maintain that a categorical label implies that there is only *one* cause of the language disorder. This is rarely the case. Although a single factor may appear in large part responsible for a language disorder, there are almost always several contributing factors.

A second critique of the etiological-categorical approach has been made by Naremore (1980), who argues that assessment and intervention are not helped by categorizing. She states that it would be difficult to find a procedure to assess a group of children defined as either mentally retarded or hearing–impaired. Within the group, assessment must be "customized" to each child with the aim of maximizing the resulting information and the understanding of that child's linguistic system and performance. The goal is to describe the child's linguistic behavior and to prescribe the specific methods and materials for improving his linguistic skills.

The Descriptive-Developmental Approach

The descriptive-developmental approach *describes* rather than classifies language disorders in children. It involves comparing the language–disordered child's ability to comprehend and formulate language with that of normal children. It assumes that a child with a language disorder needs to learn what the normal child needs to learn at some point in development (Naremore, 1980). McCormick and Schiefelbusch (1984) summarize this point of view:

> There is every reason to think that children with deficient language: (a) need language learning experiences as rich as those provided normal language users, (b) will attend to, understand and talk about many of the same objects, events and relations as typical learners, and (c) want and need to experience the same control over their environment as their more competent peers at the same stage of development. (p. 36)

According to the descriptive-developmental approach, a language disorder is "any disruption in the learning or use of the conventional system of arbitrary signals used by persons in the environment as a code for representing ideas about the world for communication" (Bloom & Lahey, 1978, p. 290). Disruptions occur either in form, content, or use, or in the interactions among them. Based on this construct, Bloom and Lahey (1978) differentiate five types of language disorders in children:

1. Children who exhibit difficulties in learning linguistic form. Included are children whose primary difficulty is in understanding and using phonological, morphological, and syntactic rules.
2. Children who exhibit difficulty in conceptualization and formulation of ideas about objects, events, and relations. Their primary difficulty is related to the semantic component—language content.

3. Children who exhibit difficulties in language use. Included are children who cannot adjust their language to meet listeners' needs, who do not use language to convey a range of communicative functions, and who have difficulties in understanding and speaking in certain contexts. Their primary deficit is in the area of pragmatics.
4. Children who exhibit difficulties in integrating form, content, and use. Bloom and Lahey (1978) termed this group of children as having association problems.
5. Children who exhibit language and communication skills that are similar in all ways to those of younger normally developing children. Delayed language development is their primary handicap.

Strengths of the Descriptive-Developmental Approach. The descriptive-developmental approach focuses on identifying the strengths and weaknesses of children with language deficits. It allows the speech and language pathologist to describe children's language behaviors and to target those areas needing remediation.

Rather than labeling a child, this noncategorical approach is instructionally relevant. It zeroes in on those areas of language that pose difficulty for the child and gives the speech-language pathologist a teaching plan and sequence.

Limitations of the Descriptive-Developmental Approach. Although the descriptive-developmental approach overcomes some of the limitations of the etiological-categorical approach, three problems still prevail:

1. It does not present the clinician with clear-cut procedures as to how to teach those areas needing remediation. While form, content, and use are useful constructs for understanding language and its disorders, the therapeutic contexts and procedures in which form, content, and use should be taught are not delineated.
2. It assumes that the administration of therapy to a language-disordered child is based on his linguistic handicap and is irrelevant to his age or total environment. The descriptive-developmental approach has been criticized by Brown and his colleagues (Brown, et al., 1976) who question whether it is useful to teach a 16–year–old mentally retarded adolescent who is developmentally a 2–year–old the same vocabulary as one might teach a normal 2–year–old. A strict adherence to the developmental approach without regard to the domestic, community, and vocational settings in which the child must ultimately function, is to Brown, et al., not educationally sound.

   Brown and his colleagues (Brown, et al., 1976) advocate an ecological perspective to intervention. The clinician is asked to search the relevant environments in which the child must function for clues as to what to teach. This might be considered the epitome of "customized therapy."
3. The descriptive-developmental approach ignores the practical problems faced by educators who require a disability label for a child prior to assignment to a special class or special services (Hobbs, 1978).

LANGUAGE DISORDERS: A DEFINITION

Because of the limitations described in both the traditional etiological-categorical approach and the descriptive-developmental approach, it is obvious that neither provides a complete definition. We present, then, ASHA's definition of language disorders as an alternative:

> A language disorder is the abnormal acquisition, comprehension or expression of spoken or written language. The disorder may involve all, one, or some of the phonologic, morphologic, semantic, syntactic, or pragmatic components of the linguistic system. Individuals with language disorders frequently have problems in sentence processing or in abstracting information meaningfully for storage and retrieval from short and long term memory. (ASHA, 1980, pp. 317–18)

According to the definition, impairment is in language comprehension (understanding), expression (formulation), or a combination of both. These deficits may be noted in listening and speaking or in reading and writing. Language–disordered children may have difficulty in processing linguistic information, organizing and storing it, and retrieving it from memory. In short, ASHA's definition informs us about three important guidelines for considering language disorders: the components of language that might be impaired, the modalities that might be impaired, and the processes that might be impaired.

SUMMARY

We began this chapter with four fundamental questions relating to the nature of language, its acquisition, and its disorders. The answers to these questions are crucial; they are the foundation upon which the remaining text is built.

Regarding language and its components, we devised a matrix for meshing language form, content, and use with phonology, morphology, syntax, semantics, and pragmatics, so that we may use the terms interchangeably. We noted the definition of language as a "dynamic system of conventional symbols that is used in various modes for thought and communication" (ASHA, 1983).

Having succeeded in defining language, we went on to explain the various approaches to language acquisition. The discussion began with the behavioral approach and proceeded through the approaches of the psycholinguistic/syntactic, semantic/cognitive, and the pragmatic. Lacking a full-blown model, we integrated the several approaches to language acquisition by suggesting that normal language acquisition is a temporal process emphasizing different dimensions of language development at different stages of chronological development. Apropos is the comment of Owens (1984) who concludes his monograph on language development by saying that "A teacher or speech–language pathologist has to rely upon many sources of information" (p. 334). These sources of information equate with the various approaches to language development. On a practical level, this means that the speech-language pathologist . . . "should be a behaviorist, a pragmatist, a cognitivist, a linguist, a developmentalist, and an optimist in order to put together an effective means of teaching language to children" (Schiefelbusch, 1978, p. 461).

A discussion of language disorders followed, with a review of two different approaches to language disorders: the etiological-categorical and the descriptive-developmental. Each approach was shown to have advantages as well as disadvantages. Unable to reconcile the differences, we presented an alternative, ASHA's approach to defining language disorders, attempting to summarize those impairments in the linguistic system that account for language disorders.

The following 11 chapters will elaborate and detail the preliminary discussions and definitions presented here. As you study the following chapters, do not hesitate to refer back to the terms and definitions outlined in this introductory chapter. This will significantly contribute to a better understanding of communication acquisition and its disorders.

STUDY QUESTIONS

1. Define these terms—speech, language, and communication.

2a. Define each of the following subsystems of language:
   a. phonology
   b. morphology
   c. syntax
   d. semantics
   e. pragmatics

2b. How do each of the subsystems above fit into Bloom and Lahey's model of form/content/use?

3. Discuss the strengths and weaknesses of each of the following perspectives in language acquisition:
   a. the behavioral perspective
   b. the psycholinguistic/syntactic perspective
   c. the cognitive/semantic perspective
   d. the pragmatic perspective

4. Compare and contrast the etiological-categorical classification of language disorders with the descriptive-developmental approaches. What are the contributions and limitations of each approach?

BIBLIOGRAPHY

The ASHA Committee on Language, Speech and Hearing Services in the Schools. (April, 1980). Definitions for communicative disorders and differences, *ASHA, 22,* 317–318.

The ASHA Committee on Language. (June, 1983). Definition of Language, *ASHA, 25,* 44.

Bates, E. (1976). *Language and Context: The Acquisition of Pragmatics.* New York: Academic Press.

Bates, E., Benigni, L., Bretherton, I., Camaioni, L., and Volterra, V. (1979). *The Emergence of Symbols: Cognition and Communication in Infancy.* New York: Academic Press.

Bernstein, D.K. (1978). *Semantic development of congenitally blind children.* Unpublished doctoral dissertation, City University of New York.

Bloom, L. (1970). *Language Development: Form and Function of Emerging Grammars.* Cambridge: MIT Press.

Bloom, L. and Lahey, M. (1978). *Language Development and Language Disorders.* New York: John Wiley & Sons.

Bowerman, M. (1974). Discussion summary—Development of concepts underlying language. In R. Schiefelbusch and L. Lloyd (Eds.), *Language*

Perspectives—Acquisition, Retardation and Intervention. Baltimore: University Park Press.

Bowerman, M. (1978). The acquisition of word meaning: An investigation in some current conflicts. In N. Waterson and C. Snow (Eds.) *The Development of Communication.* New York: John Wiley & Sons.

Braine, M. (1963). The ontogeny of English phrase structure: The first phrase. *Language, 39,* 1–13.

Brown, L., Nietupski, J., and Hamre-Nietupski, S. (1976). The criterion of ultimate functioning and public school services for severely handicapped students. In M.A. Thomas (Ed.), *Hey, Don't Forget About Me!* Reston, VA: The Council for Exceptional Children.

Brown, R. and Bellugi, U. (1964). Three processes in the child's acquisition of syntax. *Harvard Educational Review, 34,* 133–151.

Brown, R. and Fraser, C. (1964). The acquisition of syntax. In U. Bellugi and R. Brown (Eds.), The Acquisition of Language. *Monographs of the Society for Research in Child Development, 92.*

Brown, R.J. and Hanlon, C. (1970). Derivational complexity and order of acquisition. In J. Hayes (Ed.), *Cognition and the Development of Language.* New York: John Wiley & Sons.

Bruner, J. (1974/75). From communication to language. A psychological perspective. *Cognition, 3,* 225–287.

Chomsky, N. (1957). *Syntactic Structures.* The Hague: Houston.

Chomsky, N. (1959). A review of Skinner's "Verbal Behavior." *Language, 35,* 26–58.

Chomsky, N. (1965). *Aspects of the Theory of Syntax.* Cambridge: MIT Press.

Cromer, R. (1974). The development of language and cognition. The cognitive hypothesis. In D. Foss (Ed.), *New Perspectives in Child Development.* New York: Penguin Education.

Cruickshank, W. (1976). *Cerebral Palsy: A Developmental Disability.* Syracuse, New York: Universsity Press.

Dore, J. (1975). Holophrases, speech acts, and language universals. *Journal of Child Language, 2,* 21–40.

Fillmore, C. (1968). The case for case. In E. Bach and R. Harmes (Eds.), *Universal in Linguistic Theory.* New York: Holt, Rinehart and Winston.

Halliday, M. (1975). *Learning How to Mean: Explorations in the Development of Language.* New York: Edward Arnold.

Hobbs, N. (1978). Classification options: A conversation with Nicholas Hobbs on exceptional child education. *Exceptional Children, 44,* 494–497.

McCormick, L. and Schiefelbusch, R.L. (1984). *Early Language Intervention.* Columbus, OH: Charles E. Merrill Publishing Co.

McDonald, E.T., and Chance, B. Jr. (1964). *Cerebral Palsy.* Englewood Cliffs, NJ: Prentice-Hall.

McLean, J. and Snyder-McLean, L. (1978). *A Transactional Approach to Early Language Training.* Columbus, OH: Charles E. Merrill Publishing Co.

Menyuk, P. (1964). Syntactic rules used by children from preschool through first grade. *Child Development, 35,* 533–546.

Miller, J. (1981). *Assessing Language Production in Children.* Baltimore: University Park Press.

Mowrer, O. (1954). The psychologist looks at language. *American Psychologist, 9,* 660–694.

Muma, J. (1978). *Language Handbook.* Englewood Cliffs, NJ: Prentice-Hall.

Mysack, E. (1971). Cerebral palsy speech syndromes. In L.E. Travis (Ed.), *Handbook of Speech Pathology and Audiology.* Englewood Cliffs, NJ: Prentice-Hall.

Naremore, R. (1980). Language disorders in children. In T. Hixon, L. Schriberg, and J. Saxman (Eds.), *Introduction to Communication Disorders.* Englewood Cliffs, NJ: Prentice-Hall.

Nelson, K. (1973 a.) Structure and strategy in learning to talk. *Monographs of the Society for Research in Child Development, 38.*

Nelson, K. (1973 b.) Some evidence for the cognitive primacy of categorization and its functional basis. *Merrill-Palmer Quarterly, 19,* 21–39.

Newport, E. (1976). Motherese: The speech of mothers to young children. In J. Castellan, D. Pisoni, and G. Potts (Eds.), *Cognitive Theory* (Vol. 2). Hillsdale, NJ: Lawrence Erlbaum.

Osgood, C. (1963). On understanding and creating sentences. *American Psychologist, 18,* 735–751.

Owens, R.E. (1984). *Language Development.* Columbus, OH: Charles E. Merrill Publishing Co.

Phillips, J. (1973). Syntax and vocabulary of mother's speech to young children: Age and sex comparisons. *Child Development, 44,* 182–185.

Piaget, J. (1964). Three lectures. In R. Ripple and U. Rockcastle (Eds.), *Piaget Rediscovered.* Ithaca, NY: Cornell University Press.

Piaget, J. (1952). *The Origins of Intelligence in Children.* New York: International Universities Press.

Piaget, J. (1954). *The Construction of Reality in the Child.* New York: Basic Books.

Rees, N. (1980). Learning to talk and understand. In T.J. Hixon, L.D. Shriberg, and J.H. Saxon (Eds.), *Introduction to Communication Disorders.* Englewood Cliffs, NJ: Prentice-Hall.

Rice, M. (1983). Contemporary accounts of the cognition-language relationship: Implications for language clinicians. *Journal of Speech and Hearing Disorders, 48,* 347–359.

Schiefelbusch, R. (1978). Summary and interpretation. In R. Schiefelbusch (Ed.), *Bases of Language Intervention.* Baltimore: University Park Press.

Schiefelbusch, R.L. and Bricker, D.D. (Eds.) (1981). *Early Language: Acquisition and Intervention.* Baltimore: University Park Press.

Schlesinger, I. (1977). The role of cognitive development and linguistic input in language acquisition. *Journal of Child Language, 4,* 153–169.

Searle, J. (1965). What is a speech act? In M. Black (Ed.), *Philosophy in America.* New York: Allen & Unwin; Cornell University Press.

Sinclair-deZwart, H. (1973). Language acquisition and cognitive development. In T.E. Moore (Ed.), *Cognitive Development and the Acquisition of Language.* New York: Academic Press.

Skinner, B.F. (1957). *Verbal Behavior.* New York: Appleton-Century-Crofts.

Snow, C. (1972). Mother's speech to children learning language. *Child Development, 43,* 549–566.

Staats, A.W. (1963). *Complex Human Behavior.* New York: Holt, Rinehart, and Winston.

Westby, C. (1980). Assessment of cognitive and language abilities through play. *Language, Speech and Hearing Services in Schools, 111,* 154–168.

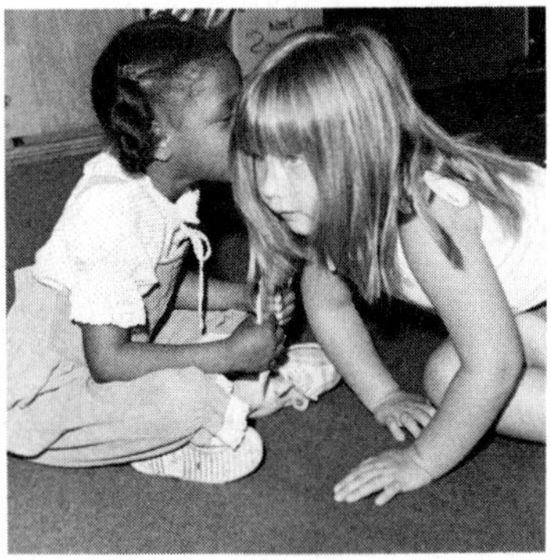

2

The Social Bases of Language Acquisition

Language codes human interaction within the social environment. During their first two years of life, children learn many behaviors that are integrated and used to communicate. Communication gradually changes, from the use of personal and idiosyncratic forms within the family, to the use of conventional forms within society (Bates, 1976; Lieven, 1977; Tiegerman & Siperstein, 1984). Children learn about the communicative *function* of language long before they learn about its linguistic *structure*.

An analysis of the development of prelinguistic behaviors highlights the social basis of the language acquisition process. Bloom and Lahey (1978) posited that prelinguistic behaviors provide the foundation for more complex forms of language. They suggested that the origin of language use begins in infancy and that certain infant behaviors are precursors to later language skills, i.e., they are "continuous with the later development of the content/form/use of language" (Bloom & Lahey, 1978, p. 76).

The sociolinguistic approach to language learning emphasizes the social-communicative functions of language (see previous chapter). The primary motivation for language development is thought to be effective communication (Bates, 1976; McLean & Snyder-McLean, 1978). The child learns to choose the form and content that will best achieve his intentions within a given communication situation. According to the sociolinguistic view, the primary context for language learning is the caretaker-child dyad.

Adult-child dyadic interaction is highly specialized for language learning. During interaction, the adult and the child negotiate the topic and purpose of communication. Although there is asymmetry in skill between the participants, there is ample evidence

---

This chapter was written by Dr. Ellenmorris Tiegerman, Adelphi University.

of reciprocity of interaction. There are features of the child's behavior that affect the language and the communication input of the adult. The attunement of the adult to the child provides the opportunity for further learning.

The processes of language learning are motivated both by the caretaker's contributions and the child's contributions. While the social environment facilitates the communication learning process, the child's organizational preprogramming imposes a bias which selects, modifies, and reorganizes the information provided in the environment (Gleitman, Newport, & Gleitman, 1984). This chapter describes the social factors that contribute to language development: maternal input, child-initiated communications, and social experiences.

MATERNAL (ADULT) INPUT VARIABLES

How adults speak to young children has been investigated by a number of researchers in recent years (Cross, 1977; Furrow, Nelson, & Benedict, 1979; Newport, Gleitman, & Gleitman, 1977; Newport, 1977). Out of this research emerges the "motherese hypothesis," which proposes that there are special properties of adult speech that play a significant role in language acquisition. According to Snow (1972), mother-child interaction represents a communication process that is sensitively attuned to the language skills of child communicators. For example, Snow suggests that the routine daily experiences of mother and child (e.g., washing, dressing, playing, and feeding) teach the child language. Within these experiences, the mother orients and regulates her speech to enhance the child's acquisition of language. Several communication and language factors provide the child with "language lessons." These are discussed by Broen (1972), Phillips (1973), Cross (1977), Remick (1972), and Snow (1977); these researchers' findings are discussed in the next section.

Complexity

A mother's language is child–sensitive in terms of its complexity; it is regulated to the child's level of comprehension. Maternal utterances, therefore, are short. They usually consist of a single clause; they are clearly enunciated; and they rarely contain a true grammatical error. Part of the facilitative effect of adult input involves the "tuning" of the adult's speech to the child's level of language development. As the linguistic structure of the child's language develops, the mother increases the syntactic complexity of her input (Snow, 1972).

Semantic Relatedness

Maternal language is child-sensitive and contextually based. The topic of conversation and the content of the interaction are determined by the child within the context. Mothers speak about the context in which the child is the focus of attention and about the child's activities. For example, if a mother sees her child playing with a large stuffed dog, she might say "nice doggie," "big doggie," or "Jimmy is playing with the doggie." This is called semantic relatedness. Snow (1977) notes that approximately 70% of mothers' speech is directly related to children's vocal, verbal, and nonverbal behavior.

Redundancy

Because maternal input relates to ongoing contextual occurrences, it tends to be redundant. A mother's linguistic message is an explanation of, clarification of, and/or comment about the child's environmental experiences. The overlapping of the linguistic with the nonlinguistic provides the young language learner with an extension of his syntactic and semantic knowledge. By coding what is occurring in the child's immediate frame of reference, the mother is providing the child with a bridge between the form and content of language. First, a mother's input provides the child with a formal code that can be used to communicate about what is happening in the context. Second, a mother's input directs the child's attention to the relevant aspects of ongoing events (e.g., agents, actions, and objects), which extends the child's semantic knowledge. Thus, by being directly related to the events in the environment, maternal input teaches the child about the overlapping relationship between the linguistic message and the nonlinguistic context. For example, if the child is pointing to a cookie that is out of reach, a mother might say, "Jeremy wants a cookie?"

Maternal Responsiveness

Another variable that contributes to the child's development of communicative behavior is the consistency in the ways in which the adult responds to the child's vocal, verbal, gestural, and/or action performances. The young communicator learns about his relationship to the environment by noting the changes created by his behavior. The consistent response or behavior from an adult or object enables the infant to note that his own behavior has a predictable effect (Beckwith, Cohen, Kopp, Parmellee,& Marcy, 1976; Bradley & Caldwell, 1976). Consider the following incident with Jeremy, a six-month-old.

Jeremy is seated in a baby-tender in the kitchen with Nana and Aunt Sue, who is a physician. Jeremy's mother is in another room of the house, when she hears Nana scream. She runs into the kitchen and finds Aunt Sue holding Jeremy upside down by his ankles. The following interchange ensues:

Nana: He's choking!

Aunt Sue: Don't get hysterical, everything is under control.

Jeremy: choke . . . choke . . . choke . . .

Nana: Do something!

Aunt Sue: What does it look like I'm doing?

In the interim, Jeremy spits up whatever is lodged in his throat. He is relaxed and returned by his mother to the baby-tender, while Aunt Sue takes care of a distraught Nana. Nevertheless, Jeremy continues to cough even though there is apparently nothing wrong with him. Everyone's response is to turn to him.

For the next several months, Jeremy continued to cough, especially in the presence of Nana, who responded consistently with additional attention and care. Nana's behavior provided the reinforcement for Jeremy's continued predictable behavior. Thus, the child's development of communication is a function of maternal response provoked by his behavior.

Bruner (1974) noted that the adult actively attempts to interpret the child's behaviors within the context: ". . . an enormous amount of consequent behavior flows from the nature of these interpretations," (p. 12). He noted that mothers provide two types of interpretations of the infant's behavior. Joint attention and reference are important parts of the mother's interpretations of the infant's behavior. One interpretation of the child's behavior involves the adult as a mediator. The adult perceives the infant's behavior as an intention to perform some action. The adult's role is to assist the infant in achieving an outcome (e.g., holding an object so the child can open it). Another form of interpretation is more concerned with the child's attention than the action. The child's gaze at an object is a signal to the adult to orient her gaze to where the child is looking; the mother then provides the child with the object. Joint attention and adult interpretation of the child's behavior help the child develop communicative behavior. Consistency of the mother's actions with objects and actions oriented to the child teaches the child to anticipate things; Bruner described this as the child's predictions of the mother's intentions. This enables the child to develop ways of signaling his own intentions. By consistently functioning as a responder/mediator when the infant initiates some behavior, the adult teaches the infant to control behavior and function as an initiator.

Reciprocity

Maternal language is sensitive to the child's independent communications. Much of the mother's behavior is directed toward eliciting responses from the infant. In treating the infant as a partner in the communication process, the mother interprets a broad range of infant behavior as communicative (e.g., yawns, sneezes, burps, and hiccups). By being responsive, the mother provides the child with role experience as a speaker. By interacting as a speaker, the mother provides the child with experience as a listener. For the infant to function as a speaker, he must learn when the conversational turn has been passed to him. The mother stimulates this learning process by making turn-taking pauses *between* utterances much longer than pauses within utterances. The mother provides these temporal lapses so that the infant learns about the speaker-listener roles (Stern, Spieker, Barnett, & MacKain, 1983). Further, the mother greatly exaggerates the terminal pitch, clearly marking the end of an utterance. This additional cue develops the infant's turn-taking behavior, later evident in conversation.

Infant studies report that the conversational nature of the mother-infant exchange occurs as early as 4 months of age (Stern, 1974; Stern, Jaffe, Beebe, & Bennett, 1974; Stern, Spieker, Barnett, & MacKain, 1983; Penman, Cross, Milgrom-Friedman, & Meares, 1983). The development of communication behaviors so early in life emphasizes their importance to the language learning process. The child's ability to interact as a speaker and as a listener forms the basic framework to communication learning. Thus, the fact that the mother modifies her speech style to encourage interaction helps us to understand the cues used by infants in language learning. She interacts with the infant with a conversational perspective and expectation. Her speech is directly related to the infant's behavior and is specifically oriented to eliciting a response from him.

In summary, there are four major implications to be drawn regarding adult language as a variable in language acquisition. One, an adult's speech to the infant learner has a much simpler structure than speech to the older language learner. An adult matches the complexity of her speech to the child's level of understanding. As the child's level of understanding becomes more sophisticated, the adult's input becomes more linguistically complex. Two, an adult's speech to the young language learner is very redundant. Three, an adult talks about what is present in the infant's immediate surroundings. Furthermore, she gives the child new and relevant information about objects and events that are directly observable to both her and the child. Four, an adult's speech encourages conversational communication.

CHILD–INITIATED COMMUNICATION

Interaction is a reciprocal process. Even the infant plays a role. Two recent studies confirm the view that the young infant is an active communicator in the interactive language learning process.

Stylistic Differences

Lieven (1977) noted a significant difference in the way two mothers communicated with their children. She showed that the mothers accommodated readily and almost naturally to the language conditions imposed by their young language learners. To the child whose style was "conversation-oriented," the mother used questions to keep the conversation going. To the child whose speech was "object- and event-oriented," the mother's comments concerned the child's environment and focused on what he was saying. This attunement of the adult communicator to the young language learner is also discussed in Barnes, Gutfreund, Satterly, and Wells (1983), who report that young children demonstrate different styles of language use. Although inadequately documented, these stylistic differences influence the input provided by adult communicators. Barnes, et al., (1983) conclude, therefore, that children facilitate changes in adult language. This, in turn, influences the future language development of children.

Gaze Behavior

One of an infant's earliest communicative acts is gazing at another human being. Mother and infant make eye contact and thereby communicate. In this first communication, both mother and child have equal control over the gaze behavior (Stern, 1974). To initiate and terminate interaction, both adults and infants effectively regulate their gaze toward or away from each other. While gazing at the infant, the mother engages in behavior unique to communication with the infant and quite different from adult communicative exchanges. Mothers sit very close to their infants, almost nose to nose, rapidly changing and exaggerating vocal variables such as rhythm, pitch, loudness, rate, and vowel production. They emphasize these vocal extremes with dramatic changes in facial expression.

The infant is not passive in this interaction. A baby's gaze has a strong effect on the mother. By regulating the gaze, the infant learns to "turn" his mother on and off. While the infant gazes at the mother, the mother does not look away. In fact, the infant is very much in control of the interaction with its mother; over 90% of all these interactions are terminated by the infant. The mother acts as if the infant were talking and responds by continuously gazing and listening.

Jaffe, Stern, and Peery (1973) propose that gazing is a prototype conversation involving mother and infant decisions as to when to look at or look away from one another. Gaze "conversation," therefore, is present long before linguistic communication is achieved.

Gaze and Vocal Behaviors

In analyzing the adult-infant "conversation," Bateson (1975) compares it structurally to the adult-adult conversation. As with adult conversations, there is near–constant eye communication and intermittent, alternating vocal communication. Thus, the mother and child maintain gaze interaction for long periods of time and alternate their vocal interchanges. In this communication interplay between the mother and infant, Bateson concludes that the mother-child communication process begins before the infant's fourth month and can be viewed as a "proto-conversation" that has definite consequences in later conversational exchanges.

Patterns of Vocal Interaction

Another factor in child–motivated variables is vocal interaction, in which there are two structurally and functionally different patterns: the simultaneous and the alternating. Mothers and infants vocalize *simultaneously* during the expression of extremely positive or negative feelings. In the alternating mode, which looks and functions like a conversational exchange, the mother and child *alternate* as speaker and listener. The presence of these two distinct patterns of vocal exchange indicates that mothers and infants engage in complex communication exchanges very early in life (Stern, Jaffe, Beebe, & Bennett, 1975). Research has further suggested that the alternating mode develops into the pattern adults use during interpersonal extremes in the affective state (Stern, Jaffe, Beebe, & Bennett, 1975).

In short, research shows that infants themselves are active contributors to the acquisition process through interaction with mother and other adults. During these early interactions, the infant learns about the communication process, including the rules for interacting with another person. The infant learns to be a speaker and a listener and to coordinate gaze, vocal, and gestural behavior into a fairly complex patterned exchange that follows the structure of adult-adult conversational exchanges (i.e., simultaneous gaze-vocal behavior followed by gaze behavior alone). We may conclude that prelinguistic patterns of behavior can be traced to early infancy, and that patterns established in this period may be reflected in later adult communicative exchanges.

SOCIAL EXPERIENCES AND COMMUNICATION LEARNING VARIABLES

Consistencies in the child's environment (objects and related actions) and the routines established in play and daily living provide a third set of factors contributing to language acquisition.

Social Play Routines

Ratner and Bruner (1978), in analyzing early children's games and routines such as peek-a-boo, reveal a highly structured pattern of mother-child exchanges containing rules that teach the infant about communication. Games like X-marks-the-spot, one-potato, patty-cake, and peek-a-boo incorporate these rules and may be considered to be of the same genre. Consider the game of X-marks-the-spot.

X marks the spot with a dot, dot, dot (tap on child's chest),
And a dash, dash, dash (draw lines across child's chest),

And a wiggle, wiggle, wiggle,
And a tickle, tickle, tickle,
And a hug
And a squeeze
And a cool mountain breeze (blow in child's face).

Four rules enhance the child's language acquisition:

1. The use of a restricted semantic format, with the adult presenting a limited number of words and semantic relationships.
2. The close relationship between what is said and what is done or performed. When mother says, "hug," she hugs the child; when she says, "squeeze," she squeezes the child. The word and the action are paired.
3. The repetition of the same words and actions each time the game is performed. The child learns the sequence of events and, eventually, predicts the next event or action.
4. A clearly defined role structure that provides for the development of speaker and listener roles.

The mother functions initially as an actor or speaker and the child functions as a recipient or listener. The mother does all of the actions to the child as she produces the verbal sequences. Ratner and Bruner report that, as the infant continues to play the game with his mother, the infant's behavior changes from passive recipient to active initiator. When the infant is between five and nine months old, he learns to be a partner in a communicative exchange, having mastered rules that include how to take turns in the exchange process and how to combine gaze, gesture, and vocal behaviors to establish, maintain, and terminate interaction. In short, the infant has become a communicator, aware of the structures of turn taking, role differentiation, and discourse components. This is in sharp contrast to the autistic language–disordered child described in Chapter 9.

Play Behaviors

Play is a mechanism for the child to learn about the world. Bruner (1969) described the play route to learning. He posited that self-initiated play stimulates learning. The ability to interact with and process reality is first related to action on or manipulation of objects within the environment. He proposes that play teaches the child about behavior not only by manipulation of objects, but by the *effect* created within the environment. As an object–manipulation experience, play teaches the child about important cognitive relationships and concepts. But it is also a social experience. The child creates a unique little world—a microcosm—to recreate the experiences he has had within the real world. Play integrates what the child has learned about objects and people.

Social Behavior and Social Interaction

In the previous sections we saw how adult-infant exchanges are communicative and social. Now we will consider to what extent and when infants are social with one another. Eckerman and Whatley (1977) provide evidence to show that infants as young as 10 months of age are socially responsive to *each other.* At 12 months, children gaze at peers, initiate interaction, and maintain exchanges with them. They also learn to discern the effect of their behaviors on others. As children develop, they become more responsive to the communicative behaviors of others, and more creative in influencing the behaviors of other social interactants.

The following incident describes this social creativity. Jeremy, a 2–year–old, is introduced to Adam, a 7–year–old autistic child who has received language therapy for several years. Jeremy speaks to Adam and moves in front of him to establish face-to-face contact. Jeremy then turns to his mother and says:

Jeremy: Mommy, Mommy, him no looka me.

Mommy: Oh? Go try again.

Jeremy returns to Adam. He starts talking to Adam in English. Adam does not respond. Jeremy then "message switches" to Spanish and again positions himself to get Adam to look at him. Again, Adam does not respond.

Jeremy: Mommy, him no looka me. Him no listena me.

Mommy: Oh (consolingly). Go try again.

Jeremy goes back to Adam, starts talking to Adam in English, then switches to Spanish, and when he does not get a response, switches to gestures. Adam still does not respond.

Jeremy: Mommy, him no looka me. Him no listena me. Him no lika me. Me no care.

Of interest here are two things: Jeremy's persistence in initiating communication and his use of different modes of communicating: gestural, verbal, and two languages. Looking, listening, and responding were behaviors that, by 24 months, Jeremy was actively using. Adam's lack of communicative behaviors disrupted the communication process.

While social behavior with peers is exhibited at about 12 months of age, researchers have found that social interaction is exhibited much earlier. At 4 months of age, infants gaze at peers as well as other adults in the environment. Gazing, touching, and vocalizing underlie the development of social behavior at this stage. At around 6 months, smiling appears as a response. As infants become more mobile (7 to 8 months), they approach, follow, and reach for adults and peers. From 9 to 12 months, children offer and take. These behaviors (summarized in Table 2–1) are important because they increase the likelihood of response from peers and adults.

TABLE 2–1
Early Interactional Behaviors

Age	*Interactional Exchange*
4 MONTHS	GAZE INTERACTION
6 MONTHS	SOCIAL SMILING
7 TO 8 MONTHS	APPROACH, FOLLOW, AND REACH
9 TO 12 MONTHS	OFFER AND TAKE
13 TO 14 MONTHS	PEER IMITATION

Adults often describe conversational exchanges between toddlers. At about 13 or 14 months, youngsters imitate each other and make noises back and forth. "With the acquisition of these component behaviors (vocal exchange, offer, approach, smile) the repertoire for social encounter is fairly complete" (Mueller & Vandell, 1976, p. 10).

SUMMARY

This chapter has described the foundations for language acquisition, beginning with the social context in which infants learn that language has a purpose: to communicate intentions. Long before the young child learns the conventional forms of language, he gazes, vocalizes, and gestures to express his intentions. These are the building blocks from which he progresses, integrating newly acquired behaviors into the communication process, until he is using conventional language forms.

The key to early communication learning is maternal input. Mothers regulate their communication to the child's particular learning style and level of understanding.

Communication grows from the mother-child relationship to child-peer relationships. Through play, the child expands his knowledge of the world about him and increases his ability to negotiate and interact with others.

Prelinguistic communicative behaviors, especially gaze behavior, are acquired early in the child-mother relationship. Gradually, these behaviors become elaborated into more sophisticated forms as seen in play, social exchange, and finally in the use of language itself.

STUDY QUESTIONS

1. How does a mother regulate her input when talking to the young language learner? How does a mother's input change as the child becomes a more sophisticated communicator?
2. What behaviors are exhibited by infants during the first 6 months that affect their mothers' interactional behaviors?
3. The adult-child interaction is in many respects different from the adult-adult interaction. What are the interaction "violations" exhibited by mothers?
4. Describe the role played by social games. How do these games facilitate language learning?
5. Describe the relationship between social play and the development of communication behaviors?

BIBLIOGRAPHY

Barnes, S., Gutfreund, M., Satterly, D., & Wells, G. (1983). Characteristics of adult speech which predict children's language development. *Journal of Child Language, 10,* 65–84.

Bates, E. (1976). Pragmatics and sociolinguistics in child language. In D. Morehead & A. Morehead (Eds.), *Normal and deficient child language.* Baltimore: University Park Press.

Bateson, M.D. (1975). Mother-infant exchanges: The epigenesis of conversational interaction. In D. Aronson & R. Rieber (Eds.), Developmental psycholinguistics and communication disorders. *Annals of the New York Academy of Sciences, 263,* 101–113.

Beckwith, L., Cohen, S., Kopp, C., Parmalee, A., & Marcy, T. (1976). Caregiver-infant interaction and early cognitive development in preterm infants. *Child Development, 47,* 579–587.

Bloom, L., & Lahey, M. (1978). *Language development and language disorders.* New York: Wiley.

Bradley, R., & Caldwell, B. (1976). The relation of infants' home environments to mental test performance at 54 months: A follow-up study. *Child Development, 47,* 1172–1174.

Broen, P.A. (1972, December). The verbal environment of the language-learning child, Monograph No. 17. American Speech and Hearing Association.

Bruner, J. (1969). Eye, hand, and mind. In D. Elkind & J. Flavell (Eds.), *Studies in cognitive development: Essays in honor of Jean Piaget.* New York: Oxford University Press.

Bruner, J. (1974). From communication to language—A psychological perspective. *Cognitive, 3,* 255–287.

Cross, T. (1977). Mothers' speech adjustments: The contribution of selected listener variables. In E.E. Snow and C.A. Ferguson (Eds.), *Talking to children.* New York: Cambridge University Press.

Eckerman, C., & Whatley, J. (1977). Toys and social interaction between infant peers. *Child Development, 48,* 1645–1656.

Furrow, D., Nelson, K., & Benedict, H. (1979). Mothers' speech to children and syntactic development: Some simple relationships. *Journal of Child Language, 6,* 423–442.

Gleitman, L., Newport, E., & Gleitman, H. (1984). The current status of the motherese hypothesis. *Journal of Child Language, 11,* 43–80.

Jaffe, J., Stern, D., & Peery, J. (1973). Conversational coupling of gaze behavior in prelinguistic human development. *Journal of Psycholinguistic Research, 2,* 321–329.

Lieven, E.V.M. (1977). Conversations between mothers and young children: Individual differences and their possible implications for the study of language learning. In E.E. Snow and C.A. Ferguson (Eds.), *Talking to children: Language input and acquisition.* New York: Cambridge University Press.

McLean, J., & Snyder-McLean, L. (1978). *A transactional approach to early language training.* Columbus, OH: Charles E. Merrill.

Mueller, E., & Vandell, D. (1976). Infant-infant interaction. In J. Osofsky (Ed.), *Handbook of infant development.* New York: Wiley Interscience.

Newport, E., Gleitman, H., & Gleitman, L. (1977). Mother, I'd rather do it myself: Some effects and non-effects of maternal speech style. In E.E. Snow & C.A. Ferguson (Eds.), *Talking to children: Language input and acquisition.* New York: Cambridge University Press.

Newport, E. (1977). Motherese: The speech of mothers to young children. In N.J. Castellan, D.B. Pisoni, & G. Potts (Eds.), *Cognitive theory* (Vol. 2). Hillsdale, NJ: Lawrence Erlbaum.

Penman, R., Cross, T., Milgrom-Friedman, J., & Meares, R. (1983). Mothers' speech to prelingual infants: A pragmatic analysis. *Journal of Child Language, 10,* 17–34.

Phillips, J. (1973). Syntax and vocabulary in mothers' speech to young children: Age and sex comparisons. *Child Development, 44,* 182–185.

Ratner, N., & Bruner, J. (1978). Games, social exchange, and the acquisition of language. *Journal of Child Language, 5,* 391–402.

Remick, H. (1972). *Maternal speech to children during language acquisition.* Paper presented at the International Symposium on First Language Acquisition, Florence, Italy.

Snow, C. (1972). Mothers' speech to children learning language. *Child Development, 43,* 549–565.

Snow, C. (1977). Mothers' speech research: From input to interaction. In E.E. Snow and C.A. Ferguson (Eds.), *Talking to children: Language input and acquisition.* London: Cambridge University Press.

Stern, D. (1971). A microanalysis of mother-infant interaction. *Journal of the American Academy of Child Psychiatry, 10,* 501–517.

Stern, D. (1974). Mother and infant at play: The dyadic interaction involving facial, vocal and gaze behaviors. In Lewis and Resenblum (Eds.), *The effect of the infant on its caregiver.* New York: Wiley.

Stern, D., Jaffe, J., Beebe, B., & Bennett, S. (1975). Vocalizing in unison and in alternation: Two modes of communication within the mother-infant dyad. In D. Aronson and R. Rieber (Eds.), Developmental psycholinguistics and communication disorders. *Annals of the New York Academy of Sciences, 263,* 89–100.

Stern, D., Spieker, S., Barnett, R., & MacKain, K. (1983). The prosady of maternal speech: Infant age and context-related changes. *Journal of Child Language, 10,* 1–16.

Tiegerman, E., & Siperstein, M. (1984). Individual patterns of interaction in the mother-child dyad: Implications for the language-disordered child. *Topics in Language Disorders, 4,* 50–62.

Vygotsky, L.S. (1976). Play and its role in the mental development of the child. In J.S. Bruner, A. Jolly, & K. Sylva (Eds.), *Play: Its role in evolution and development.* New York: Basic Books.

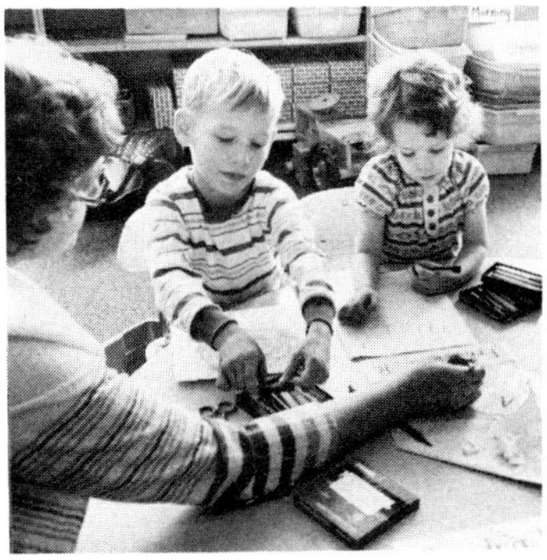

3

The Cognitive Bases to Language Development

Language is a system of components that interface to form a complex code. As a system, language should also be viewed "holistically" in terms of nonlanguage aspects of development (i.e., cognitive and social) that affect the language learning process. Cromer (1981) noted that, to understand language acquisition as a learning process, one must understand the way various developmental aspects influence one another. The degree to which language is acquired relates to the operational integrity of the general developmental system. Thus, language as an integrated system is part of a larger developmental "whole."

The previous chapter described the development of communication during social interaction, noting that language has a purpose—communication. The communicative purpose is acquired very early during the developmental process. Communication dialogue and interaction eventually lead to the child's development of communicative intentions and the use of conventional behaviors (i.e., behaviors mutually agreed upon between mother and child) that signal communication. Just as language has function, it also has form. Not only must children learn about the communicative function of language, they must learn as well the form to express their communications. An important contribution to the developing relationship between communicative function and form involves the emergence of symbols.

During the communication period from 9 to 13 months, children learn to use conventional forms of vocal and gestural behavior. As children's social experiences expand, the forms of communicative behaviors come to approximate more closely the formal code used in their culture and society. An important landmark in this progres-

This chapter was written by Dr. Ellenmorris Tiegerman, Adelphi University.

sion is the discovery that things have names. When children realize that a symbol can be substituted for its referent, communication changes qualitatively to include a symbolic form. This mental imagery or symbolic activity consists of an internalized concept of the perceptual, tactile, auditory, and action patterns related to an object in a child's interactions with it.

During the first 24 months, children learn about the communicative, linguistic, and nonlinguistic aspects of their environment. The nonlinguistic aspects of the environment provide children with direct physical experience concerning objects, actions, and people. The children's manipulations with the content of their world teach them about the relationships among people and actions and among actions and objects. This enables children to learn about how the world is organized. Their nonlinguistic experiences in the environment also contribute to the development of symbols. This chapter describes the nonlinguistic environmental experiences that affect cognitive development.

A DEVELOPMENTAL MODEL

Viewing language as part of a larger developmental model implies that the various developmental areas interface with one another; that developmental changes in one area affect occurrences in other areas; and that behaviors are shared or appear across developmental areas. The question that still needs to be answered concerns how information is shared across areas or systems. Perhaps humans possess a general learning system that looks something like a DNA molecule.

Developmental Components

In Figure 3–1, the individual strands represent various developmental components (i.e., cognition, play pragmatics, and so forth). The components intertwine, share information, and continue to develop by incorporating the shared information. In addition, during the course of the child's development, the components continue to interface.

Figure 3–1. The Interchange of Information at Various Points in Development

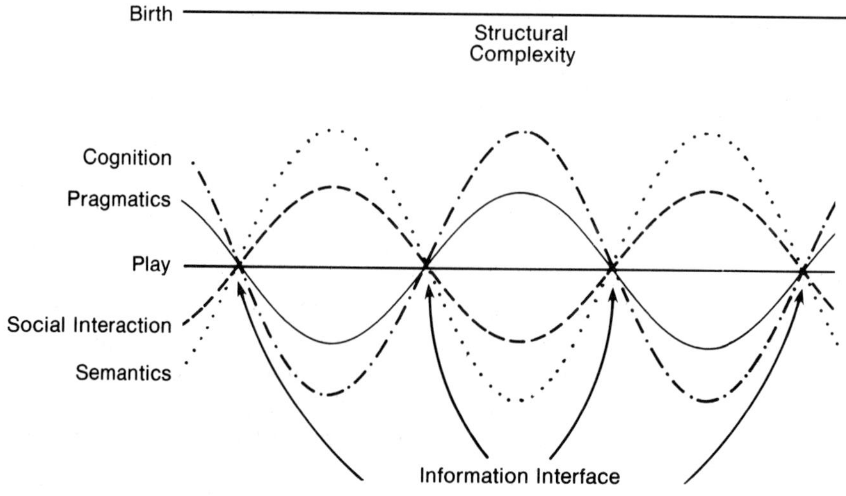

The development of each component (e.g., pragmatics) involves the integration of information from other components (e.g., social interaction, play, cognition). Thus, the manipulation of objects affects children's cognitive development. In addition, early social interactions and exchanges affect the development of pragmatic intentions. Cognition, pragmatics, play, and semantics are viewed as interrelated aspects of development. "Lack of development in any one aspect directly affects growth in all of the others" (Morehead & Morehead, 1974, p. 153).

Component Relationships

In this model, the individual learning components are operative at birth as separate and distinct areas, but they interface during development. Any two components (e.g., cognition and pragmatics) can be described as interdependent, that is, all of the components are separate areas derived from and mapped onto a more basic system, instead of being dependent on, or derived from, one another. This interdependence suggests that language is derived from broader cognitive capacities. Thus, cognitive ability would be a more basic and primary process than language, providing the foundations for language development and ultimately directing language development.

Certainly, further research will provide insight into the language learning process from birth. The purpose of the present discussion is to emphasize the function and significance of a developmental model. Several issues are presented next to highlight possible differences in the relationship between cognition and language.

COGNITION AND LANGUAGE

Various cognitive theories propose that the normal child comes to the learning environment with different types of structural and processing equipment. Common to these differing cognitive theories is the need to explain how normal children organize and code environmental experiences. This gradual process codes perceptual and conceptual patterns of social interaction into linguistic forms. Children learn to use a representational form of behavior that enables them to interact with other communicators in society.

The Strong Cognition Hypothesis

Cognition has been defined as the process of knowing and includes factors such as awareness, perception, conceptualization, and judgment. The relationship of language development to cognitive development has been an area of debate among child development specialists. There are those who claim that cognition is both necessary and sufficient for language development. This viewpoint has been termed the strong cognition hypothesis (or cognition–first hypothesis) and is discussed more fully by Rice (1980). Evidence for this point of view has been provided by many researchers including Piaget (1962), Slobin (1973), Sinclair–deZwart (1973), and Morehead and Morehead (1974).

The strong cognitive hypothesis proposes that language development is directed by perceptual-conceptual structures. The underlying contention is that language is a subsystem within a broader symbolic capacity. This symbolic capacity, in turn, depends on the development of sensorimotor intelligence. As a result, the strong cognitive hypothesis proposes that (*a*) language depends on cognitive development, and (*b*) cognitive abilities precede linguistic abilities.

Cognition Directs Language Learning

During the sensorimotor periods (birth to 24 months), children learn to experience the environment. This learning is an active process; children learn by doing. Because language is the end product of sensorimotor experience, children acquire language, which is a representational system, only when the cognitive structures have developed as a foundation. "Thus, language emerges as a means of representing already acquired knowledge" (Morehead & Morehead, 1974, p. 155).

Language, then, as a representational system, indicates that children can represent objects, actions, and events by other forms. The development of representational forms of interaction, specifically words and gestures, occurs at the close of the sensorimotor period. In addition, representational behavior is the result of sensorimotor experiences. By manipulating and experiencing agents, actions, and objects, children develop a mental image of the agent, action, or object. The representational form—the word—is related to the child's experience of an object and the immediate context within which the object was experienced.

Children develop a concept by experiencing a relationship between an object, an action performed on an object, the agent performing the action, the effect of the action on the environment (i.e., the change created), and the context characteristics. The *word,* what it means, and how it is used, is related to the child's concept of the experiences. It should not be surprising that children's word meanings are limited, because their experiences in the world are limited.

As children's experiences enlarge their perceptions and concepts of agents, actions, and objects, changes occur in their word meanings. Children's early words are used to code events in the present tense—not past or future events. The early words are often described as being "context bound," that is, denoting a specific situation or a single object.

Let us consider Jeremy's use of words at the age of 14 months.

> Jeremy carried a pacifier around with him for some 24 months. At 14 months he referred to his pacifier as a /bibi/. Although he was offered a wide range of pacifiers, especially when this bibi became rather "tired," he resolutely stated, "No. Bibi." Jeremy used several other words at this time to refer to specific objects, just as /bibi/ referred to one and only one pacifier.

Thus, the strong cognitive hypothesis holds that cognitive development precedes linguistic development and that cognitive abilities provide the underpinnings for language development.

PIAGET AND THE STRONG COGNITIVE HYPOTHESIS

Although some researchers have discerned problems in Piaget's theory of language development (Cairns & Cairns, 1976), the cognitive learning model has a great deal of support because it closely relates language and conceptual development. For many speech-language pathologists, special educators, and psychologists, Piagetian theory is holistic, explaining how language develops in relation to cognition, play, and social interaction. It describes development as a complex learning process with stages of skills that correspond to the interrelationships that occur across these components. Central to Piaget's theory of cognitive development is the description of development as the interaction of interdependent systems or processes. It is this interrelationship among systems (i.e., perception, cognition, play, language, communication, social interaction, and imitation) that results in normal learning and development.

Developmental Processes

Piaget (1968) hypothesized that cognitive development proceeds as children interact with their environment. The theory stresses the children's active role in organizing their environment. For Piaget, intellectual development parallels the stages of mental development. Intelligence is described as two-fold: adaptation and organization. The two processes of adaptation are assimilation and accommodation. Assimilation involves the incorporation of the environment into present patterns of behavior. When children carry out an action sequence (e.g., grasping a cup), they have assimilated reality to the action scheme. Accommodation involves a change in scheme as a function of the environment. When a child changes the action scheme to conform to the environment (e.g., grasps the cup more tightly when lifted from the high chair), she has modified her behavior to fit reality. These processes enable children to accommodate their performance to environmental and contextual changes, which are in turn incorporated for use in other situations. These processes help children develop a complex repertoire of behaviors for solving problems as the contexts change. Intelligence is a system of hierarchical organizations that do not become fully operational until the end of a long developmental process. Finally, according to Piaget, cognitive development results from *interaction* among genetic programming, physical maturation, environmental experience, and self-regulation.

Piagetian Principles

Some important aspects of Piaget's theory include:

1. Distinct periods of development are postulated to be universal and sequentially invariant
2. Biological structures focus and direct the infant's learning
3. The child learns through experience and interaction with the environment
4. The child must learn to act upon and transform the environment to know reality
5. Physical knowledge is learned by experiencing actions and object characteristics
6. Perception (i.e., sensory processing, sensory reorganization, sensory exploration) is an active rather than a passive learning process
7. Perceptual development permits the development of symbolic representational systems
8. Language is part of and is one form of symbolic functioning
9. Cognitive structures and their development underlie the acquisition of language
10. Symbolic functioning includes all mental behavior concerned with aspects of reality that are not immediately present
11. Language differs from other forms of symbolic functioning because it is a social communication system rather than an isolated internal system (i.e., imagery)

TABLE 3–1
Piaget's Stages of Development

Stages of Cognitive Development	Corresponding Chronological Age
I Sensorimotor	Birth to 24 months
II Preoperational (1 thought)	2 to 7 years
III Concrete operations	7 to 11 years
IV Formal operations	11 to 14 years

12. Language as a social system is the end result of communicative, cognitive, social, play, and imitative development
13. Language, as a symbolic function, represents the child's reality—the child's experiences (Morehead & Morehead, 1974)

Piaget described four stages of cognitive development and their associated developmental ages.

The Principle of Distancing

The "principle of distancing" underlies the developmental changes that occur during Piaget's sensorimotor period. Piaget described the development of language as being based within the sensorimotor period (birth to 24 months). The distancing principle provides an explanation for the unique progression of accomplishment in which children learn to control their actions and the actions of others.

At first, only reflexes are manifested. These reflexes undergo modifications with experience; movements are brought under the infant's voluntary control. During this period, children free themselves from the physical constraints of gravity, maturation, space, and time. They gradually learn to overcome these constraints of space and time to develop the ultimate form of distancing—symbolic or representational behavior. Actions are directed toward objects and events, and intentionality of action emerges. Children learn and use means–to–end sequences to explore new objects and situations. New means are invented in goal–oriented activities. The ability to represent the environment or reality in another form (deferred imitation, symbolic play, imagery, language) enables children to separate an object or event from its referent in the immediate context. Representation allows children to symbolically remove the object or event from its time and physical place. The ability to represent reality permits children to free themselves from the immediate present.

Sensorimotor Period (birth to 24 months)

The sensorimotor period consists of six substages:

Substage 1 (birth to 2 months)—Infants' behavior is controlled by involuntary reflexes. As these reflexive behaviors begin to change, children develop more voluntary control of their behavior. The infants are active learners; as they gain more motor control, they attempt directly to apply patterns of movements to the environment.

Substage 2 (2 to 4 months)—These applications of movement to the environment often bring an unanticipated result that provides an important source of learning for the infants. To recreate the environmental response, infants repeat their behavior over and over. In directing their behavior to the environment, infants also learn to coordinate visual, auditory, and tactile sensations with motor activity such as sucking, crying, and grasping.

Substage 3 (4 to 8 months)—Infants' ability to crawl and stand gives them a new perspective of their environment. In directing their behavior to objects, infants begin to note the effect created by their actions. They develop an object class and differentiate themselves from other objects in their environment. The development of an object concept eventually results in object permanence. Thus, when an object leaves the infants' sight, they will look for it.

Substage 4 (8 months to 1 year)—Infants coordinate their actions in different ways to develop new action patterns, eventually becoming able to determine which action (means) results in a particular goal (end). The infants learn to direct their behavior to achieve a goal; the means now precedes the end. Becoming increasingly mobile, children develop intentional and anticipatory behaviors interacting with objects and people. They learn that other people can be an important source of action, further differentiating themselves from others.

Substage 5 (1 year to 18 months)—Children actively pursue novelty, exploring objects in their environment to discover their properties. In order to expand this physical knowledge, they vary their actions on objects and observe the effects. By the end of this stage, the child exhibits "adultomorphisms" (i.e., relational knowledge enabling them to use objects in a way that is similar to adult use (Morehead & Morehead, 1974)).

Substage 6 (18 months to 2 years)—This stage marks the end of the sensorimotor period and the transition to the next stage. By representation, children now can manipulate reality internally. They become able to find new means to achieve a goal not only by external or physical activity, but also by internalized processes. They may achieve a goal by sudden comprehension or insight (Piaget & Inhelder, 1969). The ability to represent objects or events and their related action patterns is the onset of symbolic behavior (Piaget, 1962).

In summary, during the sensorimotor period, the child progresses from reflexive, involuntary behavior to physically generated, intentional behavior to internally (i.e., symbolic) generated intentional behavior.

Illustrative of this process is an incident involving Jeremy when he was 16 months of age. At the end of Substage 5, Piaget described the development of relational knowledge; children can now manipulate objects in ways that they observe others doing around them. This relational knowledge is evidenced by performing "adultomorphisms."

> Jeremy had a babysitter, who spoke to him only in Spanish. When she scolded him, she would shake her head and finger at him and say "No toca (touch)! No toca!" One evening, Jeremy's mother heard some noise in the kitchen and proceeded to look for Jeremy. She peeked into the kitchen to see Jeremy open a drawer and take out two cooking mitts, which he put on. Chattering away, he opened the oven, took out a pan, and slammed the door shut. He put the pan on the stove, took off the mitts and threw them back into the drawer. While shaking head and finger, he said "No! No! No!"

This is a typical incident for the child at this substage of development. What does it indicate? The adultomorphism indicates that the child has the ability to integrate, within his world and his experience, complex sequences of behavior that he has observed within his environment. Here Jeremy was recreating a situation that he had experienced with his babysitter—a situation that was both meaningful and memorable to him.

Language During the Sensorimotor Period

If language is one form of representational behavior, what are the other forms of representational behavior? Language is a social system; it serves a social and interactional function. Language enables children to distance themselves in time and space by referring to objects and events that are not immediately present. Thus, language development depends on underlying cognitive structures.

Several components are important to understanding children's language abilities during the first 24 months of life. First, from a cognitive perspective, children's language is concrete or contextually based because their mental operations are concrete. During the sensorimotor period, children tend to talk about the here and now. Their cognitive abilities, according to the strong cognitive hypothesis, determine their language abilities. Children who cannot talk about past or future events cannot cognitively separate themselves, objects, or actions from the immediate context. At this stage, children can talk about only what is happening and what they are doing right now. Changes in language development, therefore, reflect changes in cognitive abilities. As children conceptually learn to reconstruct past actions, they use words to refer to those actions, and to evoke their recurrence in the present and immediate context. Thus, children talk initially about their own actions and eventually about the performance of other agents outside the boundaries of the present place and time.

PLAY

The importance of object manipulation and play interaction has been described in the development of learning and social skills in the normal child. Piaget (1962) noted that, to know the environment, it is necessary to manipulate and control it. In the process of manipulating the environment, children discover properties of objects and how objects interrelate. For example, children can understand *in* only from objects that allow putting in (e.g., a mouth or a cup, but not a table). Reality is based upon children's physical knowledge, which is based upon direct interactional experience.

Social Interaction

Aside from the development of physical knowledge, objects also play an important role in the emergence of both social behaviors and interactions (Mueller & Vandell, 1976). Mueller and DeStefano (1973) have theorized that objects may be so important in development because they provide a basis for social interaction. Infants may notice a peer manipulate objects, inviting their mutual investigation of how objects and people interact. This theory explains why a majority of early social contacts in normal childhood include objects. Durfee and Lee (1973) found that, in 6–to–9 month–old children, at least 60% of the contact sequences with others involved inanimate objects.

Eckerman, Whatley, and Kutz (1975) noted that objects seemed to "act as vehicles" for various forms of interaction.

Play and Cognitive Development

Clune, Paolella, and Foley (1979) suggested that there may be a relationship between play and cognition (intellectual and mental development). Play assessment may provide an indirect way of measuring the child's cognitive abilities, which cannot be determined by standardized tests. The advantage of using play as a measure is that it provides a quantitative and objective means of evaluating children.

Westby (1980) indicated that symbolic play skills provide a basis for assisting cognitive development. She noted that some cognitive skills consistently precede or coincide with certain communication and language performances. She also maintained that there is a relationship among language, cognition, and play. She developed a scale that describes symbolic play stages for evaluation purposes, demonstrating how play performances integrate with language structures and how play-language performances change in developmental complexity. The underlying premise is that cognitive structures provide the foundation for language learning. This cognitive view of language development proposes that cognitive training can advance language development—not the other way around. Play might serve two functions. First, play experiences may provide a means of developing the sensorimotor prerequisites (i.e., cognitive skills) necessary for language acquisition. Westby suggested that the speech-language pathologist may be able to stimulate cognitive development by facilitating sensorimotor experiences through play. Second, play assessment permits the professional to perform two clinical functions, evaluation and remediation.

Garvey (1974) noted that play progression parallels Piaget's stages of cognitive development (see Table 3–2). First, play with objects and peers is imitative and repetitive. Second, normal children develop a variety of responses to objects and peers (e.g., feed baby, diaper baby, wash baby, put baby to bed). They also develop play performances, which are functionally related to the object itself. Third, normal children during play evidence communicative structures, such as turn-taking, which are an integral part of the social exchange process.

TABLE 3–2
Garvey's Play Stages

	Normal Child Play Performances	*Impaired Child Play Performances*
STAGE I:	play with objects and peers, imitative and repetitive play performances	limited manipulation repertoire, lack of interest in peer interaction, fixation with one kind of manipulation
STAGE II:	differential responses to objects and peers, play performances which are functionally appropriate, knowledge of object within context	lack of differential response across objects and contexts, level shift from repetitive manipulation to differential manipulation does not occur
STAGE III:	communicative structures in play interaction, play as a social exchange process	no development of communicative behaviors, no social interaction, no social play exchange

From Garvey, C., Some properties of social play. *Merrill Palmer Quarterly, 20,* 163–80.

Play and Learning

Michelman (1976) hypothesized that children learn and experience through play. As they become involved in play, their gaze is spontaneously associated with action manipulations. Thus, play interaction integrates two behavioral performances—gaze and manipulation. This gives children the opportunity to observe the effects of their play manipulations. Michelman further proposed that play provides an interactional learning experience that is basic to cognition and language. Vygotsky (1976) argued that play is important in the development of normal children because it is a natural context for interaction. Play provides a structure for dyadic interaction (e.g., adult-child and/or child-child interactions). Finally, play is an integrative experience which is active and continuous.

Symbolic Play

The use of the symbol in play has important implications for the development of preconceptual thought and words in language (Furth, 1969). In play, symbolic knowledge allows children to know objects in more than one way. Children establish a relationship between an absent object (bed) and a symbolized object (shoe box). Symbolic play allows children to transform reality by assimilation to their own needs (e.g., a shoe box becomes a bed and a tissue becomes a cover). During play, children integrate their action patterns with a symbolic language that is developed to fit the needs of the situation. The play situation centers on the children's interests, and it permits them to reenact their environmental experiences. The symbolism of play allows children to exercise and practice their internalized language within an environment that they create and control. "Rather than simply recalling an interesting or impressive event, the child has need of a more direct symbolism (play) which enables him to relive the event", (Piaget & Inhelder, 1969, p. 60).

PREREQUISITES TO LANGUAGE DEVELOPMENT

A variety of developmental models describe the interdependence of language, cognition, and social development and attempt to show how these components interact. These models share an underlying assumption that the components do, indeed, interact. Interaction of components, as noted earlier, may occur in several different ways. Interaction in a model in which there is an interdependent relationship between components suggests separate areas that interface and are derived from a more basic area (Shared Base Model, see Figure 3–2a).

Interaction in which there is a dependent relationship between components suggests that one area requires input from another (Direct Causal Model, see Figure 3–2b). The strong cognitive hypothesis proposes a developmental dependence between language and cognition: that language as a system requires input from cognition. Many researchers argue that early social and cognitive developments prepare children for later developments in language (e.g., Bloom & Lahey, 1978; Bruner, 1975). Developmental continuity can explain the emergence of symbols and, thus, the acquisition of language.

A prerequisite to language development is defined as a "structure in one system that provides input to the structure of a second system" (Bates, Benigni, Bretherton, Ca-

Figure 3–2. Shared Base and Direct Causal Models

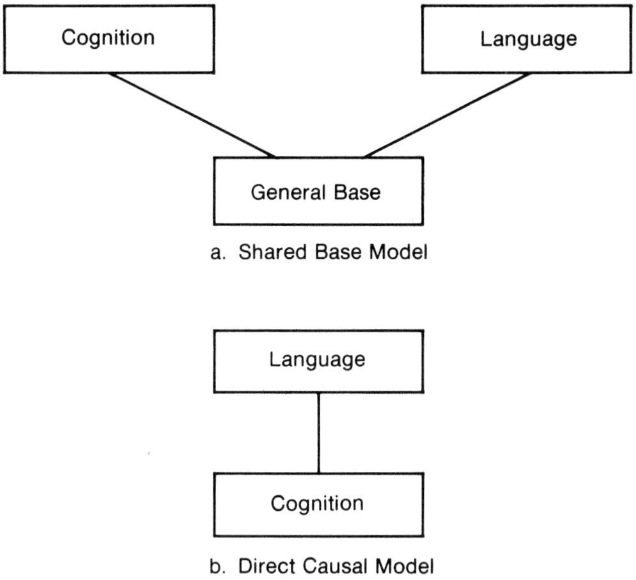

maioni, & Volterra, 1976, p. 14). The notion of skills or structures prerequisite to language echoes the strong cognitive hypothesis that cognitive underpinnings precede developments in language. The issue of preprequisites presents several problems in light of recent research investigations.

Cause and Effect

The traditional notion of prerequisites to language development focuses on a causal relationship between cognition and language. A causal relationship would indicate a pattern in which linguistic developments could be directly tied to nonlinguistic developments. For example, the children come to use names (e.g., bed) as they develop object permanence. In fact, the relationship of object permanence to language has been questioned by several investigators (Cornell, 1978; Moore, 1973). At this point, causality has been difficult to prove. In order to determine whether cognitive developments provide the underpinnings for language developments, the appearance of these skills must be identified in the child's behavior. So, for object permanence to play a role in the development of language, object permanence must at the very least, appear as a skill in the child's repertoire before language. For many years the relationship between object permanence and language was assumed. Several researchers have suggested that object permanence may not be a necessary prerequisite for the early development of words (Brown, 1973; Bates et al., 1979). The use of words seems to appear *before* Piaget's substage 6, object permanence. The present issue involves an attempt to determine the developmental relationship between cognitive abilities and linguistic skills.

TABLE 3–3
Development Skills

Age	*Cognitive Substage*	*Social/Communicative Substage*
1 (birth to 2 months)	exhibits reflexive behavior only actively attempts to direct actions develops action schemas	responds to human voice distinguishes between different sounds (speech and environmental noise) produces vowel-like sounds
2 (2 to 4 months)	repeats action patterns (primary circular reaction) coordinates sensory schemas coordinates motor schemas imitates vocal utterances	develops gaze interaction patterns coordinates gaze and vocal patterns orients head to speaker smiles at speaker produces pitch patterns
3 (4 to 8 months)	crawls and stands develops object class and concept focuses on effect of his own actions (secondary circular reaction) develops concept of object permanence differentiates between self and other objects in environment has large repertoire of action schemas	smiles and waves to continue a social exchange imitates some sounds responds to his name responds socially to others participates in routine games varies pitch, volume and rate
4 (8 months to 1 year)	coordinates action schemas in novel ways to form new schemas applies old schemas (means) to acquire a goal (end) develops intentional and anticipatory behavior sees other people and objects as sources of action can establish a correspondence between his own behavior and the behavior of a model appears to imitate systematically	sustains a social or a nonsocial goal; interchanges and recombines his various schemes for social or nonsocial goals develops protoimperative and protodeclarative—i.e., intentional communication plays action games interacts with peers uses social gestures and conventional behaviors imitates adult speech if sounds are in his repertoire
5 (1 year to 18 months)	actively pursues novelty perceives himself as source of action exhibits relational knowledge imitates words or actions in adult behavior modifies imitation to achieve a closer behavioral correspondence	interrupts interactions with objects; uses social signals to obtain adult assistance follows simple motor directions indicates preferences for people produces words and begins to combine word utterances likes social activities (games, music, dancing) plays alone and with peers points to objects when named (body parts, familiar objects, toys)
6 (18 months to 2 years)	manipulates reality internally internalizes action schemas can re-present objects or events—i.e., onset of symbolic behavior re-presents objects or events in play (make-believe or pretend behavior) uses symbol in play and imagery	engages in pretend play and parallel play communicates feelings and interests directs the action of others uses short phrases sings and hums parts of songs imitates adults in the environment

Adapted from Owens (1984), Bates, Benigni, Bretherton, Camaioni, & Volterra (1977), Morehead & Morehead (1975), and Piaget & Inhelder (1969).

Correlation

Researchers use a correlational analysis when they wish to determine the strength and direction of a relationship in a set of data or to assess whether an association occurs among variables. Correlation does not imply cause and effect. If two variables (object permanence and language) are correlated, the only permissible interpretation is that they corelate, or vary together. Another way to express the relationship would be to say that as object permanence moves in one direction (i.e., develops), language tends to move in the same direction (for a positive relationship). However, one variable (object permanence) does not cause the other (language) to vary. Although many of the sensorimotor studies are correlational in nature, only a limited number of sensorimotor abilities appear to be closely correlated with language development. Even correlations between Piaget's cognitive stages during the sensorimotor period and communication-language behaviors have not yielded consistent patterns.

Reconsidering Relationships

Several studies indicate that Piaget's sensorimotor substage 6 is not a necessary prerequisite for language development. Part of the problem here concerns the varying definitions of language. Bates, Benigni, Bretherton, Camaioni, and Volterra (1977) highlighted this issue when they noted that the first word or intentional act did not "just spring forward fully formed" (p. 251). Gradual changes, or transitions, occur in conventional behavior as children learn to integrate communicative function and form.

Initially, wordlike vocalizations may accompany gestures as children point to an object. Around 10 or 11 months, children use objects to obtain adult attention (i.e., showing and giving). The use of objects to obtain adult attention is termed the *protodeclarative.* The use of adults to obtain objects is referred to as the *protoimperative.* The protodeclarative carries the same communicative intent that later is recognized as labeling. The protoimperative scheme also leads later to more sophisticated expression of the imperative intent. In the final step, children may use referential words that suggest the object intended (e.g., "moo-moo" to indicate cow). The point is that children are communicative, social, and intentional long before they are linguistic.

Several researchers stress the notion of prerequisite cognitive *and* social schemes which are gradually combined into complex communicative sequences during the stages of sensorimotor development (Sugarman, 1973). Bruner, for example, suggested that the semantic structure of language (e.g., actor/agent and recipient) is derived from the nature and structure of social interaction. So, children learn about speaker and listener roles during communicative interchanges with adults. The language to express these roles is based on, or mapped onto, the child's developing social knowledge.

Because the issues of interdependence and interaction present more questions than answers, it might be helpful to consider when different skills appear developmentally across several areas (Table 3–3). How these areas interface presents some important questions for future investigations of a child development model.

SUMMARY

Cognitive processing provides a general developmental framework which describes how children organize the "raw data" of their experiences. Sinclair-deZwart (1973) suggested that cognitive structures composed of systems of actions are established during the first 2 years of life:

> These systems constitute the basis for many different types of cognitive structures, as much for the construction of logico-mathematical knowledge as for knowledge of the physical world and for the understanding and use of linguistic structures (p. 24).

Thus, children enter the environment structured and organized to learn about agents, actions, and objects. Cognitive theorists such as Piaget argue that properties and concepts are developed through children's active explorations of the environment.

In addition, cognitive theories attempt to explain how language is acquired and how language form and use relate to cognitive structures. Piaget proposed that cognitive structures provide the underlying bases for language development. However, recent research questions the cause-effect relationship between cognition and language (Bates, Benigni, Bretherton, Camaioni, & Volterra, 1979). This has important implications for the development of a more holistic approach to learning.

STUDY QUESTIONS

1. Describe the strong cognition hypothesis.
2. Describe the relationship between cognition and language according to Piaget.
3. Describe the sensorimotor period and how language develops.
4. Discuss the proposal that the child comes to environment structured and organized to learn. How does this change over time?
5. Why is it important to approach the area of child language development from a holistic orientation?

BIBLIOGRAPHY

Bates, E., Benigni, L., Bretherton, I., Camaioni, L., & Volterra, V. (1979). *The emergence of symbols: Cognition and communication in infancy.* New York: Academic Press.

Bates, E., Benigni, L., Camaioni, L., & Volterra, V. (1977). From gesture to the first word: On cognitive and social prerequisites. In M. Lewis & L. Rosenblum (Eds.), *Interaction, Conversation and the Development of Language* (pp. 247–307). New York: Wiley.

Bloom, L., & Lahey, M. (1978). *Language development and language disorders.* New York: Wiley.

Brown, R. (1973). *A first language: The early stages.* Boston: Harvard University Press.

Bruner, J. (1975). The ontogenesis of speech acts. *Journal of Child Language, 2,* 1–19.

Cairns, H., & Cairns C. (1976). *Psycholinguistics.* New York: Holt, Rinehart & Winston.

Camaioni, L., Volterra, V., & Bates, E. (1976). *Comunicazione nel primo anno di vita.* Turin, Italy: Boringhieri.

Clune, C., Paolella, & Foley, J. (1979). Free-play behavior of atypical children: An approach to assessment. *Journal of Autism and Developmental Disorders, 9,* 61–72.

Cornell, E. (1978). Learning to find things: A reinterpretation of object permanence studies. In L. Siegel & C. Brainerd (Eds.), *Alternatives to Piaget.* New York: Academic Press.

Cromer, R. (1981). Developmental language disorders: Cognitive processes, semantics, pragmatics, phonology and syntax. *Journal of Autism and Developmental Disorders, 11,* 57–74.

Durfee, J., & Lee, L. (1973, August). *Infant-infant interaction in a daycare setting.* Paper presented at the meeting of the American Psychological Association, Montreal.

Eckerman, C., Whatley, J., & Kutz, S. (1975). Growth of social play with peers during the second year of life. *Developmental Psychology, 11,* 42–49.

Garvey, C. (1974). Some properties of social play. *Merrill Palmer Quarterly, 20,* 163–180.

Michelman, S. (1974). Play and the deficit child. In M. Reilly (Ed.), *Play as exploratory learning.* Beverly Hills, CA: Sage.

Moore, M. (1973). *The genesis of object permanence.* Paper presented at meeting of Society for Research in Child Development.

Morehead, D., & Morehead, A. (1974). From signal to sign: A Piagetian view of thought and language during the first two years. In R.L. Schiefelbusch & L.L. Lloyd (Eds.), *Language perspectives—Acquisition, retardation, and intervention.* pp. 153–190. Baltimore: University Park Press.

Mueller, E., & DeStefano, C. (1973). *Sources of toddlers' social interaction with their peers* (Tech. Rep. No. 73–8). Boston: Psychology Department, Boston University.

Mueller, E., & Vandell, D. (1976). Infant-infant interaction. In J. Osofsky (Ed.), *Handbook of infant development.* New York: Wiley Interscience.

Owens, R. (1984). *Language development.* Columbus, OH: Charles E. Merrill.

Piaget, J. (1962). *Play, dreams and imitation in childhood.* New York: Norton.

Piaget, J., & Inhelder, B. (1971). *Mental imagery in the child.* New York: Basic Books.

Piaget, J., & Inhelder, B. (1969). *The psychology of the child.* New York: Basic Books.

Rice, M. (1980). *Cognition.* Baltimore, MD: University Park Press.

Rice, M. (1980). *Cognition to language: Categories, words, meanings and training.* Baltimore, MD: University Park Press.

Sinclair, H. (1979). The transition from sensorimotor behavior to symbolic activity. *Interchange, 1,* 119–126.

Sinclair–deZwart, H. (1973). Language acquisition and cognitive development. In T.E. Moore (Ed.), *Cognitive development and the acquisition of language.* New York: Academic Press.

Slobin, D. (1973). Cognitive prerequisites for the development of grammar. In C.A. Ferguson & D.I. Slobin (Eds.), *Studies of child language development.* New York: Holt, Rinehart & Winston.

Sugarman, S. (1978). A description of communicative development in the prelanguage child. In I. Markova (Ed.), *The social context of language.* New York: Wiley.

Vygotsky, L. (1976). Play and its role in the mental development of the child. In J.S. Bruner, A. Jolly, & K. Sylva (Eds.), *Play: Its role in evolution and development.* New York: Basic Books.

Westby, C. (1980). Assessment of cognition and language abilities through play. *Journal of Language, Speech and Hearing Services in the Schools, 11,* 154–168.

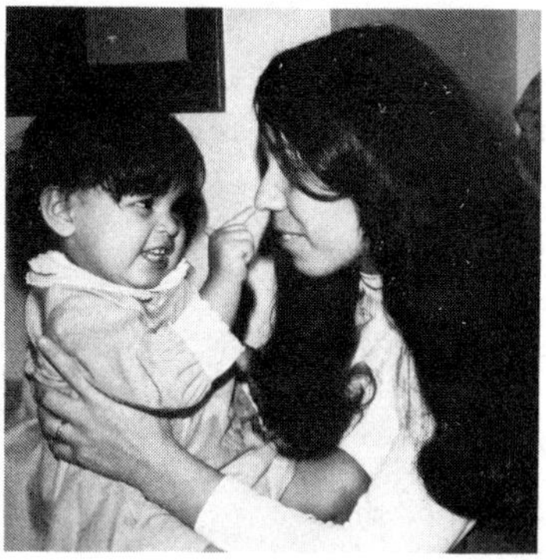

4

Early Language Development

From a developmental perspective, it is important to understand that communication *precedes* and facilitates speech and language behavior. The motive for language learning is effective communication. During the first 24 months of life, communicative intentions are coded by a variety of forms; gradually, these early intentions attain a linguistic form. Language is a system that codes a social process and exchange. It is a system that is learned in the social context. (McLean & Snyder-McLean, 1978). The child's "conquest" of the social context involves a pursuit of efficient and effective forms of interactional behavior.

This text describes language acquisition in terms of synthesis of several dynamic aspects: the social variable, the cognitive variable, and the linguistic variable. Two of these aspects, the social variable and the cognitive variable have been considered. In this section, I will discuss the third—language development.

Children learn about the conventions that code social interaction, social communication, and finally, linguistic communication. The central question for this chapter is how the child functions as an active language learner in the pursuit of rule-governed knowledge.

COMMUNICATION DEVELOPMENT

Research has shown that communicative intent appears prior to the development of speech. The child expresses his interactional intentions initially by combining gaze, gesture, and vocal behaviors. Gradually these communicative forms of behavior be-

---

This chapter was written by Dr. Ellenmorris Tiegerman, Adelphi University.

come word-like utterances as the child acquires the speech forms of his linguistic environment. Bates (1976) suggested that semantics and syntactics are derived from pragmatics: "Semantics emerges, developmentally and logically, from pragmatics, in much the same way that syntax has been shown to emerge from semantic knowledge" (p. 420). Pragmatics involves the use of language within context. The child learns to use various forms of behavior to carry out a communicative function. Thus, the early appearance of communicative acts provides a developmental timeline across which various components of language are acquired.

Communicative Intentions

Greenfield and Smith (1976) noted that children's first words are not referential in the sense that they do not refer to or name an object or event. The word accompanies an act, but does not represent or stand for a particular object, "any more than the act of pointing itself represents the thing to which it refers" (p. 425). It was already discussed that, according to Piaget, words become symbolic and representational at the end of the sensorimotor period (substage 6, 18 to 24 months). Long before children develop symbolic skills, they use words. How are these words used? From birth to 24 months, children use many forms of behavior (vocal, gestural, and lexical) to signal interaction. These signals of/for interaction can be called speech acts. The speech act occurs within the social context; it refers to the act that the speaker intends to carry out. Children may express many different intentions: request, command, question, and so forth, within the social context. During the first 24 months, the important issue concerns the acquisition of speech acts; specifically, how the child learns to code various intentions (See Table 4–1).

Infants and toddlers can use vocal and gestural behaviors to signal their intentions long before they develop word abilities. Table 4–2 illustrates some of these intentions.

Notice that at 9 months, the child was able to indicate a variety of communicative intentions by combining vocal, gestural, and gaze behaviors. Bates, Benigni, Bretherton, Camaioni, and Volterra (1979) state,

> We can infer the onset of intentionality from at least three types of evidence: changes in eye contact and checks for feedback, alterations in signalling until the goal is reached, and changes in the shape of signals toward a form that is appropriate only for communicaton. . . . It is sufficient to note that the relatively sudden onset of intentional, conventional communication around 9 months seems to be related to some other developments in learning how to get things done in the world. (p. 38)

TABLE 4–1
Acquisition of Speech Functions

Substages	*Intention to Communicate; Communicative Functions*	*Conventional Coding of Ideas; Semantic Functions*	*Conventional Coding of Forms and Structures; Syntactic Structures*
I	No	No	No
II	Yes	No	No
III	Yes	Yes	No
IV	Yes	Yes	Yes

From Bloom and Lahey, 1978

TABLE 4–2
Prespeech Communication

Communicative Intentions (9 months)	*Behavioral Form*
Request	Vocal: *eh;* reaches hand out in direction of object; alternates gaze back and forth from object to adult
Demand	Vocal: *eh, eh, eh* (staccato vocalization getting progressively louder and higher); alternates gaze between object and adult; reaches hand in direction of object, opening and closing hand.
Attention Getters	a. Coughs; gazes at adult b. Vocal *eh* (drawn-out production); pulls on adult leg; gazes at adult
Rejection	Pushes object away with hand; averts gaze
Initiating Ritual Play	a. Pokes chest and gazes toward adult (X-marks-the-spot game) b. Claps hands and gazes toward adult (patty-cake game) c. Puts hands up and gazes toward adult (hurrah game)

The child's ability to communicate intentions precedes the development of linguistic language structures, which are symbolic-representational forms. During this period of prelinguistic behavior, the context plays an important role in assisting the mother to interpret the child's intentions. The change from prelinguistic to linguistic forms can be viewed as a transition from idiosyncratic communication to symbolic communication (Bates, 1977). Once children develop linguistic structures, the conventional form of the language of their society, they can be understood with less and less contextual support (Bruner, 1974).

Communication Stages

The development of language use results from the interaction of the child and the context. The child learns how to create change within the context by combining and recombining behaviors in different ways. Bloom and Lahey (1978) hypothesized three chronological levels in the development of language use. The *first stage,* infancy, involves gradual changes of reflexive types of behavior, such as crying, to achieve ends; these are called primary forms. Infant behavior is initially directed by basic biological and physiological needs. These physiological states determine the strength, form, and direction of the behavioral acts. Gradually, there is a modification in the involuntary reflexive behaviors to voluntary motor acts, permitting infants to control their behavior more directly. The same behavior (e.g., crying) is used to meet several needs in different situations. Crying signals several affective states or needs: hunger, distress, and fatigue. There is not yet a repertoire that includes a variety of communicative behaviors.

At the *second stage,* children use some of the vocalizations, gestures, and movements that are standard to their culture. At this stage, they have only a limited repertoire of forms. However, they demonstrate the ability to combine and recombine the forms that they do have to express different communicative functions. They begin to evidence awareness of the conventional forms that signal intentionality and result in communication with the adult. For example, pointing is a conventional form of behavior. This one form, this one behavior, can be used to convey different messages; it can be a request ("Give me that.") or an attention directive ("Look at that cup.")

At the *third stage,* children express the same message in different ways. They take into consideration the social variables (i.e., listener, context, and so forth) which affect the form of the message. At this stage, children learn that there are alternative means to achieve the same purposes; they "learn when and how to say what to whom." They learn to suit the message to the social requirements of the listener, the situation, and the purpose of the interaction. The extent to which children adapt their use of language to the rules related to the social context, defines their skill as effective communicators (Bloom & Lahey, 1978, p. 203).

Consider the following incident with Jeremy (48 months) and Jonathan (15 months), in which Jeremy shares his observations on social interactional rules.

Monday

Jonathan is playing with Super Dog.

Jeremy: Jonathan, gimme that.

Jeremy pulls Super Dog away from Jonathan.

Jeremy: Say, "Please."

Jonathan: Eh.

Jeremy: Okay, here.

Tuesday

Jonathan goes to Nana and points to Super Dog on the shelf.

Nana: You want Super Dog?

Jonathan: Eh (continues pointing).

Jeremy: Yes, he wants Super Dog. He can have it; he said, "Please."

Nana leaves the room. Jeremy and Jonathan are alone together.

Jeremy: Jonathan. Jonathan, look at me.

Jonathan: (Jonathan looks at Jeremy).

Jeremy: Jonathan, when you talk to Nana you have to remember to say, "Please." She turns her ears off if you don't say, "Please."

Several interesting aspects within the above incident highlight some of the social and pragmatic learning that occurs during this process. First, Jeremy at 48 months was very aware of the "how to" part of talking to adults. In terms of the previous description, Jeremy had mastered several conventional forms of the same message. In his experiences and interactions with his Nana, he had learned that certain forms of a message achieved a certain effect, whereas other forms did not. Notice that he did not use the same form with Jonathan; with Jonathan it was not necessary to say "please." It is also clear that Jeremy was passing on his knowledge to Jonathan. In addition, Jeremy was able to interpret Jonathan's intentions from his (Jonathan's) vocal and gestural behavior. So, not only did Jeremy provide Jonathan with some advice about Nana, but he (Jeremy) also interpreted Jonathan's behavioral intentions for Nana.

The incidents also highlight some differences between the 48-month-old and 15-month-old child. With a very limited repertoire of vocal and gestural performances, Jonathan could express a variety of intentions. At 48 months, Jeremy could analyze and interpret differences in listeners and contexts to alter the form of his message. Thus, Jeremy was aware that there were alternative means for achieving the same purpose in different situations (Bloom & Lahey, 1978).

PRELINGUISTIC COMMUNICATION

Bates, Camaioni, and Volterra (1975) suggested that there are three stages in the development of communication, corresponding to Austin's (1962) perlocutionary, illocutionary, and locutionary functions. In the perlocutionary stage, from birth to about 10 months, children are not aware of the communicative impact of their behaviors. When they point at or reach for an object, they do not look at the adult for assistance, nor do they use objects to get the adult's attention. Their signals are perlocutions that create an effect but are not recognized by the speaker and the listener as a communicative act.

In the illocutionary stage, from 10 to 15 months, children develop prototypes of communicative acts. The protoimperative is the intentional use of an adult as a mediator to obtain a desired object. The protodeclarative is the intentional use of an object to gain an adult's attention. The children's signals are illocutions, conventional social acts (combined vocal and gestural performances) that are recognized by the speaker and the listener as a communicative act. It is the intention and the awareness of the child in relation to the adult that shifts the nature of the child's act from perlocution to illocution. These intentional communications do not necessarily involve speech. The cognitive prerequisite for intentional communication is Piaget's sensorimotor stage 5. Particularly relevant to the development of these gestural performances is the development of means-end relations in which the child acquires new action schemas to achieve specific goals.

The locutionary stage begins when the infant uses words to refer to environmental objects and actions. Bates (1977) noted that the appearance of words corresponds to Piaget's sensorimotor stage 6, which involves the capacity for mental representation and the use of symbols. The referential use of words coincides with the nonlinguistic developments of stage 6. The locutionary stage represents the final stage of functional communication development. It is the stage in which conventional word forms are used with or without gestures to achieve communicative intentions. Initially, these communicative functions were accomplished by gestures or word-like sounds and gestures. There is a gradual transition from one stage to another as the child learns to develop the conventional forms and structures that are part of language (i.e., phonology, pragmatics, syntax).

Finally, the child must learn about the effect, planned or unplanned, of having used a sentence—the listener's reaction to the speaker's intentions. The speaker's intention is a speech act, a performative or illocutionary force associated with an utterance (i.e., a question, a command, a request). The child must learn how the listener responds to the speech act or illocutionary "force."

Social Functions of Language

Children learn in infancy that vocalizations and gestures can perform certain functions for them. Although these vocalizations and gestures do not conform to the sounds and structures of the adult model, they have meaning in the functions they serve for children. Children evidence functions of language long before they develop conventional form and structure. Halliday noted that "from the functional point of view, as soon as there are meaningful expressions there is language" (1975, p. 6).

The first function Halliday identified in his son at 9 months was the "interactional" or "me and you function of language" as the child used sounds and gestures to interact with others in the environment (Table 4–3). The second function at 9 months was the "personal function" in which the child expressed feelings such as interest, annoyance, and anger. By 10 months, two more language functions could be identified, still without the child using the forms and structures of conventional language. The child's creative and idiosyncratic sounds, gestures, and movements, though lacking conventional form, still conveyed meaning and communicative intention. These were *instrumental functions,* whereby the child obtained objects and actions, and the *regulatory functions,* whereby the child manipulated the behavior of others. The distinction between the instrumental and the regulatory functions concerns the individual providing the service for the child. With the regulatory function, a specific person must provide the object and act for the child. With the instrumental function, anyone can provide the object or action.

In the *heuristic* (tell me why) *function,* the child uses language to explore the environment. In the early stages, children demand to be told the names of objects. In the *imaginative* (let's pretend) *function,* children use language to create their own environment and for sound-play and story telling.

Integrating Components

As children develop, the forms they use to express the functions of language become more conventional. During infancy, they gaze and vocalize. During the latter part of the first 12 months, they add gestures in imitation of adults in their environment. Finally, they speak in words indicating the acquisition of conventional forms and structures of the language. At this point, the child is able to interface form, content and use—the three components of language. Consider Jeremy at 28 months in terms of the categories just described (Table 4–4).

The Adult's Role

The context assists with the adult's interpretation of the child's speech acts. The interpretive process involves the adult's underlying assumption that the child is an active communicator. With this assumption, the adult attempts to determine the child's meaning by fitting together the limited pieces or forms: context, gesture, vocalization, intonational pattern, and word. This interaction facilitates and stimulates further exchange between the adult and the child.

TABLE 4–3
Halliday's Phase I Functions

I	*Interactional*	the "me and you" function
II	*Personal*	the "here I come" function
III	*Instrumental*	the "I want" function
IV	*Regulatory*	the "do as I tell you" function
V	*Heuristic*	the "tell me why" function
VI	*Imaginative*	the "let's pretend" function

Halliday, 1975

TABLE 4–4
Interfacing Form, Content, and Use

Pragmatic Function	*Form*	*Gesture/Action*	*Context*
I Interactional	"Hi"	Gestures with hand and approaches adult	Greets Mommy as she enters room.
II Personal	"No like bed"	Shakes head repeatedly	Jeremy is placed in crib.
III Instrumental	"Cookie"	Points to object	Points to cookie jar.
IV Regulatory	"Open"	Gives object	Gives closed jar of bubbles to Mommy.
V Heuristic	"Pig?"	Points to picture	Mommy and Jeremy are looking at a book.

LINGUISTIC COMMUNICATION

Children's earliest intentions to communicate relate to themselves; they talk about themselves and their needs. As they experience the world, they come to learn about *other* agents, actions, and objects. They develop broad categories for these, reflecting the relationships they see among agents, actions, and objects: possession ("Jeremy book"), negation ("No juice"), and recurrence ("More cookie"). At this point, children can talk about occurrences that do *not* concern their own needs (Jeremy: "Jonathan hat"). The next step is the gradual development of linguistic structure and form that match the cultural environment. There is a gradual progression from communicating intentions to ideas and then learning the structural forms to express those ideas (i.e., pragmatic intentions (pointing to cookie), to semantic notions (pointing to and saying "cookie"), to linguistic structures (pointing to and saying "I want that cookie").

The Embedded Word

During the linguistic stage, children use words, but are presyntactic insofar as they use only one word at a time. At this point, the content of the communicative act is expressed by a word form combined with other forms. The word forms are clarified and supported by gestures, intonational patterns, and context. The word forms are embedded within a broader communication schema.

Table 4–5 describes the child's single-word utterance (i.e., form) in terms of its content and use. Early in the child's language development (12 to 24 months), the

TABLE 4–5
Single-word Utterance in Terms of Content and Use

Pragmatic Functions	*Forms*	*Content*
I Interactional	"Hi."	Greeting
II Personal	"No!"	Rejection
III Instrumental	"Cookie."	Recurrence
IV Regulatory	"Open."	Action
V Heuristic	"Pig?"	Object

single-word message represents a complex ability to integrate various aspects of language. The word (cookie) conveys a message (recurrence: more cookie) for a social purpose (you give me).

LEXICAL DEVELOPMENT AND CONCEPT FORMATION

Semantic-Feature Hypothesis

Semantic development relates to the rules that govern the meaning or content of words or grammatical units. Meaning is an arbitrary system; the actual words or forms used by speakers represent ideas or concepts about objects and events, *not* the objects or events themselves. As children continue to experience reality, their ideas and concepts about objects and events change.

Clark (1973) described how referential word meanings develop. A word which names an object or referent in the environment has referential meaning. The object consists of many features and characteristics. Children must determine which features are critical or criterial in establishing a category for this referent. It has been found that at an early stage of lexical development, children make errors in referent identification, which are often referred to as overextensions. These overextensions are the result of using a limited set of semantic features. Children identify the most salient characteristic(s) or feature(s) and determine that this is what the word refers to or means. The universal examples of children who call all men "dada" and all four-legged creatures "doggie" exemplify the problems. When doggie means four-leggedness, the child has a narrower meaning and is utilizing fewer semantic features than the adult in defining the word. The word means something different to the child than it does to the adult.

Overextensions and Underextensions

Initially, children utilize one or two features and gradually add semantic features until their meaning for the word matches the adult meaning. Overextensions are noticeable between 12 and 30 months; their occurrence relates to vocabulary development. When children note a new object, they assign a label based on their established semantic system. When the adult provides the child with a word or label, such as *doggie,* the word does not indicate to the child which characteristic to attend to: shape, color, size, texture, movement, sound, or four-leggedness.

During the first language learning year, 12 to 24 months, children make noticeable errors in referent identification. Let's consider an incident that occurred quite frequently with Jeremy:

Jeremy: (Looking at a set of animal pictures) Mommy, a big pig.

Mommy: No, that is an elephant. See, the elephant has a long trunk (pointing to the elephant's trunk in the picture).

Jeremy: Like a long nose? (pointing to Mommy's nose).

Mommy: Yes, the elephant has a long nose (squeezing Jeremy's nose).

Jeremy: Little pig no has long nose.

Mommy: That's right.

Jeremy: No worry little piggy, you get bigga, you get bigga nose like Mommy.

In the process of developing meaning, children formulate certain hypotheses about underlying concepts and apply their concepts to new examples. Through this application procedure, children acquire knowledge about objects that belong and do not belong within a particular conceptual category. Overextension in child language has been more frequently cited than underextension. An overextension is a meaning that is broader than the adult's meaning (e.g., calling all men "daddy"). An underextension is a meaning that is more restricted than the adult's meaning (e.g., "bibi" referring to one and only one pacifier).

Bloom (1973) suggested that the extension process follows a developmental pattern. Initially, the concept is loosely associated with the referent, resulting in unsystematic overextensions. This is followed by a period of underextension in which the concept is applied correctly but in a very restricted manner.

Functional-Core Hypothesis

Nelson (1974) proposed another theory that described the development of child meaning. Children develop their word concepts based on active or functional characteristics related to the object rather than perceptual features. Children's definitions are based on function—something they do with the object (e.g., something they wear or eat). Nelson suggested that perceptual features (i.e., semantic-feature hypothesis), represent static components that are too abstract for young children. This hypothesis complements Piaget's theory concerning the development of physical knowledge. The functional-core hypothesis suggests that children's early explorations of object functions through direct manipulation provide the basis for concept formation. Cognitive aspects of early child development are related to semantic language development.

Prototype Hypothesis

Bowerman (1978) has summarized problems related to both the semantic-feature and functional-core hypotheses. She suggested that each hypothesis is too limited to explain the child's development of meaning. She suggested instead that children develop a prototype against which all other exemplars are compared. The prototype represents an underlying concept of "chairness," and other objects are contrasted with this stored mental representation. The closer the exemplar is to the prototype concept, the greater the likelihood that it will be called by that name.

In summary, children learn word meanings gradually. Their initial use of a word is often at variance with the adult's use, reflecting their narrow frame of reference. Children use a variety of hypotheses in attempting to define a word within new contexts. One hypothesis proposes that meaning is based upon knowledge of the object and the way it is used in the environment; as experience expands, meaning develops.

Adult Input

The adult's input or corrections (i.e., "that's a cow, not a dog") provide children with new semantic or criterial information that can be used to define and identify the object. Given the fact that adults and children have different semantic systems (the "word" has a different meaning to adults and children), how do they understand each other? The environment and context play an important supporting role in establishing, maintaining, and clarifying communication between adults and children. In developing word meanings, children rely on the perceptual and functional characteristics of an object.

This reliance on the context permits adults to understand children's meaning of the word. Thus, in attempting to understand children's meanings, adults anlayze *what* the children *say* within the framework of *what* is *happening.* This dependence on context lasts until children develop the ability to ask questions (i.e., What's that?) about the new experiences they encounter.

SEMANTIC DEVELOPMENT

The development of meaning has been described in terms of semantic characteristics, which are closely related to children's perceptual and functional notions of the environment. Children's experiences with agents (people), actions (doing and manipulating), and objects enable them to develop relationships between and among these basic components. There are many *similarities* across environmental contexts in terms of people, their manipulation of objects and the objects manipulated by child and adult, so that many theorists have highlighted the semantic universals in child language development. These experiences result in the development of semantic relationships that express how the object relates to the agent (i.e., possession) or how an object or action is noted again and again (i.e., recurrence). Because there is such consistency across environments, children of various cultures who speak different languages develop the same semantic relationships. The result is that all children learn to express the same ideas about agents, actions, and objects. There are, of course, certain experiential differences across cultures and environments. These differences might explain why children code different occurrences within their environment (i.e., there are some important individual differences in learning).

Table 4–6 illustrates how different environments and experiences can affect the content of a child's language. Notice that although Jeremy and his friend Jason (both 30 months) have different-looking lexical corpora, they were expressing the same semantic functions.

Table 4–6 does not represent a complete corpus for these children either in terms of all of the semantic categories developed by 30 months, or all of the lexical entries in each of the categories. It is important to note that these two children came from rather

TABLE 4–6
Universality of Semantic Functions

Semantic Function	*Jeremy*	*Jason*
Object	ball, shoe, binky, cup, boat, car, put-put (piggy bank)	Snoopy (cup), ball, yacht, Mercedes, put-put (plane—i.e., family's airplane)
Action	up, throw, open, give	fly, throw, swim, ski, give
Agent	Mommy, Nana, Poppy, Mimi	Miss Ann (governess), Henny (maid), Mother, Father, Grandmother
Recurrence	more	again, another
Negation		
a. Rejection	no	no
b. Cessation	no	stop

TABLE 4–7
Semantic Functions and Lexical Examples

Semantic Functions	*Lexical Entries*
Object	ball, cup, dog, hat, juice
Action	up, push, open, drink, eat
Agent	Mommy, Poppy, Jonathan-baby
Possession	me dog, Nana hat, Poppy ball
Recurrence	more cookie, cookie, cookie
Locative-state	dog bed
Locative-action	binky (pacifier) mouth
Negation	
a. Rejection	no
b. Cessation	stop
c. Disappearance	all gone

different environments. They were, therefore, coding different objects, actions, and agents, but developing the same semantic relations or categories. Remember that children talk about, or code, their immediate experiences. Children talk about what they experience, what they know. Notice that Jason's "put-put" is his father's private plane. The counterpart for Jeremy is a piggy bank. Here, the boys were using the same form to refer to different referents. In the case of Jeremy's "Nana" and Jason's "Grandmother," they were using different forms to refer to the same referent.

Although there are many differences in terms of specific lexical entries within each semantic category, the general categories that children learn are universal across languages and cultures. In addition, the ideas about the world, expressed by the use of these semantic relationships, are universal. Table 4–7 presents some of the semantic functions developed by children with examples of each category from Jeremy's productions. It is important to remember that the context helps the adult to determine what the child is referring to. *What* is happening in the situation helps the adult determine *what* the child means. By combining children's lexical productions with their vocal and gestural behaviors within a context, the adult formulates a gestalt about what they are talking about.

PHONOLOGY

Phonology is that aspect of linguistic form which governs the relationship of sounds within a language. As a part of early linguistic learning, it is important because infants begin to vocalize and to use sounds as part of the communication process during the first 9 months of life. It should be noted from the outset that child phonology cannot be described independently of the total developmental process. A description of components is an arbitrary separation but necessary for explicative purposes.

Phonological development is dependent upon several factors in child development:

1. Physical structural changes which affect sound production abilities
2. Integration of sound production (not phoneme production) with communication
3. Integration of sound production (phonemic production) with semantic meaning
4. Progressive development of phonemic structures and phonological rules

Prelinguistic Sound Production

Although infants are uniquely attuned, or perhaps preprogrammed to perceive various phonemes in language, they cannot produce a wide range of speech sounds (Elmas, 1971). The structure of an infant's mouth and throat simply does not permit it. A relatively large tongue fills the oral cavity, limiting its movement and therefore the production of sounds.

The earliest sounds are all vowels or vowel-like in quality. At 6 months, the baby utters and repeats syllable sequences, initiating the babbling period. Jakobson (1956) noted that the babbling stage begins with undetermined sounds, which are neither consonants nor vowels, and ends with a distinct separation. During the first 12 months, the form of sound production changes to express communicative intentions. Children learn to use sounds as well as gestures to communicate their intentions.

Once the semantic system develops, the form of the sound system changes to the use of phonemic structures. The progression proposed is that phonemic development is linked or tied to semantic development. Phonology is part of the child's developing linguistic system. It is rule-governed as the other components of language are rule-governed. The phonetic abundance of babbling gives way to phonemic restriction with the advent of the semantic stage. The phonological system interfaces with the semantic and syntactic components to result in language—a symbolic social system.

Jakobson and Halle (1971) suggest that children first acquire sounds that are universal to all languages along with sounds having simpler articulatory movements and fewer distinctive features. Sounds that are unique to the native language are acquired later with the more difficult sounds. Chapter 5 presents normative data describing the sound acquisition process and the characteristics for identifying children who are developmentally delayed in phonological productions.

Distinctive Feature Theory

According to the distinctive feature theory, phonemes are characterized by elements which enable one phoneme to be distinguished from another. For example, the difference between /p/ and /b/ relates to voicing; /b/ is a voiced sound, whereas /p/ is voiceless. The /d/ and /n/ sounds are produced in the same way (tongue tip-alveolar ridge), but /n/ has nasal support. Similarly, /t/ and /n/ are also tongue tip-alveolar ridge productions, but /t/ is voiceless whereas /n/ is voiced and nasalized. There is a two-feature difference between /t/ and /n/.

The appealing aspect of the distinctive feature theory is that a limited number of sound characteristics can be used to describe the phonemes of various languages (Jakobson & Halle, 1956). Although several distinctive feature systems describe phonemes, the core of the approach is the same. Phonemes are described by means of their presence (+) or absence (−) on a given set of features. For example, the phoneme /n/ may be described by the following features:

Code	*Feature*
+	Voicing
+	Consonantal
+	Anterior
+	Coronal

Code	*Feature*
+	Continuant
+	Nasal
−	Strident
−	Vocalic
−	Lateral

As with phonology, the distinctive feature theory provides a developmental schedule or sequence for the acquisition of features associated with articulatory characteristics. Table 4–8 presents a feature acquisition sequence, indicating that the features acquired earlier within the phonological system are less complex than the features acquired later.

Phonological Processes

Emphasis on previous approaches to sound acquisition centered on the child's learning of sounds and features. Another more recent theory focuses on rules for learning words—phonological processes. Strategies or rules for learning words were originally described by Francescato (1968). Building on this early work, other researchers elaborated phonological rules or processes that account for the sound sequences which children produce in their first words (Ingram, 1974; Klein, 1978; Smith, 1973). Children learn the sounds of a language not as separate entities, but in relation to one another within the framework of the word. Phonological processes have been identified as regularities in the ways in which children change the target production of syllables in their attempts to produce words. These phonological processes are described in greater detail in the next chapter.

Menn (1976) has suggested that phonological development involves the child's active discovery of patterns in linguistic input. Children use these patterns to attempt new words and to analyze adult input for new structures. Phonological development is the interaction between the child's inventory of stored perceptual and productive strategies and the ongoing incidental input. This interactionist-discovery theory assumes that children invent a set of phonological *rules* that reduce the linguistic input to a manageable and producible level.

Fey and Gandour (1982) suggested that the form of the rules used by children reflects the specific developmental relationship between a developing phonological

TABLE 4–8
Feature Acquisition Sequence

Order of Acquisition	*Feature*	*Complexity*
Early ↓ Later	Voicing Nasality Stridency Continuancy Place	Less ↓ More

system and articulatory control. Thus, children's phonological knowledge must be viewed in terms of phonetic output and production limitations. Correct phonological output and production finally occur when children possess both the necessary control over the articulatory mechanism and the perceptual awareness that a phonological contrast must be coded.

In summary, phonological development is rule-governed and consistent. All children learning a language acquire the phonemes of the language in an ordered and predictable sequence. Phonemes are not acquired until the semantic component is operative. Thus, the sounds produced during the babbling period are not phonemes and are not indicative of phonological progression, although they serve a communicative function. The functional purpose of the sounds produced during the babbling period remains controversial. It is not clear what the relationship is between the sounds produced during the babbling period and the phonological acquisition period. Phonological acquisition is accomplished over several years; therefore, substitutions appear as part of the normal acquisition process. Finally, recent theories suggest that phonological processes underlie the development of phonemes. An understanding of the normal phonological process is necessary if phonological impairments are to be identified.

Form and Function: Interaction and Integration

At a later stage, between 12 and 24 months, children express semantic relationships by integrating phonology with pragmatics. The complexity herein is that, while all of the sounds of the language are in the process of being acquired, lexical items are added to semantic categories. Note Jeremy's semantic categories and his phonological system at 14 months (Table 4–9).

At this point, the child's phonological system begins to include word-like vocalizations which add to the context of language and contribute to communication clarification. For an adult who is not familiar with the child's phonological system, the child's speech productions are difficult to understand without this contextual support. This difficulty is frequently evident when an adult comes in contact with a 14-month-old. Consider the following exchange with Jeremy.

TABLE 4–9
Normal 14-Month Semantic and Lexical Systems

Semantic Function	*Lexical Entries Described Phonologically*
Object	/bə/ ball
	/bibi/ binky pacifier
	/də/ dog
	/gʌgʌ/ cup
Action	/ʌbi/ up
	/fo/ throw
Agent	/mamă/ Mommy
	/papă/ Poppy
	/nænæ/ Nana
Recurrence	/mɔI/ more

Jeremy: /Da/ (Grandpa)
Grandpa: (No response)
Jeremy: /Da/ (louder and more insistent)
Grandpa: (No response)
Jeremy: /Da/ (plus a yank on Grandpa's arm)
Grandpa: Hmm? (looking at Jeremy)
Jeremy: /Gi bibi/ (pointing to binky pacifier on a cluttered table)
Grandpa: What does he want?
Mommy: (answering from another room) He wants his pacifier.
Jeremy: /bibi, bibi, bibi, bibi/ (jumping up and down)
Grandpa: Where is it?
Mommy: Dad, where is he pointing?
Grandpa: Oh, I see it.

Is there a first word? The one-word stage really represents a combination of lexical, vocal, and gestural forms that are used to communicate a message (Table 4–10). Given the gradual changes in form and function, there is not a first word.

As children acquire more of the phonemes of their language, speech production more closely approximates the phonological system and children become more intelligible. The phonological system interfaces with the semantic system. The one-word stage begins to highlight this interface.

As noted earlier, adults interpret children's messages as complex wholes, relying on the combination of lexical, vocal, and gestural behavior and context to understand the message. Adults' "liberal" or "rich" interpretations of children's meanings usually involve the assumption that children mean more than they actually say. Children are viewed as active communicators who have something meaningful to contribute to the social exchange process. The following interaction between Grandpa and Jeremy demonstrates the multifaceted nature of communication even at this developmental stage.

Jeremy: /Da kʌm/
Grandpa: Jeremy wants Grandpa to come?
Jeremy: /Kʌm, kʌm/ (Jeremy gesturing for Grandpa to approach)
Grandpa: Okay, what do you want?
Jeremy: /Mi duθ/ (pointing to refrigerator)

TABLE 4–10
Progression Toward Combining Lexical, Vocal, and Gestural Forms

Developmental Period	*Descriptive Form*	*System*
0–12 months	Vocal behavior	Suprasegmental
	Gestural behavior	Kinesis
	Pragmatic functions	Communication
12–24 months	Phonemes	Phonological
	Lexical items	Semantic
24–36 months	Lexical combinations	Syntactic

Grandpa: You want me to give you something? (Grandpa does not understand what /duθ/ is)
Show Grandpa what you want. (Grandpa opens the refrigerator)

Jeremy: /Duθ/

Grandpa: Jeremy wants milk?

Jeremy: /No duθ duθ duθ/ (pointing)

Grandpa: Oh, you want some juice! (taking the container out and pouring juice in a cup)
Here's the juice (giving the cup to Jeremy).

Jeremy: /Duθ/ (pointing to the cup that he now holds)

What seems to occur first is the development of a communication system. Children learn about the interactional and exchange process and learn progressive forms to code the communicative exchange. During the first period (0 to 12 months), they learn to combine vocal and gestural forms to communicate a message. During the second stage (12 to 24 months), they begin to code some of their ideas and experiences by using the phonemes within the language. Finally, they learn to combine lexical items. This gradual progression indicates children's ability to develop the conventional structures of their language system. As they learn to approximate more closely the sounds and words of their language, they learn to formulate or generate an idea by using a more conventional or sophisticated form.

In summary, children first learn to code communication exchanges. They then learn to code ideas which represent semantic relationships. Finally, they develop the syntax of their language. This communication system permits children to channel their ideas into conventional forms.

SUMMARY

This chapter has presented some of the more recent viewpoints regarding early language development. By viewing language development as a gradual and changing process, speech-language pathologists have an expanded and detailed knowledge of how language develops relative to other developmental areas. This development has implications for the language-disordered child and the content of the therapeutic programs developed.

Early language development involves the integration of a number of components: phonology, pragmatics, semantics, and syntax, to form a socially accepted code. In addition, the language-learning process interfaces with other aspects of child development: social learning, play, and cognition. How these various aspects of development affect one another is being investigated. Language acquisition follows an orderly developmental progression and is, therefore, predictable. Next, language is a social process. Children learn about the communicative aspects of interaction before they learn about the linguistic aspects of interaction. Finally, the normal developmental model can provide important insights into the nature and structure of training for the language-disordered learner.

STUDY QUESTIONS

1. Explain the viewpoint that normal children are communicative long before they are linguistic.
2. Describe the relationship between intentionality and reference. How do children express their intentions during the prelinguistic period? How does this change during the linguistic period?
3. Explain how children's meanings are closely related to their experiences with objects and events. How do their meanings change over time?
4. What is the difference between pragmatic and semantic functions?
5. Describe how form and function interface during the first 24 months.

BIBLIOGRAPHY

Austin, J. (1962). *How to do things with words.* London: Oxford University Press.

Bates, E. (1976). Pragmatics and socialinguistics in child language. In D.M. Morehead & A.E. Morehead (Eds.), *Normal and deficient child language.* Baltimore: University Park Press.

Bates, E., Benigni, L., Bretherton, I., Camaioni, L., & Volterra, V. (1977). From gesture to the first word: On cognitive and social prerequisites. In M. Lewis & L. Rosenblum (Eds.), *Interaction, conversation, and the development of language* (pp. 247–307). New York: Wiley.

Bates, E., Benigni, L., Bretherton, I., Camaioni, L., & Volterra, V. (1979). *The emergence of symbols: Cognition and communication in infancy.* New York: Academic Press.

Bates, E., Camaioni, L., & Volterra, V. (1975). The acquisition of performatives prior to speech. *Merrill-Palmer Quarterly, 21,* 205–226.

Bloom, L., & Lahey, M. (1978). *Language development and language disorders.* New York: Wiley.

Bowerman, M. (1978). The acquisition of word meaning: An investigation in some current conflicts. In N. Waterson & C. Snow (Eds.), *The development of communication.* New York: Wiley.

Bruner, J. (1974). From communication to language—A psychological perspective. *Cognitive, 3,* 255–287.

Chomsky, N., & Halle, M. (1968). *The sound pattern of English.* New York: Harper & Row.

Clark, E. (1973). What's in a word? On the child's acquisition of semantics in his first language. In T.E. Moore (Ed.), *Cognitive development and the acquisition of language* (pp. 65–110). New York: Academic Press.

Clark, E. (1974). Some aspects of the conceptual bases for first language acquisition. In R. Schiefelbusch & L. Lloyd (Eds.), *Language perspectives—Acquisition, retardation and intervention* (pp. 105–128). Baltimore: University Park Press.

Elmas, P., Siqueland, E., Jusczyk, P., & Vigorito, J. (1971). Speech perception in infants. *Science, 171,* 303–306.

Fey, M., & Gandour, J. (1982). Rule discovery in phonological acquisition. *Journal of Child Language, 9,* 71–82.

Francescato, G. (1968). On the role of the word in first language acquisition. *Lingua, 21,* 144–153.

Greenfield, P., & Smith, J. (1976). *The structure of communication in early language development.* New York: Academic Press.

Halliday, M.A.K. (1975). *Learning how to mean—Explorations in the development of language.* London: Edward Arnold.

Ingram, D. (1974). Phonological rules in young children. *Journal of Child Language, 1,* 97–106.

Jakobson, R., & Halle, M. (1956). *Fundamentals of language.* The Hague: Mouton.

Jakobson, R., & Halle, M. (1971). Phonemic patterning. In Bar-Adon & Leopold (Eds.), *Child language*. Englewood Cliffs, NJ: Prentice-Hall.

Jakobson, R. (1971). Why "Mama" and "Papa"? In Bar-Adon & Leopold (Eds.), *Child Language*. Englewood Cliffs, NJ: Prentice-Hall.

Klein, H. (1978). *The relationship between perceptual strategies and productive strategies in learning the phonology of early lexical items*. Unpublished doctoral dissertation, Columbia University.

Leonard, L., Rowan, L., Morris, B., & Fey, M. (1982). Intraword phonological variability in young children. *Journal of Child Language, 9,* 55–70.

Lieberman, P. (1968). Primate vocalizations and human linguistic ability. *Journal of the Acoustic Society of America, 44,* 1574–1584.

Menn, L. (1976). Evidence for an interactionist–discovery theory of child phonology. *Papers and Reports on Child Language Development, 12,* 169–177.

Menyuk, P. (1971). *The acquisition and development of language*. Englewood Cliffs, NJ: Prentice-Hall.

McLean, J., & Snyder-McLean, L. (1978). *A transactional approach to early language training*. Columbus, OH: Charles E. Merrill.

Nelson, K. (1974). Concept, word, and sentence: Interrelations in acquisition and development. *Psychological Review, 81,* 267–285.

Smith, N. (1973). *The acquisition of phonology*. Cambridge: Cambridge University Press.

Stern, D. (1971). A microanalysis of mother-infant interaction. *Journal of the American Academy of Child Psychiatry, 10,* 501–517.

Stern, D., Jaffe, J., Beebe, B., & Bennett, S. (1975). Vocalizing in unison and in alternation: Two modes of communication within the mother-infant dyad. In D. Aaronson & R. Rieber (Eds.), *Developmental psycholinguistics and communication disorders: Annals of the New York Academy of Sciences, 263,* 89–100.

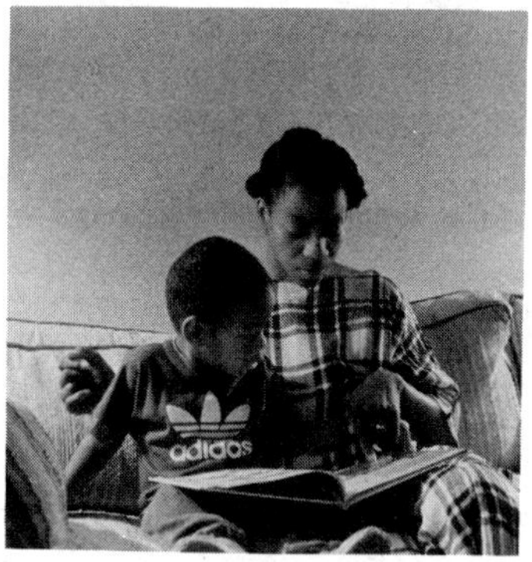

5
Later Language Development

The previous chapters traced the origins of early communicative functions and the coding of early semantic relationships. Maternal input, social interaction, play, and cognitive development all play a dynamic role in early language development. Although children come to the language acquisition process biologically equipped to learn language, the role they play is an active one. Their eye-gaze behaviors, gestures, interactions with caretakers, and attempts to affect the behavior of others are significant for understanding the origins of early child language as well as for later language learning.

Although a large body of literature focusing on children's development of syntax emerged in the 1960s, more recent research emphasizes the influence of semantics and pragmatics on syntactic development. Researchers argue against viewing syntactic development in isolation (Bloom & Lahey, 1978; deVilliers & deVilliers, 1978). Attention to the meanings children convey in their utterances and to the social purposes of child language is considered crucial (Bates, 1979; Bloom & Lahey, 1978; McLean & Snyder-McLean, 1978; Rees, 1978). Syntax, semantics, and pragmatics essentially operate together and must be treated as such in the theoretical description of language development and in assessing and planning language intervention programs (Bloom & Lahey, 1978; Lund & Duchan, 1983; McLean & Snyder-McLean, 1978). However, for the purpose of analysis and study, I will treat each separately and point out their interrelationships where appropriate.

Four aspects of later language learning are the focal points of this chapter:

This chapter was written by Dr. Deena Bernstein, City University of New York.

1. Development of syntactic forms, including increased use of morphological endings and various sentence types
2. Phonological growth
3. Development of meaning
4. Elaboration of pragmatic skills, including greater use of more sophisticated and varied communicative functions and discourse skills

Five basic questions guide the material presented in this chapter:

1. What makes some linguistic forms and communicative functions easier to acquire than others?
2. What plans or strategies do children use to discover the meaning and form of language?
3. What is the role of spontaneous imitation in language learning?
4. Does parental reinforcement or correction contribute to language development?
5. What linguistic forms, meanings, and communicative functions do children learn in the preschool and later school years?

Although the questions are complex and the data needed to answer them incomplete, I will present the current research findings. I will look not only at what children learn and how they go about learning it, but also at some of the factors that determine the course they follow as they expand and elaborate their linguistic skills.

LATER LANGUAGE DEVELOPMENT: AN OVERVIEW

What changes are observable in children's language in the preschool years? As children advance from simple one- and two-word utterances, their utterances become longer and more complex. Children gradually elaborate the way they say things by adding more detail. In terms of syntactic development, they add and fill in words and word endings which were missing in their early utterances. These take the form of articles (*a, the*), prepositions (*in, on*), pronouns (*I, he*), auxilliary verbs (*is, are*), noun endings (such as *-s*, which indicates plurality), and verb endings (such as *-ed*, which indicates past tense). The inclusion of these forms into children's speech makes their utterances seem more like adults' and less like a telegram. Their utterances begin to lose their telegraphic quality as they progress from "More milk" to "I want more chocolate milk," or "Mommy car" to "Mommy is going in the car."

In the early preschool years, children's vocabulary continues to grow and they learn many new word meanings. They learn new concepts and how to code these concepts linguistically. They also learn how to transform their ideas into sentences, and they begin to use a variety of sentence types. By the age of 4, most children's syntax is adult-like (Menyuk, 1977). Their utterances contain expanded noun and verb phrases (Gimme the big red ball; He pushed me down the steps); negative sentences (I won't do it.); Yes/No questions (Can you cut the cake?); and, *Wh*-questions (What will I do later?). Passive constructions (The boy was hit by the car.); causal constructions (He didn't get a prize because he was bad.); conditional constructions (If I'll do my homework, I'll get to watch T.V.); and, temporal constructions (When he will come, he'll get a surprise.) are also evident. They learn more complex ways to use language socially, and they begin to develop discourse skills such as participating in conversations, telling stories, giving instructions, and providing descriptions about objects, events, and people. By the time children enter the 1st grade, they are able to use language for a variety of functions: to contribute new information on a topic (Bloom, Rocissano, & Hood, 1976); to describe objects, events, past experiences, and plans (Moerk, 1975); and to use language to demonstrate, instruct, imagine, and reason (Tough, 1977).

Last, in the preschool years, children progress from talking about events in the "here and now" to talking about events in the "there and then" (Lucariello & Nelson, 1982). Young children generally talk about events and objects that are present in the immediate context. They refer to what they are doing or another person is doing in the immediate environment. Also, maternal input to younger children focuses on events and objects in the immediate environment. As children develop cognitively, they begin to refer to people, objects, actions, and events that are displaced in terms of time and place. They talk about past and future events and about objects and activities in the absence of external props or contextual support. How early this ability emerges is being studied (Lucariello & Nelson, 1982).

Although children's language has reached a measure of complexity by the age of 5, much communicative development is yet to come. Vocabulary continues to grow throughout the school years. The use of nonliteral language such as jokes, riddles, and metaphors (Nippold, Leonard, & Kail, 1984) begins to appear in middle childhood along with the comprehension of sentences which contain verbs such as "promise" or "ask" (Chomsky, 1969). Ambiguous sentences that allow for more than one interpretation, such as "The lamb is too hot to eat," are understood a bit later, during middle childhood and early preadolescence (Shultz & Pilon, 1973; Wiig, Gilbert, & Christian, 1978). Complex sentences which contain subject complements (The possibility that he may go on safari frightens me) or sentences which contain subject relative clauses (The man who smashed the car left the scene of the accident) appear during preadolescence (Hass & Wepman, 1977).

Pragmatic skills of children also continue to develop beyond age 5 into adolescence. For example, children entering kindergarten do not use indirect requests or hints to achieve a desired response, object, or action, while school-aged children do. Consider the differences in the use of language by a 2-year-old, a 5-year-old, and an 11-year-old in the same context:

CONTEXT: (A plate of cookies)
2-year-old to adult: Gimme cookie.
5-year-old to adult: Can I have a cookie, please?
11-year-old to adult: My, those cookies look good!

The 2-year-old directly requests the object, the 5-year-old politely requests it, while the 11-year-old hints at the request.

Even in light of the fact that language development continues as children mature cognitively and socially, a good deal of language learning has been mastered by the time the child enters the 1st grade. Just how complex a normal 5-year-old's language can be is underscored in the following incident.

> In a course entitled Language Development and Disorders of Children, students were asked to observe, record, and analyze the language of a 2- to 2½-year-old normal child. The assignment included two parts: (*a*) computing the average number of morphemes used by the child (called MLU—mean length of utterance), and (*b*) recording the language forms and functions used by the child. Both of the above measures were to be used by the college student as an index of the subject's overall language development. (Greater detail about MLU is provided later in this chapter. In addition, Chapter 6 discusses how to compute an MLU and how to analyze the language sample of language-disordered children.)
>
> The class followed the instructor's advice and studied 2- to 2½-year-old subjects, with the exception of one student who had a 6-year-old brother and chose him as her subject. At the end of the semester when the assignment was due, the student approached the instructor in desperation and exclaimed, "This assignment has been very difficult. I never realized how complex a 6-year-old's language could be. I should have chosen to do my report on a 2-year-old!"
>
> The student in this incident was overwhelmed by three things: first, the sheer volume and length of the language produced by a normal 6-year-old; second, the complex syntax of her subject's language sample; and third, the variety of pragmatic functions and discourse skills evidenced by the 6-year-old, necessitating analysis using a variety of taxonomies.

THE "COURSE" OF LANGUAGE DEVELOPMENT

Research findings on the course of language acquisition agree that children learn the simplest communicative functions and linguistic forms first and more complex ones later on. Complexity has been talked about in two ways. The first involves the mapping of children's ideas onto language, or cognitive complexity, for it deals with what children know. Cognitive complexity, in part, sets the pace for language acquisition as discussed in Chapter 3. The second involves the acquisition of various linguistic forms available within a language, or linguistic complexity, and has been used, in part, to explain what makes one syntactic form easier to acquire and another more difficult. Linguistic complexity will be discussed more fully in the following section.

Linguistic Complexity

Speakers of a language intuit that some linguistic forms are more complex than others. Long sentences are usually more complex than shorter ones; sentences which contain many clauses are more complex than sentences with only one clause.

Our intuitions about what appears to be complex in language are confirmed when we examine the way adults modify the language directed to their young children. Studies of maternal input (Ferguson, 1964; Newport, 1976; Snow, 1972) reveal that when parents talk to their young children, they reduce the complexity of what they say both in content and in length. The following exchange between a mother and her 18-month-old child demonstrates this point. (Details regarding maternal input are provided in Chapter 2.)

Mother: Jimmy, look.
Look (pointng to a coat on a chair).
Look over there (continuing to point).
Good, get your coat.
Right, your coat (continuing to point).
On the chair (pointing again).
Bring it to Mommy (gesturing).
Right, get your coat,
Bring it to Mommy.
Good boy. Let's put it on.
Put one hand in here.
Put the other hand in here.
Good boy.
Mommy is zipping it up.
All finished.
Now we're going bye, bye.

Let us consider the same mother giving instructions to Lisa, her 4-year-old.

> Mother (is in the kitchen and calls to Lisa, who is upstairs in her room): Lisa, Lisa. Get your coat on. It's in Jimmy's room on the dresser. Hurry up. It's late and I've got to pick Dad up at the train station.

Look at the differences between the two exchanges. When the mother was talking to her 18-month-old, she repeated the same utterance many times; and, by gesturing and pointing, she made use of the nonlinguistic context so that her child might understand her. The language directed by the mother to her 4-year-old, however, was more complex. It was uttered in the absence of gestures and contextual support. She used more complex syntax and the sentences were longer. As children's linguistic comprehension becomes more sophisticated, maternal input to them also becomes more complex (Moerk, 1974).

It is also interesting to note that even when older children (4-year-olds) talk to younger children (2-year-olds), they modify and simplify their language to them. Apparently, being sensitive to the linguistic level of younger children is a skill that even 4-year-olds seem to have mastered (Gellman & Shatz, 1974).

To linguists, the term *linguistic complexity* or *formal complexity* has a specialized meaning. A linguistic system is considered more complex if it contains rules to which there are exceptions. Linguistic systems that contain rules that have no exception are considered less complex. Put another way, the fewer the exceptions to the rule, the less complex the system.

For example, the past tense in English is considered more complex than the expression of possession because the formation of the possessive requires the knowledge of only one rule to which there are no exceptions. That rule states that possession is expressed by adding the suffix *-'s* to any noun. The formation of the past tense requires knowledge of a linguistic rule and also knowledge about when that rule should be violated. The rule for past tense in English is expressed by adding the suffix *-ed.* But there are exceptions, as in *went, took, taught,* and *ran.* In short, the expression of possession is regular, whereas the expression of the past tense is not. It is the irregularity of the past tense formation which makes it more complex. Linguistic complexity, then, will determine the time it takes to acquire a given linguistic form.

Language Acquisition Strategies

Clark and Clark (1977) provided an alternative explanation to why some syntactic forms are acquired before others. According to them, the determining factor is the "degree of fit" between the linguistic forms to be acquired and the processing strategies of children. Slobin (1973) has labeled early processing strategies *operating principles.* To Slobin, all children come to the task of language learning equipped with these operating principles. Some principles or strategies fit some linguistic forms, but not others. For example, one operating principle states, "Pay attention to the ends of words." Armed with this strategy, children pay attention to suffixes before they pay attention to prefixes. Because children pay attention to the ends of words almost naturally, they will find it easier to acquire suffixes. Because there is a match between the linguistic form and the operating principle, suffixes such as *-ing* or plural *-s* (which are found at the ends of words) will be acquired before prefixes such as *un-* (as in unhappy, unable) or *im-* (as in immature, impossible) which are at the beginnings of words. Prefixes appear to be linguistically more complex than suffixes, because there is a mismatch between the operating principle and the linguistic form. Conversely, suffixes appear to be simpler structures than prefixes, because there is a fit between the linguistic form and the operating principle.

Slobin's Operating Principles. After examining over 40 languages, Slobin (1973) confirmed that all children use processing strategies or *operating principles* to discover the structure of the language they are acquiring. These six strategies are used to discover the semantic coherence of utterances and their surface forms. They are universal and are used by children as they struggle to master syntax. Principles 1, 2, and 3 are concerned with the "mapping of ideas onto language," ensuring that language makes sense. These are the *semantically* based strategies. Principles 4, 5, and 6 are concerned with how to segment or divide up the speech stream and keep track of different linguistic forms. These strategies are called *segmentation strategies.*

Strategy 1: Look for systematic modification in word forms. From the earliest stages of language learning, children are confronted with variability in word forms. Managing this variability is crucial. It is accomplished by looking for systematic modifications in words. Using this strategy, children determine that there is a common element to the words *walk, walked,* and *walking*—the root word *walk.* Similarly, there is a common element to the words *book* and *books*—the root word *book.* Children learn that the mapping of the sequences of sound for *walk* and *walking* or *book* and *books* is the same by "tuning in" to the nonlinguistic context in which these words are used. Although there are a number of words which sound the same, such as *mat* and *match,* or *fee* and *feet,* children do not confuse the two because adults do not use these pairs of words in the same context. Both the similar sound pattern and the nonlinguistic context are crucial cues. By using them, children begin to make sense out of the utterances they hear.

Strategy 2: Look for grammatical markers that clearly indicate the underlying meaning. With this strategy, children look for regularities in language which will clearly mark particular meanings. Grammatical markers such as the suffix *-s* which notes plurality, or the suffix *-ed* which notes past tense serve this function. Children search for a one-to-one mapping between an idea and the linguistic form which expresses it. For example, English-speaking children go through a stage in which they use *only* the *-ed* form to mark the past tense. This form is used even when an ungrammatical word is produced. It is not uncommon for 2- or 2½-year-olds (and even older children) to say *goed, holded,* and *breaked.* In doing so, children reflect the strategy of looking for grammatical markers which simply map an idea (in this case, the past tense) and a linguistic unit (the morphological *-ed* ending).

Strategy 3. Avoid exceptions. The search for regularity and predictability of linguistic forms aids children in their mastery of syntax. For many months (and possibly years), rules internalized by children are applied in a consistent fashion. The realization that exceptions to rules are not merely permitted but are necessary comes with linguistic maturity.

Numerous examples of the "avoid exception" strategy are available. The mastery of the past tense form is most illustrative. (See Table 5–1.)

In Stage I, the present rather than the past tense is used. At Stage II, the past tense is correctly used. However, at Stage III, the child seems to have regressed, by adding the suffix *-ed* to the root word *eat.* This behavior clearly conforms to the strategy of seeking consistency and avoiding exceptions. The result, however, is an ungrammatical production. What appears to be an error at Stage III is no more than the overgeneralization or overuse of a rule the child has mastered. By Stage IV, the child recognizes the need to make rather than to avoid exceptions, and the irregular tense begins to emerge.

Strategy 4: Pay attention to the ends of words. To attend to word endings is one of the earliest strategies used by children. It helps them identify suffixes that alter the meanings of word stems. For example, the suffix *-s* when added to a noun indicates plurality (e.g., cat–cat*s*). Similarly, the addition of *-ed* to a verb indicates past tense (e.g., walk–walk*ed*). Using a segmentation strategy, the child learns to divide the speech stream and isolate surface forms which signal meaning. The importance of the nonlinguistic context cannot be minimized. The information at the ends of words is salient to children only in a meaningful context. Children will learn that there is a commonality between *tree* and *trees,* and between *play* and *played,* but not between *cat* and *catches.* The processes of segmentation and mapping go hand in hand as children learn which word forms are variants of one another and what changes can be made in the formation of words.

TABLE 5–1
The Mastery of Past Tense

Stage	*Verb Tense Use*	*Example*
I	Little or no use of past tense	eat cookie
II	Sporadic use of irregular form Appropriate use of past tense	ate cookie
III	Use of regular suffix *ed* for *all* past tense forms. Systematic overgeneralization and apparent regression noted	eated cookie
IV	Correct use of irregular and regular past tense forms	ate cookie

Strategy 5: Pay attention to the order of words and morphemes. This strategy guides children's comprehension and production of language until after the preschool years. Even before children produce full-blown utterances, their three- and four-word utterances contain a word order that resembles that produced by adults. Consider the following utterances produced by a 2½-year-old child and his 5½-year-old sibling.

CONTEXT: 2½-year-old and 5½-year-old watching baseball game on television

2½-year-old: Man hit ball.

5½-year-old: Yeah, Reggie Jackson swung high and hit the ball to right field.

Although the 5½-year-old's utterance is longer and more complex, the utterance of the 2½-year-old contains the same basic word order as that of his older sibling. By attending to word order, children are provided with clues for identifying the grammatical relations of a sentence, such as its subject, predicate, and recipient object of the action. Mastery of the basic grammatical relations of Subject-Verb-Object (S-V-O) is guided by the word-order strategy and emerges early in child language.

So powerful is the word-order strategy that preschool children misinterpret reversible passive sentences such as "The boy was pushed by the girl" to mean "The boy pushed the girl." For preschoolers, the clue to who did what to whom comes from the order of the words in the sentence. Preschoolers interpret reversible passive sentences in an actor-action-receiver relationship using the order in which the words were mentioned to understand their meaning (Fraser, Bellugi, & Brown, 1963). As they develop, children will come to know that the passive verb construction requires an order reversal of actor and receiver.

Paying attention to the order of words and morphemes also encourages children to keep track of whether a grammatical morpheme is a suffix or a prefix. Children rarely, if ever, add a suffix to the beginning of a word or a prefix to the end of a word.

Strategy 6: Avoid interruptions or rearrangement of linguistic units. The following questions produced by a 3½-year-old child demonstrate this strategy:

CONTEXT: Mother and child are watching a man operating a bulldozer at a construction site.

Child: Mommy, what the man is doing?

CONTEXT: Mother and child are in the playground. All the children have balls to play with except one boy.

Child: Mommy, why he has no ball?

CONTEXT: Mother is busy packing a suitcase for Daddy.

Child: Mommy, where Daddy is going?

The form of the above *Wh-* questions (questions which begin with the word *how, who, what, where, when,* or *why*), is typical for a 3½-year-old. In all the questions the child did not rearrange the linguistic units to produce a grammatically correct question form. The child simply attached a *Wh-* element to a basic sentence type in order not to interrupt the linguistic units. It is not until later that children rearrange linguistic units, and, in the case of *Wh-* questions, invert the subject of the sentence and the auxiliary form. (Children's acquisition of questions is discussed later in this chapter.)

Preschoolers also avoid interrupting the main thrust of a sentence to include additional information. For example, when asked to imitate a complex sentence such as "The girl who hit the ball ran away," preschoolers often leave out the relative clause (who hit the ball) altogether and will say "The girl ran away." Older children understand that switching word order as well as interrupting linguistic units is necessary to produce grammatically correct *Wh-* questions and complex sentences.

The operating principles outlined by Slobin (1973) are early processing strategies which children use to discover the structure of language. Gradually the early processing strategies evolve into later processing strategies of a more complex nature.

Later Processing Strategies. Clark and Clark (1977) have outlined a series of strategies that adults use to comprehend language. Three of these strategies will aid understanding the linguistic deficits of older language-impaired and learning-disabled children, specifically, their difficulty in applying these strategies to oral or written language comprehension.

Strategy 1: Look for a definite noun phrase that refers to entities you know and replace the interpretation of each noun phrase by a reference to that entity. Example: Bob and Jane climbed Mt. Blanc last winter. He surveyed the peak, and she climbed it.

By itself, the second sentence is meaningless. We do not know to whom or what *he, she, the peak,* and *it* refer. This strategy instructs us how and where to find meaning, namely to search the prior linguistic context (sentence 1) to derive the correct interpretation of the present linguistic context (sentence 2). By identifying the correct noun phrase which is linked to *he, she, the peak,* and *it,* we are able to understand the second sentence. This strategy has been called *tying the sentence to context strategy* or *a discourse strategy.* Closely related is the strategy in which the listener uses given information from the discourse to define newer information.

Strategy 2: Look for given or old information to precede new information. Example: Joan and Jim meet on a street corner. The following discourse ensues:

Joan: I saw Tom yesterday. He's leaving for Africa tomorrow.
Jim: Oh, I'm happy for him. He needs a vacation.

In the example, the old or given information in Joan's first utterance is that Jim, the listener, knows who Tom is. The new information is about what Tom will be doing—Tom's forthcoming trip. The listener also knows that the pronoun *he* refers to *Tom* because it follows in this discourse. It is clear that Joan's information regarding Tom's forthcoming trip was news to Jim. (Note Jim's first utterance, "Oh?".) Next, Jim provides new information of his own—that Tim is in need of some time off. Notice also that Jim's use of the pronouns *him* and *he* clearly refers to *Tom,* who was the subject or topic of conversation in Joan's previous utterances. Through the use of this strategy, the listener groups sentences together in order to integrate older information with new information. New information is that which is not apparent from the context. The old information (either previous knowledge or a previous sentence) helps define the new. Clark and Clark (1977) termed this the *given-new strategy.*

Strategies 1 and 2 instruct the listener to attend to both the linguistic and nonlinguistic context to comprehend the speaker's meaning. Because of the need to rely on the previous discourse and the social context to understand the sentences in the examples given, Strategies 1 and 2 can be thought of as pragmatically based comprehension strategies. (Chapter 6 treats the assessment of pragmatically based strategies.)

Strategy 3: Look for the order of mention of clauses to match the order of events of occurrences, but watch for exceptions. Example: Touch your toes before you touch your nose.

The order of the clauses in the sentence matches the order in which the events should take place. Touching your toes, which is mentioned first, would be event 1, and touching your nose would be event 2. This sentence conforms to the first half of the strategy. Now consider the second half of the strategy, *but watch exceptions,* in light of the following sentence: Before you touch your nose, touch your toes. The order of mention of clauses does not match the order in which the events should take place. The event mentioned second (touch your toes) should precede the event mentioned first (touch your nose). This strategy has been termed the *order of mention strategy.* The difficulty older learning-disabled children experience in applying this strategy is reported by Wiig and Semel (1984).

THE "HOW" OF LANGUAGE ACQUISITION

In the following sections, we will examine imitation, reinforcement, and parental corrections. We will focus on assessing their contribution, if any, to language learning.

The Role of Spontaneous Imitation

It has often been said that language is learned by imitation. A closer look at this popular idea reveals that imitation has only a limited role in language acquisition. Imitation may be questioned on two grounds. First, if children learned language by imitating what they heard, they would produce only those utterances which they had heard. Yet we know that children produce utterances which they have never heard before. For example, utterances like "Allgone Daddy" (as Daddy leaves for work) or "Allgone dirty" (as Mommy removes a dirty diaper) are not uncommon in young children's speech. Second, children's early utterances contain systematic errors. These are linguistic productions that they never could have heard, such as "tooths," "sheepses," "I goed," or "He taked it away from me." These errors are common; they indicate, as explained earlier, that children learn a syntactic rule and overgeneralize its application.

Nevertheless, children's imitative utterances provide a measure of their linguistic functioning. Studies of children at the two-word utterance stage indicate that their imitations are systematic and are either on par with their spontaneous speech, or simpler. For the most part, content words, words most recently heard, or the stressed elements of a sentence are retained in their imitations (Ervin-Tripp, 1964). Elements such as articles, prepositions, and auxiliary verbs, which are absent from their spontaneous speech, are also absent in their imitative production. Ervin-Tripp argued that imitation by children does not imply a faithful reproduction of what they hear, but rather the production of what they know. What is already known about the form and structure of their language serves as a filter for what is imitated. In short, children will imitate only those forms which they know. (For a discussion on the use of elicited imitation for assessment purposes, see Chapter 6.)

Bloom, Hood, and Lightbown (1974) found that although children vary greatly in the amount of their imitation, their imitative utterances contain only those structures which appear in their spontaneous utterances; a finding similar to that of Ervin-Tripp (1964). They concluded that imitation is used by children primarily for acquiring new vocabulary words, but not for acquiring new or more complex syntax.

Imitation and Communication. Children's communicative intentions also play a role in their ability to imitate. A sentence is imitated more easily when it reflects the child's own intentions to communicate information. For example, Slobin and Welsh (1973) described a child they named Echo, who could utter some fairly long and complex sentences spontaneously, but could not repeat those sentences when asked to do so later.

CONTEXT: Echo and her father at the breakfast table
Echo: If you finish your eggs all up, Daddy, you can have your coffee.

Echo's utterance contains 14 morphemes and the conditional construction *if,* making her utterance fairly complex. Immediately after she produced this utterance, Echo's father asked her to repeat it.

Father: Say, "If you finish your eggs all up, Daddy, you can have your coffee."
Echo: After you finish your eggs all up, then you can have your coffee.

On the whole, Echo's imitative production may be considered successful. The meaning or semantic intent as well as the length was preserved even though the temporal (*after-then*) clause was substituted for the conditional clause (*if*). Ten minutes later, when Echo was again asked to repeat the sentence, she produced the following:

Father: Say, "If you finish your eggs up, Daddy, you can have your coffee.
Echo: You can have coffee, Daddy, after.

In this case, the imitation is not successful because the meaning, the length, and the syntactic complexity have been significantly altered. Presumably, because the utterance was devoid of communicative intention, Echo missed the mark. Slobin and Welsh (1973) pointed out that, because children are rarely asked to imitate utterances which reflect their own communicative intentions, imitation does not normally provide a means for learning linguistic devices that express these intentions.

R. Clark (1977) suggested that children imitate adult utterances when they fail to understand portions of the adult's message. Consider the following dialogue between a mother and her normal 2-year-old:

CONTEXT: Mother and child looking at a picture book. Mother is pointing to the pictures.

Mother: Oh, Jimmy, look. Look at the doggie; he's crawling under the fence.
Jimmy: Under fence.
Mother: See, he's wagging his tail.
Jimmy: Waggin' tail.
Mother: Oh, what do you think is happening here?
Jimmy: Happenin' here.

It appears that the child did not understand everything that he was imitating. It is also doubtful that he understood everything that his mother was saying. To use Clark's (1977) term, the child *plagarized* the final portions of his mother's utterances.

Ramer (1976) hypothesized that these plagarisms serve a communicative function. She speculated that when young children don't understand the language directed to them, they imitate what they have heard, in order to keep the interaction going. By imitating a previous utterance, children indicate to the adult that they are attending to the speaker and wish to serve as a respondent in a turn-taking role. Ramer argued that imitation is an early conversational strategy which the child uses for communicative purposes.

The Role of Reinforcement and Parental Corrections

Parental approval and disapproval provide another possible explanation about how children learn language forms. According to this view, the learning of grammatical utterances by children is a function of parental approval and disapproval. Children are positively reinforced or rewarded when their utterances are grammatically correct. Parents disapprove and correct utterances which are grammatically wrong. Research findings, to date, pose problems to the acceptance of this point of view.

For example, it has been shown that parents pay little attention to *how* children say things, that is, to their grammar or syntax. They are more interested in *what* their children say, that is, the meanings they convey in their utterances. In a study of parental approval and disapproval, Brown and his colleagues (1969) confirmed that parents tend to correct the semantic or truth value of their children's utterances and their pronunciation rather than their syntax. The following dialogues illustrate a parent's attempt to correct semantic and pronunciation errors (Brown, Cazden, & Bellugi, 1969).

CONTEXT: Child pointing to a picture of a horse
Child: Doggie.
Adult: No, that's a horse.
CONTEXT: Child pointing to a picture of a lighthouse
Child: That's the animal farmhouse.
Adult: No, that's the lighthouse.
Adult: Where is your coat?
Child: I tooked it upthtairs.
Adult: Upstairs, say, "upstairs."

The parent corrects the child's pronunciation of *upstairs,* but does not correct the child's grammatical mistake "tooked." Brown and Hanlon (1970) suggested that even blatant grammatical errors will go uncorrected by parents, as long as what the child says is true.

In a startling study, Nelson (1973) revealed that parental disapproval might even inhibit children's linguistic development. She found that children whose mothers selectively reinforced good and bad pronunciation and word choices developed more slowly than those whose mothers were generally more accepting of their lexical choices and pronunciation.

On the whole, parents do not "tune in" to their children's syntactic productions, nor do parental corrections provide the means for children to learn the more complex linguistic structures used by adults. Moreover, an attempt by parents to correct their children's syntactic mistakes which are normal for their stage of linguistic development is usually doomed to failure. The following dialogue demonstrates the fruitless efforts of Braine (1971) to correct the grammar of his $2^1/_2$-year-old daughter.

CONTEXT: Breakfast table
Child: Want other one spoon, Daddy.
Father: You mean, you want *the other spoon.*
Child: Yes, I want the other one spoon, please, Daddy.
Father: Can you say, "the other spoon?"
Child: Other, one, spoon.
Father: Say . . . "Other."
Child: Other.
Father: Spoon.
Child: Spoon.
Father: Other spoon.
Child: Other spoon. Now, give me the other one spoon, Daddy.

McNeill (1966) also reported on a mother-child interaction which vividly illustrates the futility of parent corrections.

Child: Nobody don't like me.
Mother: No, say "Nobody likes me."
Child: Nobody don't like me.
Mother: No, say "Nobody likes me."
Child: Nobody don't like me.

After repeating this dialogue seven more times, the mother finally says:

Mother: No! Now listen carefully! Say, "Nobody . . . likes . . . me!"
Child: Oh! Nobody don't *LIKES* me!

The evidence against the role of parental approval and disapproval in normal children's learning of syntax seems to be best summarized by Clark and Clark (1977): "Correcting children's syntax is very hard work" (p. 336).

The Child As a Scientist

Learning models which rely solely on imitation and reinforcement to account for language development place children in a passive role. They are seen as reactors rather than actors. (For a review of the behavioral model of language development, refer to Chapter 1.) Anyone who has watched children try to master the linguistic system cannot miss the sense of trial and error and the active role the child takes. Piaget and his colleagues stressed the need to view children as investigators of the world, as explorers actively engaging in finding solutions to problems. From the utterances they hear, children form hypotheses about the structure of their language. Some of his hypotheses are correct, but others are not. (Recall children's consistent use of overgeneralized forms such as "comed" and "broked.") Children test their hypotheses against the language they hear and refine them until they conform to the adult rules.

The active role taken by children in constructing the rules of their language can be seen when examining the findings of a classic study conducted by Berko (1958). Berko hypothesized that, if children formulated rules for constructing words which indicate plural or past tense (as in cat*s*, push*ed*), they should be able to use these rules and apply them to words which they had never heard before. Berko constructed a series of nonsense drawings depicting strange animals and people doing odd actions. For example, the experimenter pointed to a picture of a bird-like creature and said, "This is a wug." She then pointed to a second picture and said, "Now there's another one. There are two of them. There are two ________." The children usually filled in the plural form wug*s*.

Using this format, Berko was able to elicit from the children constructions such as "he ricked" (indicating their knowledge of the rule for forming past tense) and the "bik's hat" (indicating their knowledge for formulating possessives). The findings clearly indicate that children construct rules and generalize them, a result which illustrates their creativity. The words of Piaget (1964) are particularly relevant here: "The goal of education is to create men who are . . . creative, inventive, and discoverers" (p. 5). Surely, there can be no better description of children as they struggle to master the language of their community.

Summary. This chapter began by asking five questions. In this section, I have addressed the first four of the five basic questions:

1. What makes some linguistic forms easier to acquire than others?
2. What are the strategies children use to figure out the structure of their language?
3. What is the role of imitation in language learning?
4. Does parental reinforcement play a role in the language learning process?

Although all the data are not complete, we can at this time hypothesize that:

1. Children are active participants in the language learning process.
2. Children first learn linguistic *forms* which more easily fit their strategies.
3. Children first learn linguistic *rules* to which there are no exceptions.
4. Children rely on similar sound patterns and nonlinguistic contexts to learn linguistic meanings and linguistic forms.

5. Parents seem to correct their children's semantic mistakes and their mispronunciations. Attempts to correct their syntax tend to be fruitless.
6. Children tend to vary in the amount of spontaneous imitation that they do. Those children who do imitate do so either to master a new vocabulary word or as a means for "taking a turn" in a conversation, not as a way for acquiring syntax.

SYNTACTIC DEVELOPMENT

This section deals with question 5—What linguistic forms, meanings, and communicative functions do children learn in the preschool and later school years? The order in which children acquire linguistic forms is examined first.

Brown's Stages

Roger Brown's pioneering work, *A First Language* (1973) demonstrated that children's acquisition of syntactic structures is not as much a function of their chronological development as the mean length of their utterances (MLU). In a longitudinal study of three children, Adam, Eve, and Sarah, Brown found that utterance length and the mastery of grammatical forms varied greatly with age. For example, Sarah and Adam progressed from an MLU of less than 2.0 to an MLU of 4.0 in 15 months. It took Eve less than 8 months to make this progress. Eve achieved an MLU of 2.75 morphemes at age 2. Adam was 3 years old and Sarah was 3 years, 5 months when their utterances reached that length. In contrast, the three children were remarkably consistent with each other in one very important way: the order in which morphological endings and function words were acquired.

According to Brown (1973), children acquire basic semantic/syntactic constructions when their MLU is approximately 1.7 morphemes (Stage I). Examples of utterances produced at this stage include "Mommy eat," "Drink milk," and "Gimme juice." When children's MLU reaches 2.25 morphemes (Stage II), their utterances include nuances of meaning. They modify their linguistic productions by including morphological endings such as *-ing,* the plural *-s,* and the prepositions *in* and *on.* Utterances such as "Jimmy eating," "Put ball in," and "See cats" are characteristic of this stage.

A burst of development occurs at Stage III. Utterance length grows to 2.75 morphemes, and children begin to use simple sentences, imperative sentences, *Wh-* questions, and simple negative sentences. Examples of utterances characteristic of this stage include, "Jimmy hit the ball," "Push the car," "Will I eat?" and "The boy is not eating." During Stages IV and V (when MLU reaches 3.5 to 4.0 morphemes), some

TABLE 5–2
Brown's Stages

Linguistic Stage	*Approximate MLU (In morphemes)*	*New Syntactic Developments*
I	1.7	Semantic/syntactic relations
II	2.25	Modulation of meaning by the incorporation of some grammatical morphemes
III	2.75	Emergence of negative, imperative, and interrogative sentence forms
IV	3.5	Emergence of complex constructions: coordination, comple-
V	4.0	mentation, relativization

Source: R. Brown. *A first language: The early stages.* Cambridge, MA: Harvard University Press, 1975.

complex constructions emerge. Noun and phrase elaborations are used, as are conjoined and complex sentences. Examples of utterances produced at these stages are "Daddy is cooking, and Mommy is writing," "I want to buy the green truck," and "Put the dog with the spots here."

Table 5–2 summarizes the syntactic achievement and the corresponding MLU which emerges at each linguistic stage. Brown's seminal findings on three subjects were confirmed by the deVilliers' and deVilliers' (1973) study involving a significantly larger number of children. In following sections, the syntactic developments which occur in Brown's Stages II through V are described in greater detail.

The Acquisition of the 14 Grammatical Morphemes

At Brown's Stage II (at approximately 2 to 2½ years of age), children begin filling out their short, immature sentences by incorporating one or more of the 14 grammatical morphemes studied by Brown. The mastery of all the grammatical morphemes, however, takes several years. Table 5–3 lists the order of emergence of these 14 grammatical morphemes.

Brown examined the possibility that those morphemes which children learned first were used more often by parents and adults. He discounted this hypothesis when he

TABLE 5–3
Order of Emergence of 14 Grammatical Morphemes

Grammatical Morphemes	*Examples*
1. Present progressive verb ending *-ing*	Mommy push*ing*. Johnny throw*ing*.
2. Preposition *in*	Put *in* box.
3. Preposition *on*	Put *on* table.
4. Plurals (regular) (*-s*)	Eat cookie*s*. More block*s*.
5. Past irregular verbs (*came, fell, broke, went*)	He *went* outside. Johnny *broke* it.
6. Possessive noun (*'s*)	Jimmy*'s* car. Mommy*'s* coat.
7. Uncontractible copula (*be* as the main verb, *am, is, are, were, was*)	He *was* bad. They *are* good.
8. Articles (*a, the*)	Billy throw *the* ball. Give me *a* big one.
9. Past regular (*-ed*)	He jump*ed*. She push*ed* me.
10. Third person singular regular	He cook*s*. Johnny go*es*.
11. Third person singular irregular	He *has* books. She *does* work.
12. Uncontractible auxiliary (*be* verbs preceding another verb: *am, is, are, was, were*)	The boys *are eating*. The baby *is crying*.
13. Contractible copula	I'*m* good. She'*s* nice.
14. Contractible auxiliary	I'*m* eating. She'*s* jumping. They'*re* playing.

Source: R. Brown. *A first language: The early stages.* Cambridge, MA: Harvard University Press, 1975.

discovered that the two forms used most frequently by parents (e.g., *a* and *the*) were acquired later than those forms which were used less frequently (e.g., *in* and *on*).

Derwing and Baker (1977) believed that phonological considerations influence early morphological use. Wells (1979), hypothesized that cognitive and semantic considerations are reflected in the order of acquisition of the grammatical morphemes. All agree that early morphological development focuses on more concrete relationships (such as plurality and possession), while later developing grammatical morphemes are more abstract. The progression from simple to complex, from concrete to abstract, is reflected in children's cognitive processing which in turn is reflected in their language development.

Other Early Morphemes. In addition to the early grammatical morphemes identified by Brown, other early morphemes were studied by other researchers. Trantham and Pedersen (1976) investigated the acquisition of pronouns. Palmer (1965) studied auxiliary verb development, and Carrow (1973) researched the acquisition of noun and adjective suffixes. These, like the grammatical morphemes, begin to develop in Brown's Stage II and continue until the age of 5 (Owens, 1984).

Phrase and Clause Development

Whereas words are made up of morphemes, sentences are composed of phrases and clauses. There are two major types of phrases: noun phrases and verb phrases. Noun phrases must contain a noun and may contain optional elements which modify the noun. In the sentence, "The girl in the red dress is pretty," there are two noun phrases: *The girl* (*girl* is the main noun) and *in the red dress*, a noun phrase which modifies the main noun.

There are four types of noun phrase modifiers:

1. *Determiners*—include articles (*a* and *the*); possessive pronouns (*my, your*); demonstratives (*this, that*); and qualifiers (*any, some*). They are always the first element in a noun phrase (e.g., *the* boy, *my* book, *some* toys).
2. *Adjectivals*—include adjectives (*little, big*); ordinals (*first, last*); and quantifiers (*two, few*). They modify nouns (e.g., *two* dresses, *big* boy).
3. *Initiators*—include *all, only, both, just,* which limit or quantify nouns and must precede a determiner (e.g., *only* the boy, *all* the girls)
4. *Postmodifiers*—modifiers that follow the main noun. They may include prepositional phrases (e.g., the toy *on the floor* is broken) and clauses (e.g., the boy *that came to my house*).

Although noun phrases emerge at Brown's Stage II, the greatest surge in their development occurs at Stage IV (Miller, 1981). Early modifier types are determiners and adjectivals, while initiators and postmodifiers are noted later in development. By late Stage IV, noun phrase elaboration appears both in subject and object positions and includes the use of almost all the modifier types mentioned previously.

In addition to noun phrases, sentences also contain verb phrases. Verb phrases must contain a main verb and may contain some optional elements. In the sentence, "The girl is pushing the boy," *is pushing* is the verb phrase. It contains the main verb *push* and the optional present progressive forms *is* and *-ing*. Optional elements of verb phrases include the *progressive construction* (e.g., *is eating*), *modals* (words that indicate mood or attitude, e.g., *may, must*), and *perfective constructions* (used to specify certain types of action, e.g., *has seen*). Verb phrase elaboration emerges at Brown's Stage II (with the marking of the present progressive) and continues through Stage V (Miller, 1981). Modals emerge at Stage IV and perfective constructions at Stage V.

In contrast to a phrase, a clause is a group of words that contains both a subject and a predicate. Some clauses can stand alone and can function as simple sentences (e.g., *Billy walks* or *Mary ate*). Sometimes a sentence contains more than one clause. Sentences which are made up of two or more main clauses which are joined as equals are called compound sentences (e.g., *John drank, and Mary ate*). They usually emerge at Brown's Stage IV (Miller, 1981).

Complex sentences are made up of one main clause (which can stand alone) and one subordinate clause. Although a subordinate clause contains both a subject and a predicate, it cannot stand alone. Note the embedding of the subordinate clause *that we bought yesterday* into the sentence "The dress that we bought yesterday is pretty." The embedding of subordinate clauses appears late in language development, usually at early Stage V. (The use of clauses in compound and complex sentences is discussed in later sections.)

Clauses can also be classified according to the nature of the verb contained in the clause (Crystal, Fletcher, & Garman, 1976). Generally, intransitive clauses (clauses containing a verb which cannot take a direct object, e.g., *The girl walked*) appear in children's declarative sentences before transitive clauses (clauses which take a direct object, e.g., *The boy drank milk*). The last type of clause to emerge is equative clauses, which contain a copula and a complement (e.g., *He is the teacher,* Dever, 1978).

Sentence Modulation

One of the most basic and elemental syntactic rules states that every sentence must contain a noun phrase and a verb phrase. Thus, the only required syntactic elements of a sentence are the subject and the predicate. By the end of Brown's Stage II or early Stage III, children have mastered this rule, enabling them to understand and produce simple, active declarative sentences such as "The boy hit the ball." Children then begin to modify this basic sentence pattern. They develop a variety of sentence types, including the negative, interrogative, and imperative sentence forms.

The Development of Negative Sentence Forms. Bloom (1970) found that children at the one- and two-word utterance stage express three semantically distinct types of negation: (*a*) *nonexistence* ("allgone juice"—when there is no more juice in the cup); (*b*) *rejection* ("no milk"—as the child rejects the offer of milk); and (*c*) *denial* ("not a book"—as mother points to a truck and says "This is a book"). Mastery of the rules which change a declarative sentence into a negative sentence, however, does not emerge until Brown's Stage III.

Klima and Bellugi (1966) traced the development of negation in Adam, Eve, and Sarah. Three phases in the acquisition of the negative construction were identified. In Phase I, the appearance of the negative element *no* at the start of the sentence indicates that children have acquired the deep structure for negation and apply it primarily for negating affirmitive sentences. In Phase II, children learn to transfer the *no* marker to its correct position before the verb in the sentence. The negative form, *not,* also appears. In Phase III, the negative contractible forms, *can't* and *don't* emerge. Table 5–4 illustrates the development of the negative sentence form.

Although most negative forms are mastered within the preschool period, indefinite negative forms such as "nobody," "no one," and "nothing" are difficult even for older school-aged children. Utterances such as "I don't got no books," or "Nobody don't goes there" are often heard in the speech of older children (and even some adults).

The Development of the Interrogative Sentence Form. There are two types of questions that can be asked: Yes/No questions and *Wh-* questions. Yes/No questions ("Do you want a cookie?") require that the listener simply answer the question with either a *Yes* or *No* word. *Wh-* questions (questions that begin with *who, what, when, where, why,* and *how*) are more complicated. They require that the listener provide further content to the speaker based on the question word that specifies the information being requested. For example, *Where* questions demand information about location; *When* questions demand temporal information; and *Who* questions demand information about people.

To form correct Yes/No questions, children must learn to invert the subject and the auxiliary verb. ("Is the boy eating?") To form correct *Wh-* questions, they must learn two operations: (*a*) to transpose the subject and the auxiliary verb, and (*b*) to add the *Wh-* form at the beginning of the sentence ("*What* is the boy eating?")

Klima and Bellugi (1966) found that children go through four phases as they develop the ability to formulate questions.

Phase 1. Use of rising intonation and some *Wh-* forms (MLU 1.75 to 2.25)
In this first phase, children typically ask Yes/No questions by adding a rising intonation to the end of their utterance. Examples of such question forms are "Johnnie eat?" "Baby drinking?" "Go outside?" To ask *Wh-* questions, children simply attach a *Wh-* word to an assertion and produce questions like "Where doggie?" and "What dat?" These *Wh-* questions are used only in routines in which children generally ask for names of objects, actions, or locations of previously present objects. The more prominent *Wh-* questions used during this phase are *Where* and *What* questions. At this stage, however, children do not respond appropriately to any of the *Wh-* questions.
Phase 2. Use of greater variety of *Wh-* questions (MLU 2.25 to 2.75)
Children at this stage continue to ask Yes/No questions by using rising intonation. Children ask *Wh-* questions by adding the *Wh-* form at the beginning of the question, but fail to use the auxiliary verb. Examples of *Wh-* questions which characterize this period are

Where my truck?
Why you pushing it?
What the man doing?

TABLE 5–4
Development of the Negative Sentence

Phase	*Description*	*Example*
I	The negative marker appears outside the sentence.	*No* the girl running.
II	The negative marker occurs before the verb.	The girl *not* running.
III	The auxiliary is added and completes the transformation to the adult form.	The girl *is not* running.

Children can give appropriate answers to *Wh-* questions asking *what, who,* and *where.*

Phase 3. Limited use of inversion (MLU 2.75 to 3.5)
At this phase, children regularly invert the subject and verb to produce Yes/No questions, but fail to do so in all *Wh-* questions. Examples of questions that characterize this period are

Will I go?
What the boy is riding?

Phase 4. Use of inversion in positive *Wh-* question (MLU 3.5 +)
In this last stage, children invert the subject and the auxiliary verb when asking positive *Wh-* questions, but still have difficulty with negative *Wh-* questions. Examples of *Wh-* questions of this period are

What is the boy eating?
Where are you going?
Why I can't do that?

Ervin-Tripp (1970) analyzed the specific order of emergence of the *Wh-* form. Her data showed that children comprehend *What, Where,* and *Who* questions before *When, Why,* and *How*—a correspondence to the production of these forms in their own speech. Ervin-Tripp explained that *What, Where,* and *Who* forms code cognitively simple ideas involving person, place and identity. *When, Why,* and *How* forms code the cognitively more complex ideas of temporal and causal relationships. The order of acquisition of questions is summarized in Table 5–5.

Another explanation for the emergence of *Wh-* questions is offered by Wotten, Merkin, Hood, and Bloom (1979). They suggested that the semantics of the verb influences children's comprehension and production of *Wh-* questions. For example, the verb *eat* is most clearly linked with the question form *What* than with *Where* or *Who.* Similarly, the verb *drive* is most logically linked with the question form *Where.* A verb which codes time, such as *finish,* would logically have as its expected question marker *When.* Wotten, et al (1979) suggested that certain verbs are expected with certain *Wh-* markers and that the development of syntactically correct *Wh-* questions is closely related to semantic considerations.

The Development of Imperative Sentence Forms. The imperative sentence requests, demands, commands, and insists that the listener perform some action. In imperative sentences, the subject "you" is understood and not included in the surface

TABLE 5–5
Order of Acquisition of Wh Questions

Type	Example
What	What is the girl eating?
Where	Where is the ball?
Who	Who is pushing the truck?
When	When will you go?
Why	Why is it dark?
How	How did it break?

form of the sentence, while the verb is uninflected. Examples of imperative sentences are "Gimme milk," "Push the truck," and "Pass the butter, please."

At the prelinguistic level, infants request and demand by pointing and gesturing. As they develop into toddlers, they begin to employ the imperative form to request, demand, and command. At Brown's Stage I, children produce forms that sound like imperatives because they often omit the subject even from sentences which require one. These early forms are not the true imperatives that begin to appear at Brown's Stage III when the omission of the subject in the surface form reflects the mastery of the rule of subject deletion for imperative sentences rather than the omission of the subject due to processing limitations.

The Development of Complex Sentences

Children begin to combine more than one semantic/syntactic relation in a single utterance when their MLU increases beyond 3.0. Their utterances reflect the elaboration or specification of agent-action-object interactions, and sentence construction advances from a linear ordering of words to a hierarchical ordering within and among sentence elements. Children learn to use complex sentences allowing the expression of old functions and new ideas with increasing clarity.

Coordination. The complex construction which emerges first in children's language is *coordination.* There are two types of coordination constructions: sentential coordination and phrasal coordination. In sentential coordination, two events are combined into one sentence by the conjunction *and* ("John went to the doctor, *and* his sister stayed home.") There are no redundant elements expressed in either phrase. In phrasal coordination, the connective *and* is also used, allowing the speaker to delete a redundant element. In the sentence, "Jane went to the movies and ate popcorn," the word *and* allows for the deletion of Jane from the second phrase (". . . and (Jane) ate popcorn.")

The earliest use of coordination by children is in stereotypic phrases ("bread and jam," "milk and cookie") which are present in young children's utterances as responses to routine questions like, "What do you want to eat?" Researchers in the early 1970s believed that sententials were less complex than phrasal coordinated sentences and were therefore acquired first. Recent studies do not confirm this order of emergence. DeVilliers (1982) found that children 2½ to 3 years of age used both sentential and phrasal coordinations appropriately when the communicative context was set up to elicit them.

Bloom, Lahey, Hood, Lifter and Fiess (1980) focused on semantic considerations in children's acquisition of coordinated sentences. They found the following order of acquisition of *and* coordinations:

1. *Additives*—the use of *and* to connect two propositions that go together
   Example: Mother is baking a cake *and* Daddy is reading.
2. *Temporal*—the use of *and* to designate a sequential ordering of events
   Example: Mommy will mix the batter *and* put it in the oven.
3. *Causal*—the use of *and* to indicate that one event led to another
   Example: She put a band-aid on *and* it made her feel better.

4. *Adversitive*—the use of *and* to indicate a contrast relationship
   Example: This goes in here *and* that goes there. (Often the connective used in this instance is *but.*)

The sequence of acquisition of coordinate constructions proposed by Bloom, Lahey, and Hood (1980) suggested that the level of cognitive development determines their use. DeVilliers (1982), however, suggested that children's learning of adaptive social strategies determines their use of coordinate constructions. Bloom's and deVilliers' views are not mutually exclusive. The learning of syntactic structures may be a function of cognitive/semantic *and* social/pragmatic constraints.

Complementation. There are several types of *complement* structures in English. Examples of sentences with complement constructions are "I want to buy a red lollipop," "Show me where this one goes," and "Look at what she's doing." In each of these sentences, the main portion of the sentence is coupled with a clause that in some way modifies the verb.

Bloom, Lifter, and Hafitz (1980) studied complement constructions and found that their order of emergence was based on the semantics of the verb. The first complements to emerge in children's speech are with *state* verbs: verbs that express a feeling or intention. *Like, want,* and *need* are state verbs and take the complement *to.* Examples of sentences using state verb complements are "I want to go home," and "I like to get dirty."

The next complement to emerge is attached to *notice* verbs. Notice verbs like *see, look,* and *watch* are followed by the complement *what,* as in "Look at what he's doing."

The third complement to emerge is attached to *knowledge* verbs like *know* and *think.* These are followed by the complement *that* or *what* as in "I know what to do," or "I think that one is good."

The last complement to emerge is attached to the *speaking* verbs, *ask, tell,* or *promise.* Speaking verbs require the complement construction *to* plus a verb. Sentences like "Ask Mary to come inside" or "John promised to leave" are examples of sentences with speaking verb complements. In keeping with her earlier hypothesis, Bloom concluded that the acquisition of complement constructions is a function of semantic constraints.

Relativization. Complex sentences can be formed by adding *relative* clauses, which restrict or qualify the meaning of another portion of the sentence. Relative clauses are of two types: objective and subjective. Objective relative clauses modify the object of the sentence as in "That picture is about some birds *that got all smeared up.*" An example of a sentence with a subject relative clause is "The girl *who lives down the block* is my cousin." Menyuk (1977) reported that object relative clauses emerge before subject relative clauses. The object relative clause develops after 5 years of age, while the subject relative clause is rare even at 7 years. DeVilliers, et al. (1979), remaining consistent with their social context/pragmatic approach, maintained that children use both subject and object relative clauses if the context is structured to demand specfication of the referent. Accordingly, if several similar objects, such as toy people, are placed in an array and each has a distinguishing feature such as hair color, clothing style, or body shape, the child will produce a sentence with a subject relative clause specifically describing each object. DeVilliers, et al., concluded that the pragmatic context influences children's use of relative clauses.

PHONOLOGICAL DEVELOPMENT

Children produce their first words with recognizable meaning between 1 and 1½ years of age. But toddlers' ability to make themselves understood is often limited by inadequate production of the sounds and the sound sequences which constitute these words. Without knowing the child or something about the nonlinguistic context, it would be difficult to recognize /doti/ for *doggie* or /dut/ for *juice.*

In order to master the sound system of the language, children must acquire an inventory of sounds. The sequence of English consonant acquisition is listed in Table 5–6.

In addition to acquiring individual sounds, children must also learn the rules which govern the position of sounds in words, *distributional rules,* and the rules for sequencing these sounds, *sequential rules.* They must learn to determine which speech sounds make a difference in meaning (Ingram, 1974). These rules are learned gradually, beginning in the early preschool years and continuing into early elementary school.

TABLE 5–6
The Age at Which 75% of Children Produced Consonant Sounds

	According to Templin (based on testing in initial, medial, and final positions)		*According to Prather (based on testing in initial and final positions only)*	
Sound	*Years*	*Months*	*Years*	*Months*
m	3		2	
n	3		2	
h	3		2	
p	3		2	
ŋ (as in si*ng*)	3		2	
f	3		2	4
j (as in *y*es)	3	6	2	4
k	4		2	4
d	4		2	4
w	3		2	8
b	4		2	8
t	6		2	8
g	4		3	
s	4	6	3	
r	4		3	4
l	6		3	4
ʃ (as in *sh*oe)	4	6	3	8
tʃ (as in *ch*urch)	4	6	3	8
ð (as in fa*th*er)	7		4	
ʒ (as in gara*g*e)	7		4	
dʒ (as in *j*udge)	7		4+	
θ (as in *th*umb)	6		4+	
v	6		4+	
z	7		4+	

Source: M.C. Templin, 1957; E.M. Prather, D.L. Hedrick, & A. Kern, 1975

Phonological Processes

As with morpho-syntactic development, children formulate and discard hypotheses regarding the rules of the sound system of the language. In examining the phonological rules used by children, linguists have noted that children simplify adult productions of a target word. The simplification "rules" used by children are called *phonological* or *natural processes.* These rules reduce the complexity of the consonant structure of a word or syllable that the child attempts to say. These are evident in children's first words and are discarded or fade out of children's speech by the age of 4. Some of the phonological processes used by children are described in the following sections (Edwards & Shriberg, 1983, Lund & Duchan, 1983).

Syllable Structure Processes. Children frequently simplify words by reducing them to either the basic consonant-vowel (CV) syllable or to CVCV structure. Four processes which accomplish this simplification are reduplication, final consonant deletion, cluster reduction, and deletion of unstressed syllables.

Reduplication—a well-known childlike pattern which usually occurs in normal children's first words. Using this process, children repeat the first syllable (which is usually the stressed syllable) and substitute it for subsequent syllables in multisyllabic words. Examples of reduplication are /kæ kæ/ for *cracker* or /dada/ for *daddy.*

Final consonant deletion—a syllable structure process in which the final consonant of a word is deleted. The result of this simplification is the production of a CV structure for a CVC word, such as /bɛ/ for *bed* or /fI/ for *fish.* Normally, this process completely disappears by the time the child is 3 to 3½ years old.

Cluster reduction—a structural simplification in which one or more consonants from a target consonant cluster are deleted. For example, the word *stop* becomes /top/ and the word *please* becomes /piz/. Cluster reduction is evident in children's speech until they are about 3 years of age.

Deletion of unstressed syllables—a simplification resulting in words like /næ na/ for *banana.*

Substitution Processes. A number of rule-governed substitutions are common in the speech of preschoolers. These substitutions are classified according to the place or manner of production of the speech sounds. Among the substitution processes are fronting, stopping, and gliding. Substitution processes are those in which one sound is substituted for another, depending on the sound's position in a word.

Fronting—one of the best known patterns in early childhood speech. Using this process, children replace palatal and velar sounds (made in the back of the mouth) with alveolar sounds (made in the front of the mouth). Examples of fronting are the production of /tΛp/ for *cup* or /dΛn/ for *gun.* Fronting of velars is usually suppressed by 2½ to 3 years of age, and velar consonants are usually established in children's speech by 4 years at the latest.

Stopping—instead of producing fricatives (sounds which are made by passing air through a narrow constriction, thereby creating a hissing sound) or affricates (sounds which combine a "popping" sound and a fricative), children substitute a plosive (a popping sound). The use of the stopping process results in productions such as /dut/

for *juice* or /ban/ for *van.* Stopping begins to disappear for most fricatives and affricates by 2½ to 3 years of age, but the emergence of the correct pronunciation of these sounds is gradual (Grunwall, 1982).

Gliding—children substitute glides (sounds which are produced during the movement of articulators from one vowel position to another) for liquids (sounds with vowel-like quality of little air turbulence). Examples of gliding are the production of /wabIt/ for *rabbit* or /yaIt/ for *light.* This process may persist for many years.

Assimilation Processes. Another group of processes are those in which two phonemes within a word become alike. Two assimilation processes are consonant harmony and prevocalic voicing.

Consonant harmony—consonants within a word become more alike in terms of place or manner of articulation. An example of consonant harmony is the production of /gɔgi/ for *doggy.*

Prevocalic Voicing—unvoiced consonants are affected by the following vowel and take on the voicing feature of the vowel. The result is the production of /dΛb/ for *tub.*

In tracing children's development of linguistic forms I have observed that they are in the direction of (*a*) lengthier utterance and (*b*) increased morphological, phonological, and syntactic complexity. I have examined children's development of different sentence types, noting semantics and pragmatic considerations. (A discussion of how to assess linguistic form is included in Chapter 6). In the following section, I will discuss semantic development of preschool and school-aged children.

SEMANTICS: THE DEVELOPMENT OF MEANING

Semantics is the component of language concerned with meaning. Without meaning there would be no point to language. People talk in order to express meaning, and they listen in order to discover the meaning of what others say.

This section will focus on recent studies concerning children's acquisition of relational, contextual, and nonliteral meanings.

The Development of Relational Meaning

The most familiar sense of meaning is lexical meaning. It is concerned with the meaning of words and the characteristics of the category to which a word applies. The development of lexical meaning has been studied most extensively at the very early stages of language acquisition and was discussed in Chapter 4. Children's lexical growth increases steadily during the preschool years; by the age of 8, children's receptive vocabulary is said to be between 6,000 and 8,000 words, while their expressive vocabulary ranges between 2,500 and 2,800 words (Berry, 1969).

In addition to acquiring lexical knowledge of words which specify referents, children acquire meanings which code relationships among people, objects, and events. These relationships can be conveyed at the word level or at the sentence level. The early relational meanings (or semantic content categories) of nonexistence and recurrence are evident early in children's language. These and other early semantic relations were discussed in Chapter 4. As children develop cognitively, the relationships they map and

TABLE 5–7
Semantic Relations Expressed by Children 2 to 4 Years of Age.

Semantic Relation	*Age*	*Example*
Coordination	2.0	My car . . . . truck.
Sequence	2.0	Bye, Bye, Mommy, Daddy, Joey.
Causality (Logical)	2.0	I can't do it. It too big.
Reasons	2.4	You hit me because you don't like me.
Temporality	2.8	Now I wash my hands, then I eat. When he goes to school he goes on the bus.
Conditionality	3.4	I wear this while walking.
Temporal Sequence	3.5 to 4.0	I will make a tree after I finish this.

Source: J.F. Miller. *Assessing language production in children: Experimental procedures.* Baltimore: University Park Press, 1981.

the forms they use to express these relationships become increasingly complex. In addition to the early semantic relations, their utterances reflect the coding of concepts of space, time, causation, and the sequencing of action. They begin to give limited reasons for their actions, and they talk not only about events in the "here and now," but also about events which are removed from the time and place of the conversation. Table 5–7 lists the semantic relations expressed by children between 2 and 4 years of age.

Recent studies have pointed to the interrelationship between the development of semantic relations and the linguistic forms used to express them. Bloom and her colleagues (1980) found that the sequence of emergence of linguistic connectives was related to the semantic relations which they express. Additive, temporal, and causal relationships emerged relatively early, while adversative and notice relations emerged later. These relationships were marked by a variety of linguistic forms, as noted in Table 5–8. The table defines the semantic relationships noted by Bloom, et al. (1980) and provides examples of each semantic category.

TABLE 5–8
Semantic Relationships Expressed by Connectives

Relationship Expressed	*Definition*	*Example*
Additive	Two events are joined without a dependent relationship.	You can run *and* I can jump.
Temporal	One element of a sentence describes an event that preceded (or followed) in time another event that is noted in the other element of the sentence.	I'm going outside *and* ride my bike. I'm going outside *and then* I'll come back.
Causal	A dependency involving two events occurs in which one is the result of the other.	Get them *because* I want it.
Adversative	The information in one element of the sentence contrasts with information in the other element(s) of the sentence.	Before I was tired, *but* now I'm not.
Notice	The first element of the sentence calls attention to a state or action in the second element of the sentence.	Watch *what* I'm doing.

Source: L. Bloom, M. Lahey, L. Hood, K. Lifter, & K. Fiess. Complex sentences: Acquisition of syntactic connectives and the semantic relations they encode. *Journal of Child Language, 7* (1980), 235–262.

The Development of Contextual Meaning

Context affects many aspects of language. The linguistic context or the discourse provides information necessary to derive intersentence meaning. The nonlinguistic context gives clues about the meaning of words whose referents shift depending on the perspective of the speaker and the timing of the utterance. I will explore the impact of context on meaning and examine children's acquisition of discourse cohesion devices and deictic terms.

Cohesive Devices. The influence of the linguistic context on meaning can be understood by examining the following sentence: He bought it.

Is it possible to derive the meaning of the sentence without knowing something about the previous linguistic context? Who is *he* and what is *it*? If the sentence occurs within the context of the following discourse, however, the meaning of *he* and *it* becomes clear.

Tom: John saw a red Jaguar at a car dealer yesterday.
Susan: What happened?
Tom: He bought it.

In the discourse, the pronouns *he* and *it* are used to refer to something that had already been identified linguistically. The use of a pronoun to refer to a previously mentioned referent is called *anaphoric reference.* Anaphoric reference as well as other linguistic devices help bind discourse so that it is better understood. Collectively, these are called *cohesive devices* because they provide the glue for intersentence meaning. They are included within the semantic component of language to highlight how meaning is derived from the linguistic context. Table 5–9 defines some cohesive devices and gives examples of each.

There is little information about the development of children's use of cohesive devices. In a seminal study, Bloom, Lightbown, and Hood (1975) found that

TABLE 5–9
Cohesive Devices

Type	*Definition*	*Example*
Anaphoric Reference	The use of pronouns or definite articles that refer to a previously established entity	Gina is sick today. *She* has the flu.
Cataphoric Reference	The use of pronouns or demonstratives that direct the listener to coming elements	After *he* warms up, John will be unbeatable.
Ellipsis	The deletion of information available in an immediately preceding portion of the discourse	Do you like to paint? I do. (like to paint)
Lexical Cohesion	The use of synonyms that refer to previously noted referents	Suddenly a lion appeared. The *beast* let out a terrifying roar.

Source: M. Halliday & R. Hasan. *Cohesion in English.* London: Longman, 1976.

2–year–olds do not use pronouns anaphorically. The children in their study used pronouns when the context gave the listener no clues about the referent (and when the use of a noun would have been more appropriate). At the same time, the children used nouns (instead of pronouns) when the referent was obvious from the context. It was concluded that the ability to recognize when it is appropriate to use pronouns anaphorically is a developmental achievement related to children's cognitive and social awareness of the linguistic context. In a related study, Tanz (1977) found that while children of 3 years of age understood the pronoun *it* when used anaphorically, the age at which they used pronouns anaphorically was not clearly determined.

Warden (1976) investigated between-sentence anaphoria. He found that by 7 years of age, children used the definite article to describe a referent that had already been mentioned. The tendency to use the indefinite article when introducing a referent appears to develop later.

Fine's study (1978) revealed that in dyadic communication, children follow up the utterances of an interactant with ellipsis more frequently than their own. In addition, Fine (1978) discovered that for children between 5 and 9 years of age, lexical cohesion usually represents no more than repeating the name of a referent in a subsequent utterance (e.g., John wanted to watch T.V. But it was broken. So John went for a walk instead). While the data on children's acquisition of discourse cohesive devices are presently limited, we expect that future research will focus on this area of language development.

Deixis. Another way in which context affects meaning is apparent in words whose meaning shifts as the nonlinguistic context changes. Consider the sentence, "I want you to go there tomorrow." The meanings of *I, you, there,* and *tomorrow* depend on who is speaking, who is listening, where the speaker and listener are when the sentence is uttered, and when the sentence is spoken. Words whose meaning and use depend on who is speaking and the time and place of the utterance are called *deictic terms.* Words like *I, you, here, there, today,* and *tomorrow* indicate the deictic relationship of person, place, and time, respectively.

Some studies have examined children's development of person, place, and time deixis. The limited data in this area indicate that it takes considerable time to master deictic terms. Although the exact ages for deictic acquisition are not specified, development sequence is (Tanz, 1980). Tanz found that children tend to acquire person deixis first: that is, deixis involving pronoun use. Spacial deixis, involving prepositions such as *in back of* and *in front of,* usually develops next. Temporal deixis is the last to emerge.

The Development of Nonliteral Meaning

Nonliteral meaning adds richness and depth to language and communicates in an indirect way what might be communicated directly. Consider the meaning inherent in the metaphor "Her eyes were ice," or in the proverb "The early bird catches the worm." Metaphors, proverbs, and jokes are examples of nonliteral language—language that doesn't mean what it says. The understanding and use of nonliteral meaning depends on the ability to disregard the literal interpretation of each word and to rely on a nonreferential, abstract, general meaning. Current research that focuses on the development of nonliteral meaning—specifically, on the understanding and use of metaphoric language, proverbs, and humor—is discussed in the following section.

Metaphoric Language. Studies dealing with children's comprehension and use of nonliteral language have focused on metaphors, which use a likeness to stand for a word, a referent, or an idea (He has a heart of stone). When metaphoric language is marked by the connectives *as* or *like,* it is called *simile* (It is as light *as* air).

The basic ability to comprehend nonliteral language emerges early, and it continues to develop with time (Nippold, Leonard, & Kail, 1984). In the development process (Winner, Rosenthal, & Gardner, 1976), young children understand cross-sensory metaphors (e.g., Her perfume was bright as sunshine) better than psychological-physical metaphors (e.g., The prison guard was a hard rock). In addition, similarity metaphors, where objects are compared on the basis of shared features (e.g., The stars are a thousand eyes) are comprehended better than proportional metaphors, where three objects are mentioned and a fourth must be inferred to complete a proportion (e.g., My head is like an apple without a core). Performance on each of the more difficult metaphoric types increases with age. Billow (1975) suggested that the precise use and understanding of metaphors are related to the cognitive attainments of adolescence. At this stage, children are able to understand that figurative language is based on a variety of links between domains.

Proverbs. Proverbs are a form of nonliteral language that are more abstract than metaphors. In a proverb, the domain that is the topic is never mentioned. Wise sayings such as "Don't put all your eggs in one basket" or "A stitch in time saves nine," mean something more general and abstract than the literal meaning of the statement. The real topic is never named. Billow (1975) found that preadolescents are generally unable to interpret proverbs and that it is not until adolescence that proverbs are understood.

Humor. We often infer information about children's semantic knowledge (or lack of knowledge) from the riddles and jokes they understand and tell. The source of humor in riddles and jokes is largely semantically based. It depends on understanding words that have the same surface form but different meanings, words which sound the same but are spelled differently (e.g., *bear* and *bare*), or words which sound the same and are spelled the same way but have more than one meaning (e.g., *glasses* or *nail*). The comprehension of humor often depends on perceiving the incongruity among the meanings of homonyms or multiple-meaning words.

Fowles and Glanz (1977) found that prior to age 6, children tell jokes in a confused manner and show no evidence of riddle structure. Between 6 and 9 years of age, children understand the frame of riddles, but not their meaning. When telling riddles, 6- to 9-year-olds delete or add portions to the riddle, making it informative rather than a riddle. When asked to explain jokes and riddles, 6- to 9-year-olds tend to be quite literal. They may identify something in the joke or riddle as funny, but do not see that it is the *language* which contributes to the humor. Note the explanation of a riddle given by a child in Fowles and Glanz's study (1977):

Question: How do you keep fish from smelling?

Answer: Cut off their noses.

Child's Explanation: It's funny because I don't think fish really have noses.

After 9 years of age, children tell riddles using the appropriate structure, and their explanation of jokes and riddles focuses on the attributes of language that contribute to the humor rather than on the nonlinguistic situation.

Jokes are another form of humor which requires suspending the usual literal meaning to appreciate the unexpected. The comprehension of jokes often depends on an incongruity or a sudden shift in perspective.

Different joke types have been identified (Lund & Duchan, 1983), and Shultz and Horibe (1974) have found an order in the acquisition of joke types. Prior to age 6, children only understand the nonlinguistic pie-in-the-face type of jokes. Between 6 and 9 years of age, children become sensitive to jokes which are based on the phonological structure of a word, or a group of words, within the utterance (Lund & Duchan, 1983).

Man: What is this?
Waiter: It's bean soup.
Man: I don't care what it's been. What is it now?

Between 9 and 12 years of age, children begin to develop an appreciation for humor that depends on a dual interpretation of a lexical item.

Question: What is black, white, and red (read) all over?
Answer: A newspaper.

After 12 years of age, children appreciate humor that involves alternative deep structure of the same surface structure.

Question: What kind of flower likes to be kissed?
Answer: Tulips (two lips).

Although research in this area is relatively new, current investigations are beginning to shed light on children's development of nonliteral meanings.

Summary. In this section, I presented current trends in the study of children's later semantic development, including the development of later relational meanings and the impact of syntax and pragmatics on semantics. I examined children's development of contextual meaning as revealed in their understanding and use of deictic terms and cohesion devices. Last, I reviewed children's understanding and use of nonliteral meaning as evidenced by their comprehension and use of figurative language and humor. (These areas of semantic development are assessed during a language evaluation and may be targeted for remediation if found deficient. For a discussion of semantic assessment, see Chapter 6.)

In the next section, I will trace the development of children's use of language in social contexts. The focus will be on preschool and school-aged children's pragmatic development.

PRAGMATIC DEVELOPMENT

During the preschool years, children's speech reflects an elaboration of communicative intent. The basic communicative functions of the earlier sensorimotor period expand. New communicative strategies and functions emerge. Children become more aware of the social context, and the linguistic forms that they use begin to vary with the changing characters of the social setting and the interactors within it. Children describe objects and events removed from the immediate context, they ask and answer questions, and they use language effectively to express their wants and needs. In addition, they become more aware of the general conditions governing cooperative conversations. They learn to stick to a topic of conversation and contribute new and relevant information to the discourse (Bloom, Rociassano, & Hood, 1976). These abilities begin in the preschool years and continue as the child matures cognitively and socially.

The development of language use in the preschool years sets the stage for the changes which take place later on. Comprehensive data are not yet available from which to draw a cohesive picture of the development of pragmatic skills past the age of 7. From the available research, however, it is clear that as children get older, they extend their repertoire of language use. They become more sensitive to what their listener needs to know. They decide what information to present. They add to their repertoire various means for conveying their intentions, and they learn how to express their intentions indirectly.

This section will deal with three aspects of pragmatic development: (*a*) the elaboration of communicative functions and strategies; (*b*) the development of communication strategies; and (*c*) the expansion of discourse skills.

The Elaboration of Communicative Function

Several studies have explored children's use of language during the preschool years. Moerk (1975) identified nine language functions used by children 2 to 5 years of age. According to Moerk, these categories account for 65% of 2- to 5-year-olds' utterances as they interact with their caretakers by:

1. Imitating
2. Asking a question
3. Expressing a need
4. Answering a question
5. Encoding from picture books
6. Describing objects or events
7. Describing own acts
8. Describing plans
9. Describing a past experience

Complementing the analysis of 2- to 5-year-olds' interactions with their caretakers is Dore's (1978) study of peer group interaction for the same age group. The communicative functions displayed by children during play were classified in three groups: (*a*) conveying content, (*b*) regulating conversation, and (*c*) expressing attitude. In Table 5–10, six communicative functions are elaborated. For each function, various specific categories are listed and examples are given. Note the wide variety of communicative functions used by the 2- to 5-year-olds and the explicitness of Dore's taxonomy.

Tough (1977) examined the communicative functions used by children 3 to 7 years of age. Her older subjects used language to think and to solve problems. They also used language to reason, to relate events to one another, to engage in complex imaginative play, and to control their own behavior. These changes in language use

TABLE 5–10
Communication Functions of Children 2 to 5 Years of Age

Communicative Functions	*Specific Categories*	*Example*
Requests information, action, or acknowledgement	Asks *Yes/No* questions, seeks *true-false* judgements about propositions	Is he eating candy?
	Asks *Wh-* questions, seeks factual information	What's next? Where are you going?
	Requests action or seeks that the listener do or stop doing an action	Why don't you get it, Come on. Look at this. Stop it.
	Requests permission	Can I put the block in?
	Asks rhetorical questions or seeks acknowledgement from the listener to allow speaker to continue	You know what?
Responds to requests	Answers *Yes/No* questions or supplies *true-false* judgements	No, he's not going.
	Answers *Wh-* questions or supplies factual information	Tomorrow.
	Agrees with or accepts previous utterance	That's right.
	Complies with or expresses acceptance, denial, or acknowledgement of a prior action or permission request	Okay.
	Qualifies or supplies unexpected information in response to question	But I wasn't the one who did it.
Describes	Identifies or labels objects, events, etc.	That's a car. There's a big truck.
	Describes events, actions, or processes	I'm making a house. He's doing it slowly.
	Describes properties or conditions	That's a truck with a crane.
	Describes location or direction	It's in here.
States facts, rules, attitudes, feelings, and beliefs	Reports time of event	It happened yesterday.
	Reports or expresses reasons, causes, and prediction	It will rain.
Regulates contact and conversation	Calls or solicits attention	Johnny, Hey!
	Indicates ostensible politeness	Please, thank you.
Miscellaneous	Protests or registers complaints about listener's behavior	Stop that.
	Jokes or displays nonbelief toward a proposition for a humorous effect	I ate the elephant.
	Claims or establishes rights	I'm first. Finders keepers.
	Teases or annoys, taunts, or playfully provokes response	You're a fatso.

Source: J. Dore, 1978; J.F. Miller, 1981

TABLE 5–11
Communicative Functions Used by Children 4 to 7 Years of Age

Function	*Uses*	*Strategies*	*Example*
Directive	Self-directing	Monitoring action	John (accompanying action): This piece goes in here—in—go in.
		Focusing control	Lisa (actions accompanying each word): I'm winding it—turn–turn.
		Foward planning	Tim: I'll roll the clay out and then put it in two piles.
	Other-directing	Demonstrating	Carol: Put the car in front of the house. That's right. Now you put your truck at the end of the street like this.
		Instructing	Bob: Put your block on top of mine, but be careful not to knock it down. Go slowly.
		Foward planning	Monica: You'll have to get the red block and put it in front of the green one; otherwise, it won't be the same.
		Anticipating collaboration	June (to Daryl, who is building sand castle): Make the castle road come on to here so it can connect with my road.
Interpretive	Reporting on present and past experiences	Labeling	That's a banana and the other one's an apple.
		Elaborating detail	I saw a lake with a lot of ducks swimming and fish jumping out of the water.
		Comparing	I've got one but it's bigger.
		Recognizing incongruity	This pie is too big to go in this little space.
		Awareness of sequence	First we went into the restaurant. I ordered a sandwich and later I had dessert.

Source: J. Tough, 1977; J.F. Miller, 1981

reflect internal cognitive and social changes. Tough (1977) classified children's language use in four major function categories: (*a*) directive, (*b*) interpretive, (*c*) relational, and (*d*) projective. Table 5–11 lists each function, outlines the strategies children use when expressing a particular function, and gives examples for each function category. Tough's classification system is noteworthy for the cognitively advanced semantic content that it captures.

TABLE 5–11
Continued

Function	*Uses*	*Strategies*	*Example*
Projective	Predicting	Forecasting events	When it will snow we'll build a snowman.
		Anticipating consequences	Mommy will be mad 'cause I lost it.
		Weighing alternatives	We can play with the dolls or the Pac Man. Which?
		Forecasting possibilities	If the roof isn't strong enough, he may fall in.
		Recognizing problems	It can't close. It's not good. It's bad.
		Predicting solution	Maybe if I go get some tape. Yep, I think that will help.
	Empathetic	Projecting into experience and into other people's feelings	She's crying because he's mean to her. She feels bad.
		Anticipating the reactions of others	He'll be mad at Johnny if he does it.
	Imagining	Reenacting	Jim (Putting two round blocks on a plate): This is your cupcake and this one's mine.
		Commenting on imagined context (building a scene through language)	Jill (Using an imaginary telephone): Quick, Bob, you must come home. Jimmy fell off a tree and broke his head. Quick, and bring the doctor, too.
		Using language for role playing	Tom (taking imaginary tickets): Where's your ticket, lad. Thank you. That will be 5 cents.
Relational	Self-maintaining	Expressing need	Look at what I can do.
		Protecting of self-interest	Stop—that hurts me.
		Justifying	Give me the yellow one so I can make a sun.
		Criticizing	Yours stinks!
		Threatening	Give it back or I'll tell the teacher.
	Interactional	Self-emphasizing	Give it to me—it's mine.
		Other recognizing	Mommy's calling me. I've got to go. Can I have my truck back, please?

Speech Act Development. Another perspective on the development of children's language use is provided by speech act theory (Searle, 1975; see chapter 4). According to Searle (1975), speech acts belong to five basic categories, each based on the speaker's intention (See Table 5–12).

Each speech act conveys a different intention on the part of the speaker but also requires something of the listener. In the case of representatives, the listener must take note of the speaker's beliefs. Directives require listeners to determine a course of

TABLE 5–12
Searle's Categories of Speech Acts

Category	*Type*	*Speaker's Intentions*	*Listener's Requirements*	*Example*
Representative	Assert State	To convey belief to the listener	To take note of speaker's belief	Tom owns a bus.
Directive	Order Command Request Plead	To get the listener to do something	To carry out action or formulate a response	Catch the ball. Does Tom own a bus? What does Tom own?
Commissive	Promise Pledge Guarantee	To commit themselves to a future action	To note new information about the speaker's intended action	I promise that Tom will own that house.
Expressive	Apologize Thank	To convey their psychological states	To note or to respond to the speaker's feelings	I'm sorry for being late.
Declaration	Marry Fire Arrest	To bring about a new state of affairs	To note or to respond to a change in the status quo	You're under arrest. I now pronounce you husband and wife.

Source: J.R. Searle. A taxonomy of illocutionary acts. In K. Gunderson (Ed.), *Minnesota studies in the philosophy of language* (pp. 344–359). Minneapolis: University of Minnesota Press, 1975.

action and to carry it out. Commissives, expressives, and declarations require listeners to take note of information reflecting the speakers' intended course of action, their feelings about some fact, or a change in the formal status of present conditions.

Researchers who have examined the use of directives by children 2 to 5 years of age (Ervin-Tripp, 1977; Mitchell-Kernan & Kernan, 1977) have revealed that children's production of directives goes through a series of stages. In the earliest stage, children are direct in their use of directives (*want, gimme*). At an intermediate stage, they use polite forms to express directives ("Would you give me?" "Please give me."). At about age 5, they produce directives in which the desired goal may not even be mentioned (e.g., My, that car is nice!!).

Grimm (1975) studied the development of directives and commissives of children 5 to 7 years of age by examining their ability to ask, order, forbid, permit, and promise. Her study showed that, while 5-year-olds managed very well in producing adequate utterances for some directives (asking, ordering, forbidding), they experienced some difficulty in producing adequate utterances to convey permission. The 7-year-olds in her study, however, did better on all four directives, but still had difficulty in making promises.

Grimm's findings may be explained in terms of the different requirements placed on speakers and listeners when producing directives and commissives. Directives place an obligation on the listener, whereas commissives place an obligation on the speaker. With directives, the listener is expected to act, refrain from acting, or provide information. The obligation is on the listener, and the speaker must simply wait for a response. Such is not the case with commissives. When speakers utter a commissive, they place themselves under an obligation. When they make a promise, *they* are the ones expected to carry it out, not the listener. Grimm's finding suggests that speech acts which place the obligation on the speaker tend to be acquired later than those that place the obligation on the listener.

These findings seem to conform with the results of the study of directives and commissives by C. Chomsky (1969). Chomsky (1969) found that children understand the directive *tell* before they understand the commissive *promise.* In her study, children under the age of 8 often assumed that the verb *promise* was a directive and interpreted it to mean *tell.* She described the following example:

Adult: Bozo promises Donald to do a somersault. Can you make him do it?

The child made Donald do the somersault and said:

Child: I promised you you can do a somersault.

Although some experimental data have been collected regarding children's understanding and use of directives and commissives, fewer data are available regarding the use of expressives. Expressives, which are often essential to the smooth functioning of society, constitute one part of language that adults seem to teach children by rote. Parents begin to insist that children at the age of 2 or 3 say "Please," "I'm sorry," "Excuse me," and "Thank you," in the appropriate contexts. In contrast to directives and commissives, expressives place no direct obligation for action on either the speaker or the listener. Although expressives may reflect the speaker's true feelings about someone or something, they reflect the feeling expected in a particular context within a given society and are therefore hard to justify and explain to children. Most parents don't try. Their concerns are usually social ones. They will say, "Say, 'thank you' to your uncle," or "Did you say, 'I'm sorry,' to your grandfather?" or "I hope you said 'please' to Mr. Wolfson," and so on. Usually it takes many years before children fully understand the social role of expressives (Berko-Gleason, 1973; Berko-Gleason & Weintraub, 1976).

The relationship between the development of speech acts and children's cognitive and social development is still being explored. Clark and Clark (1977) concluded that speech acts are acquired in the following order: (*a*) directives, (*b*) commissives, (*c*) expressives, and (*d*) declarations. Future research should help corroborate this order.

The Development of Communication Strategies

As children mature, they slowly adapt their language to the needs of the listener. With the realization that other people's perspectives must be taken into account, *presuppositional ability,* comes the emergence of new communication strategies. By the time children reach the concrete operational stage, they perceive the needs of their listeners and make *un*differentiated adaptations in their communication to satisfy those needs. In settling peer disputes, for example, children give reasons for disagreements involving their own feelings and beliefs about an event or an action. In the stage of formal operations, children adapt to their listeners' needs in a differentiated manner by negotiating, justifying, and stating reasons for their positions. These often involve accounting for another person's perspective. Table 5–13 summarizes the different communication strategies utilized by children in the preoperational, concrete, and formal operations stages.

TABLE 5–13
Communication Strategy Development: An Overview

Cognitive Period	*Strategy*	*Examples*
Preoperational		
Early	Self-oriented perception Nonadaptation to listener	Context: Jim and John in sandbox. John wants to play with the pail and shovel. Jim is playing with it. John: Gimme pail and shovel!
Late	Perception of listener Nonadaptation to listener	Context: Sue and Jean are in the yard. Sue has been riding the bike for 5 mins. Jean: Now *I* want to ride the bike!
Concrete	Perception of listener Undifferentiated adaptation to listener	Context: Bill and Sam are in the playground. Bill: Please, pretty please, can I try your baseball glove? Context: Linda borrowed Stacy's pen. Linda: I'm sorry I broke your pen.
Formal	Perception of listener Differentiated adaptation to listener needs	Context: Jason and Peter are on the playground. Jason: If you'll let me try your mitt, I'll let you try my head-to-head Coleco football (Jason takes the game out of his pocket.) Context: Lisa has returned from school. Her mother is upset. Lisa: I know you're upset, but the English teacher assigned us a composition about El Salvador for tomorrow, and I stopped off at the library to get some books to do the research.

Source: E.H. Wiig. *Let's talk inventory for adolescents.* Columbus, OH: Charles E. Merrill, 1982.

The Development of Discourse Skills

This section deals with children's expansion of discourse skills. The focus will be on conversation and narratives, two areas of pragmatic development which researchers are actively investigating.

Conversation. The rules of conversation are a skill all children must master. Conversations usually occur between two or more people in face-to-face interaction. Certain parts of a conversation are topic-oriented. Others involve management of the conversation itself. Management devices are units which alter the conversation and include:

1. Conversation openings—Hi! What's new? Do you have a sec?
2. Conversation closings—Bye! Got to go. See you later.
3. Repairs—No, what I meant was. . . . That's not what I said. That one, not this one.
4. Turn exchange—John, what do you think?
5. Topic change—Speaking of dresses, I went shopping yesterday and saw Sue. Sue is looking great. She cut her hair.

In addition to management devices, there are rules which regulate the content and manner of conversations. Grice (1975) and Lakoff (1973) have outlined two general conditions which appear to govern conversations: the obligation to be clear and informative and the obligation to be polite. By following these rules, people are able to communicate their perceptions of social relationships and to carry on an intelligent exchange. In short, skilled conversation is in part a function of abiding by conversational rules. Although research has provided knowledge about the roots of conversation (eye gaze, turn taking, play routines), the ages and stages at which different conversational rules are learned have yet to emerge.

Narratives. By the time children command a small linguistic repertoire, language assumes a social and communicative role. Children learn how to transform ideas into sentences and to communicate information through narratives. As toddlers, children are exposed to narratives or stories in picture books and television. They begin to relate stories early in the preschool years. By 1st grade, demands are placed on them to relate narratives: "show and tell," relating vacation activities or holiday experiences, or retelling a story previously heard. These are activities common to all 1st- and 2nd-grade children and are later given to them in the form of written assignments. "My summer or winter vacation," "How I spent the holidays," or a synopsis of a book or a story are frequently assigned topics for speeches and compositions.

Narratives are a form of discourse. They contain sentences and statements which are logically connected to reflect causal and temporal relationships. They also contain principles and structure which give them cohesiveness. One perspective on the nature and structure of narratives is seen in the work of Stein (1978), and Stein and Glenn (1979). Stein and Glenn (1979) suggested that stories are combined by various categories, or units, and rules. Category definitions and rules of the story grammar model, as outlined by Johnston (1982), are shown in Table 5–14.

According to Stein and Glenn (1979), there is an internal structure to stories, and competent storytellers structure their information in a form which guarantees the full understanding of the story. They sequence and organize events in time and space so that the consequential nature of the story is ensured.

When children hear stories in which the informational sequences are inverted (for example, they are told the consequence unit before the initiating event), they remember them less well than if the story were told to them in the order given by the model. If children are given individual narrative statements and asked to make up a story, the sequence of their stories correlates highly with the sequence predicted by the story

TABLE 5–14
Story Grammar Model

STORY = Setting Unit + Episode Structure
- *Setting Unit*—introduction of main characters, protagonist, context of time and place
- *Episode Structure*—initiating event + internal response + plan + attempt + consequence + reaction unit
  - *Initiating Event*—action or occurrence which influences the main characters
  - *Internal Response*—characters' motivations, thoughts, and feelings about the initiating event
  - *Plan Unit*—protagonist's intended action or verbal responses to the initiating event
  - *Attempt Unit*—protagonist's actions in pursuit of the goal
  - *Consequence Unit*—outcome of the attempt; success or failure of the protagonist
  - *Reaction Unit*—protagonist's response to the outcome

Source: N. Stein. In J. Johnston, Narratives: A new look at communication problems in older language disordered children. *Language, Speech, and Hearing Services in Schools, 13* (1982), 144–155.

grammar model. Also, when asked to retell a story, children are most likely to include a setting, initiating event, and consequence unit.

Although children use the schematic knowledge of story grammars to understand stories and to formulate narratives, there are developmental differences between the abilities of younger and older children to formulate these narratives. The following characteristics are more likely to be found in the stories of older children:

1. Greater detail in the setting information
2. More complex episode structure
3. More concern with motivations, thoughts, and feelings of the character
4. Less unimportant or extraneous detail in general; greater detail in the internal response unit
5. Greater information regarding changes in time and place
6. Fewer unresolved problems
7. Greater adherence to the story grammar model (Clancy, 1979; Kernan, 1977; Stein & Glenn, 1979)

Greater complexity, more attention to motivations, thoughts, and details, as well as attention to the needs of the listener to know about sequences of time and place, are characteristic of the narratives of older children. These developments in children's narratives are the result of their cognitive development and social awareness. By the time children are 10 years old, their stories include an established protagonist, a clear problem to be solved, an action to be pursued, and consequences or outcomes of the action, as well as statements regarding their attitude or evaluation of the story.

SUMMARY

Children's language development is indeed a multifaceted and complicated process. Although there are common developmental patterns, there are variances in children's language acquisition which account for their respective differences. Children have unique predispositions from birth and different cognitive, social, and linguistic experiences. In a similar vein, the rate of learning linguistic forms differs among children.

In this chapter, I analyzed the process of language development. Children's utterances are observed to increase in length and complexity. From an MLU of 2.0 and continuing beyond an MLU of 4.0, children simultaneously learn several linguistic subsystems. They develop grammatical morphemes, acquire a variety of sentence types, and master the phonological system. They acquire more abstract meanings and the ability to map these onto linguistic structures. Last, children elaborate their use of language to suit a variety of social contexts. Although each component of language was discussed separately, in the real world, language form (phonology, morphology, and syntax), content (semantics), and use (pragmatics) are interrelated in development.

I conclude this chapter on later language development with a quotation from Rees (1980).

> For professionals in the area of communication disorders, it is recognized that only the most complete understanding possible of the nature and growth of child language will suffice as basic information with which to approach clinical problems. Normal language development provides not only the base of reference against which to evaluate the communicative functioning of the clinical subject, but also guidelines for assessment and intervention. (p. 38)

Information about normal language development provides the speech-language pathologist with a framework for understanding the assessment and remediation of language disorders in children. Because new knowledge is continuously emerging about the stages, strategies, and processes of normal language development, what we "do today will be replaced tomorrow by wiser principles and improved techniques" (Rees, 1980, p. 38).

STUDY QUESTIONS

1. What are operating principles? How do they help children learn language?
2. How does the notion of systematic overgeneralization aid us in viewing the child as a hypothesis builder and tester?
3. Discuss the contribution of imitation in language development.
4. As children develop linguistically, their utterances become more complex. Discuss this statement as it relates to phonological, syntactic, semantic, and pragmatic development.
5. What linguistic changes occur at each of Brown's Stages I through V?

BIBLIOGRAPHY

Bates, E. (1979). *The emergence of symbols.* New York: Academic Press.

Berko, J. (1958). The child's learning of English morphology. *Word, 14,* 150–177.

Berko-Gleason, J. (1973). Code switching in children's language. In T.E. Moore (Ed.), *Cognitive development and the acquisition of language* (pp. 159–167). New York: Academic Press.

Berko-Gleason, J., & Weintraub, S. (1976). The acquisition of routines in child language. *Language in Society, 5,* 129–136.

Berry, M.F. (1969). *Language disorders of children.* Englewood Cliffs, NJ: Prentice-Hall.

Billow, R. (1975). A cognitive developmental study of metaphor comprehension. *Developmental Psychology, 11,* 415–423.

Bloom, L. (1970). *Language development: Forms and functions of emerging grammars.* Cambridge, MA: MIT Press.

Bloom, L., Hood, L., & Lightbown, P. (1974). Imitation in language development: If, when, why. *Cognitive Psychology, 6,* 380–420.

Bloom, L., & Lahey, M. (1978). *Language development and language disorders.* New York: Wiley.

Bloom, L., Lahey, M., Hood, L., Lifter, K., & Fiess, K. (1980). Complex sentences: Acquisition of syntactic connectives and the semantic relations they encode. *Journal of Child Language, 7,* 235–262.

Bloom, L., Lifter, K., & Hafitz, J. (1980). Semantics of verbs and the development of verb inflection in child language. *Language, 56,* 386–412.

Bloom, L., Lightbown, P., & Hood, L. (1975). Structures and variation in child language. *Mono-*

graphs of the Society for Research in Child Development, 40.

Bloom, L., Rociassano, L., & Hood, L. (1976). Adult-child discourse: Developmental interaction between information processing and linguistic knowledge. *Cognitive Psychology, 8,* 521–552.

Braine, M. (1971). On two types of models of the internalization of grammars. In D. Slobin (Ed.), *The ontogenesis of grammar* (pp. 153–167). New York: Academic Press.

Brown, R. (1973). *A first language: The early stages.* Cambridge, MA: Harvard University Press.

Brown, R., Cazden, C., & Bellugi-Klima, U. (1969). The child's grammar from I-III. In J. Hill (Ed.), *Minnesota symposia on psychology* (Vol. 2). Minneapolis: University of Minnesota Press.

Brown, R., & Hanlon, C. (1970). Derivational complexity and order of acquisition. In J. Hayes (Ed.), *Cognition and the development of language* (pp. 155–207). New York: Wiley.

Carrow, E. (1973). Test of auditory comprehension of language. Austin, TX: Urban Research Group.

Chomsky, C. (1969). *The acquisition of syntax in children from 5 to 10.* Cambridge, MA: MIT Press.

Clancy, P. (1979). The development of narrative discourse in Japanese. *Papers and Reports in Child Language Development # 17* (pp. 41–48). Stanford University, Department of Linguistics.

Clark, E., & Clark, H. (1977). *Psychology and language: An introduction to psycholinguistics.* New York: Harcourt Brace Jovanovich.

Clark, R. (1977). What's the use of imitation? *Journal of Child Language, 4,* 34–358.

Crystal, D., Fletcher, P., & Garman, M. (1976). *The grammatical analysis of language disability: A procedure for assessment and remediation.* London: Edward Arnold.

Derwing, B., & Baker, W. (1977). The psychological basis for morphological rules. In J. Macnamara (Ed.), *Language learning and thought* (pp. 85–110). New York: Academic Press.

Dever, R. (1978). *TALK: Teaching the American language to kids.* Columbus, OH: Charles E. Merrill.

deVilliers, P. (1982). *Later syntactic development: The contribution of semantics and pragmatics.* Paper presented at New York State Speech-Language-Hearing Association Convention.

deVilliers, J.G., & deVilliers, P.A. (1978). *Language acquisition.* Cambridge, MA: Harvard University Press.

deVilliers, J., Tager-Flusberg, H., Hakuta, K., & Cohen, M. (1979). Children's comprehension of relative clauses. *Journal of Psycholinguistic Research,* 499–518.

Dore, J. (1978). Requestive systems in nursery school conversations: Analysis of talk in its social context. In R. Campbell & P. Smith (Eds.), *Recent advances in the psychology of language: Language development and mother–child interaction* (pp. 271–292). New York: Plenum Press.

Edwards, M.L., & Shriberg, L. (1983). *Phonology: Applications in communicative disorders.* San Diego: College Hill Press.

Ervin-Tripp, S. (1964). Imitation and structural change in children's language. In E. Lenneberg (Ed.), *New directions in the study of language* (pp. 163–169). Cambridge, MA: MIT Press.

Ervin-Tripp, S. (1970). Discourse agreement: How children answer questions. In J.R. Hayes (Ed.), *Cognition and the development of language* (pp. 79–107). New York: Wiley.

Ervin-Tripp, S. (1977). "Wait for me to roller skate". In S. Ervin-Tripp & C. Mitchell-Kernan (Eds.), *Child discourse* (pp. 165–189). New York: Academic Press.

Ferguson, C.A. (1964). Baby talk in six languages. *American Anthropologist, 66,* 103–114.

Fine, J. (1978). Conversation, cohesive and thematic patterning in children's dialogues. *Discourse Processes, 1,* 247–266.

Fowles, B., & Glanz, M.E. (1977). Competence and talent in verbal riddle comprehension. *Journal of Child Language, 4,* 433–452.

Fraser, C., Bellugi, U., & Brown, R. (1963). Control of grammar in imitation, comprehension and production. *Journal of Verbal Learning and Verbal Behavior, 2,* 121–135.

Gelman, R., & Shatz, M. (1977). Appropriate speech adjustments: The operation of conversational constraints on talk to 2-year-olds. In M. Lewis & L. Rosenblum (Eds.), *Interaction, conversation, and the development of language* (pp. 27–61). New York: Wiley.

Grice, H.P. (1975). Logic and conversation. In P. Cole & J.L. Morgan (Eds.), *Syntax and semantics* (Vol. 3, *Speech Acts,* pp. 41–58). New York: Seminar Press.

Grimm, H. (1975, September). Analysis of short-term dialogues in 5-7 year olds: Encoding of intentions and modifications of speech acts as a function of negative feedback. Paper presented at the Third International Child Language Symposium, London.

Grunwell, P. (1982). *Clinical Phonology.* Rockville, MD: Aspen Publications.

Halliday, M., & Hasan, R. (1976). *Cohesion in English.* London: Longman.

Hass, W., & Wepman, J. (1974). Dimensions of individual differences in the spoken syntax of school children. *Journal of Speech and Hearing Research, 17,* 455–469.

Ingram, D. (1974). Phonological rules in young children. *Journal of Child Language, 1,* 97–106.

Johnston, J. (1982). Narratives: A new look at communication problems in older language disordered children. *Language, Speech, and Hearing Services in Schools, 13,* 144–155.

Kernan, K. (1977). Semantic and expressive elaboration in children's narratives. In S. Ervin-Tripp and C. Mitchell-Kernan (Eds.), *Child discourse* (pp. 91–103). New York: Academic Press.

Klima, E., & Bellugi, U. (1966). Syntactic regularities in the speech of children. In J. Lyons & R. Wales (Eds.), *Psycholinguistic papers* (pp. 183–208). Edinburgh: Edinburgh University Press.

Lakoff, R. (1973). The logic of politeness; or minding your p's and q's. In C. Corum, T. Smith-Clark, & A. Weiser (Eds.), Papers from the Ninth Regional Meeting of the Chicago Linguistic Society, University of Chicago, Department of Linguistics, Chicago.

Lucariello, J., & Nelson, K. (1982, March). Situational variation in mother-child interaction. Paper presented at the Third International Conference on Infant Studies, Austin, TX.

Lund, N., & Duchan, J. (1983). *Assessing children's language in naturalistic contexts.* Englewood Cliffs, NJ: Prentice-Hall.

McLean, J., & Snyder-McLean, L.K. (1978). *A transactional approach to early language training.* Columbus, OH: Charles E. Merrill.

McNeill, D. (1966). Developmental psycholinguistics. In F. Smith & G. Miller (Eds.), *The genesis of language: A psycholinguistic approach* (pp. 15–84). Cambridge, MA: MIT Press.

Menyuk, P. (1977). *Language and maturation.* Cambridge, MA: MIT Press.

Miller, J.F. (1981). *Assessing language production in children: Experimental procedures.* Baltimore: University Park Press.

Mitchell-Kernan, C., & Kernan, K. (1977). Pragmatics of directive choice among children. In S. Ervin-Tripp and C. Mitchell-Kernan (Eds.), *Child discourse* (pp. 189–208). New York: Academic Press.

Moerk, E.L. (1975). Verbal interactions between children and their mothers during the preschool years. *Development of Psychology, 11,* 788–794.

Moerk, E.L. (1974). Changes in verbal child-mother interactions with increasing language skills of the child. *Journal of Psycholinguistic Research, 3,* 100–116.

Nelson, K. (1973). Structure and strategy in learning to talk. *Monographs of the Society for Research in Child Development 38* (Serial No. 1–2).

Newport, E. (1976). "Motherese": The speech of mothers to young children. In N.J. Castellan, D.B. Pisoni, & G.R. Potts (Eds.), *Cognitive theory* (Vol. 2, pp. 177–219). Hillsdale, NJ: Lawrence Erlbaum.

Nippold, M., Leonard, L., & Kail, R. (1984). Syntactic and conceptual factors in children's understanding of metaphors. *Journal of Speech and Hearing Research, 27,* 197–205.

Owens, R. (1984). *Language development.* Columbus, OH: Charles E. Merrill.

Palmer, F. (1965). *The English verb.* New York: Lungmans.

Piaget, J. (1964). Development and learning. In R.L. Ripple & V.N. Hardcastle (Eds.), *Piaget rediscovered* (pp. 1–5). Ithaca, NY: Cornell University Press.

Prather, E.M., Hedrick, D.L., & Kern, A. (1972). Articulation development in children aged two to four years. *Journal of Speech Hearing Disorders, 37,* 55–63.

Ramer, A. (1976). The function of imitation in child language. *Journal of Speech & Hearing Research, 19,* 700–717.

Rees, N. (1980). The nature of language. In T. Hixon, L. Shriberg, & J. Saxman (Eds.), *Introduction to communication disorders* (pp. 2–41). Englewood Cliffs, NJ: Prentice-Hall.

Searle, J.R. (1975). A taxonomy of illocutionary acts. In K. Gunderson (Ed.), *Minnesota studies in the philosophy of language* (pp. 344–359). Minneapolis: University of Minnesota Press.

Schultz, T.R., & Pilon, R. (1973). Development of the ability to detect linguistic ambiguity. *Child Development, 44,* 728–733.

Shultz, T.R., & Horibe, F. (1974). The development of the appreciation of verbal jokes. *Developmental Psychology, 10,* 13–20.

Slobin, D.I. (1973). Cognitive prerequisites for the development of grammar. In C.A. Ferguson & D.I. Slobin (Eds.), *Studies of child language development* (pp. 175–208). New York: Holt, Rinehart & Winston.

Slobin, D.I., & Welsh, C.A. (1973). Elicited limitations as a research tool in developmental psycholinguistics. In C.A. Ferguson & D.I. Slobin (Eds.), *Studies of child language development* (pp. 607–619). New York: Holt, Rinehart & Winston.

Snow, C.E. (1972). Mother's speech to children learning language. *Child Development, 43,* 549–565.

Stein, N. (1978). *How children understand stories: A developmental analysis* (Technical Report No. 69). Center for the Study of Reading, University of Illinois, Urbana-Champaign.

Stein, N., & Glenn, C. (1979). An analysis of story comprehension in elementary school children. In R. Freedle (Ed.), *New directions in discourse processing* (pp. 53–120). Norwood, NJ: Ablex.

Tanz, C. (1980). *Studies in the acquisition of deictic terms.* Cambridge, England: Cambridge University Press.

Templin, M.C. (1957). *Certain language skills in children: Their development and interrelationships.* Minneapolis: University of Minnesota Press.

Thrantham, C., & Pederson, J. (1976). *Normal language development.* Baltimore: Williams & Wilkins.

Tough, J. (1977). *The development of meaning.* New York: Halstead Press.

Warden, D. (1976). The influence of context on children's use of identifying expressions and references. *British Journal of Psychology, 67,* 101–112.

Wells, G. (1979). Learning and using the auxilliary verb in English. In V. Lee (Ed.), *Language development* (pp. 250–270). New York: Wiley.

Wiig, E. (1982). *Let's talk inventory for adolescents.* Columbus, OH: Charles E. Merrill.

Wiig, E.H., Gilbert, M.F., & Christian, S.H. (1978). Developmental sequences in the perception and interpretation of lexical and syntactic ambiguities. *Perceptual and Motor Skills, 46,* 959–969.

Wiig, E.H., & Semel, E. (1984). *Language assessment and intervention for the learning disabled.* Columbus, OH: Charles E. Merrill.

Winner, E., Rosenthal, A., & Gardner, H. (1976). The development of metaphoric understanding. *Developmental Psychology, 12,* 289–297.

Wotten, J., Merkin, S., Hood, L., & Bloom, L. (1979). *Wh-* questions: Linguistic evidence to explain the sequence of acquisition. Paper presented to the Society for Research in Child Development, San Francisco.

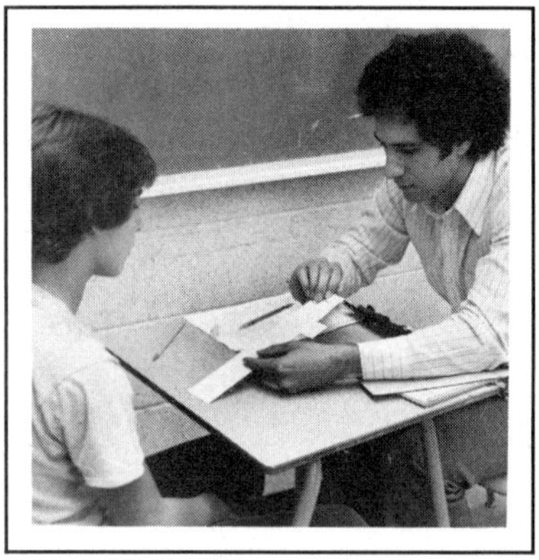

6

Assessing Children With Language Disorders

As speech-language pathologists, we are responsible for identifying children with language disorders and for designing and implementing effective intervention programs for them. In order to fulfill these responsibilities, we must obtain accurate information about a child's language and language-related abilities, interpret that information, and use it to make decisions about the need for and focus of intervention. Thus, assessing a child's language and communication behaviors is a very important aspect of meeting our professional responsibilities.

The task of assessing children's language would be relatively simple if language were easily quantified like height or weight. However, language is not a unitary dimension which can be measured with a yardstick or scales. It is multidimensional, complex, and dynamic; it involves many interrelated processes and abilities; and, it changes from situation to situation. As Miller (1981) pointed out, the elusive nature of language makes it very difficult to measure and quantify. The task is complicated further by the range and variety of behaviors exhibited by children with language disorders. Every child that you evaluate will have a unique pattern of language abilities and deficits. For example, one child may have an adequate vocabulary and good communication interaction skills, but may have severe deficits in the use of grammatical morphemes and syntactic structures. Another child may be able to produce a variety of grammatically acceptable sentences, but may use many nonspecific terms like "that one," "it," and "the thing," because she has trouble retrieving the appropriate words for objects, people, and events. One of the challenges in assessment is to reveal and describe the unique pattern of language behaviors for each language-disordered child.

This chapter was written by Dr. Sharon James, Syracuse University.

Although the nature of language and the heterogeneity of the population complicate the crucial task of assessment, we can meet the challenges of this task by having an open and curious mind, developing keen observational skills, and maintaining current information about language theory and research. As Siegel and Broen (1976) pointed out, "The most useful and dependable 'language assessment device' is an informed clinician who feels compelled to keep up with developments in psycholinguistics, speech pathology, and related fields, and who is not slavishly attached to a particular model of language or of assessment" (p. 75). The task of assessing children's language and communication is not only our professional responsibility—it also is one of the most creative and exciting facets of our work.

This chapter is designed to introduce the nature and scope of the assessment task rather than to provide all of the information necessary for carrying out an in-depth language assessment. I will explore the following major questions:

1. *Why* do we assess a child's language and communication abilities?
2. *What* aspects of the child's functioning will we assess?
3. *How* will we assess those aspects?
4. *How* will we interpret and use the results of our assessment?

Although I will focus on assessing children behaviors, I will touch on other aspects of development that need to be considered in evaluating a child. It is crucial to remember that a child's communicative functioning involves not only language knowledge and skills, but also cognitive and social abilities. We also may be concerned with a child's physical status and motor abilities and with those environments in which the child spends a good deal of time. These pieces of information may be especially important in choosing assessment procedures and in designing effective intervention programs. We will not need to obtain information in all of these areas for every child we assess; however, we will need to be prepared to assess whatever areas are relevant for a particular child.

PURPOSES OF ASSESSMENT

The nature of the information to be obtained and the methods used to obtain that information will be influenced greatly by the purpose of assessment. There are three major purposes for assessing children's language behaviors:

1. Identifying children with language disorders
2. Designing appropriate language intervention programs
3. Monitoring changes resulting from intervention

The first step in meeting the purpose of identification is to locate those children who may have language deficits so that they can be evaluated further. This step involves some sort of screening procedure. Within many school districts, the speech-language pathologist is responsible for carrying out brief evaluations of the language abilities of all preschool or kindergarten children served by that district. Those children who perform below a given acceptable level for their age or grade level are recommended for more comprehensive evaluations. Another important screening device consists of referrals from adults, such as a parent or teacher, who interact with a child. These individuals have numerous opportunities to observe the child's language behaviors and, therefore, often pick up subtle indications of a language disorder which might be missed in a brief screening procedure.

Regardless of how the child with a potential language problem is located, the second step in identification is to determine whether the child actually has a language disorder. Might we expect this child to continue developing language normally or may some intervention be required to facilitate language development? In order to answer this question, we must obtain information about the child's language behaviors which can be compared to developmental data from normal children. We want to know if the child's language behaviors are age-appropriate and, if they are not, which areas of language functioning are involved.

Once a child is identified as demonstrating a language disorder, we will be concerned with the second purpose for language assessment: designing an appropriate language program. For this purpose, we need a detailed description of the child's understanding and use of all components of the language—phonology, syntax, semantics, and pragmatics. We may need to obtain information about other behavioral areas, such as cognitive abilities, and about the child's environment and interpersonal relationships. Those behaviors which we focus on in assessment will depend on the child's performance during the evaluation. For example, if the child demonstrates good syntactic comprehension, but has trouble using various syntactic and grammatical structures, we will want an in-depth analysis of his syntactic production in various situations.

The kind of in-depth information needed for intervention may require a number of observations of the child's language behaviors. We may need to see the child in group or classroom situations as well as in individual interactions; we may need to observe the child at home or at nursery school. Many times, some of this information will be obtained once intervention has begun. Hubbell (1981) has argued that we may learn more about children's language abilities by observing their language behaviors during therapy than by continuing preintervention evaluation indefinitely. It is important to keep in mind that assessment and intervention are not two distinct activities. All good intervention programs involve ongoing assessment.

The third major purpose of language assessment is to monitor change resulting from intervention. Throughout the intervention process, we will be observing and recording the child's language behaviors so that we can modify our intervention goals and strategies as needed. For example, if the child is not making progress toward one of the goals that we established initially, we may want to try a different approach for teaching the target behavior. Once a target behavior has been mastered, the short-term goals will be expanded to introduce a new target behavior. Such adaptations in goals and approaches require that we continually assess changes in the child's language behaviors. We also will be concerned with whether the child is generalizing new language behaviors to situations that have not been a specific part of the intervention program. In other words, is the child using the knowledge gained in the teaching context in natural communication contexts? Generalization of target behaviors is the true measure of the success of any language intervention program (Miller, 1978). To assess generalization, we must observe the child in a number of different communication situations or contexts. This issue is discussed in more detail in chapter 7.

DIMENSIONS OF ASSESSMENT

After determining the major purpose for the language assessment, we need to consider what we are going to assess. Because language and communication assessment is concerned first and foremost with a child's knowledge and use of language, we will focus on language behaviors. However, we are concerned with the whole child. Therefore, we must look for and note all behaviors that provide information about the child's cognitive, social, and motor abilities. Also, we sometimes find ourselves responsible for assessing some children who are preverbal, who have not begun comprehending or producing language. In these cases, we must focus on early cognitive and communicative behaviors rather than on language.

Early Cognitive and Communicative Behaviors

Increasing numbers of speech-language pathologists are responsible for assessing preverbal children. Obviously, we cannot assess language comprehension and production in a child who has not yet developed any knowledge of the language system. For these children, we need to assess behaviors which seem to be precursors to language development.

Those infant behaviors which have been suggested as precursors to language fall into two types: social behaviors and cognitive behaviors. Several investigators have proposed that language develops from the early social interactions between infants and their parents (Bates, 1979; Bruner, 1975, 1977; Lewis, 1978; Stern, 1977). These behaviors include eye contact; mutual gaze at an object; covocalizations; interactional games, such as peek-a-boo; and conventional social actions, such as the child's waving bye-bye and giving or showing an object to an adult. At first, these interactions are initiated by adults, but they become increasingly child-initiated. In assessing a preverbal child, therefore, we begin by seeing if the child will engage in interactions which we initiated. We also note whether the child initiated any of these interactions with parents or other adults in the immediate environment.

Cognitive behaviors proposed as precursors to language include some of the sensorimotor concepts described by Piaget (1952). Bates (1979) and Steckol and Leonard (1981) have reported that the two sensorimotor cognitive concepts most closely related to language development are means-ends relations and schemes for relating to objects. Means-ends behaviors are those actions that are intended to achieve a goal, such as obtaining an object that is out of reach. Children's early means-ends behaviors involve using their own familiar actions as a means (reaching for and grasping an object), while later means-ends behaviors involve developing novel ways of achieving a goal, such as using an external object (e.g., a stick) to get an unreachable toy. This nonverbal ability has been suggested as a precursor for language, because language is a verbal means to an end.

Schemes for relating to objects are the actions that children engage in when they are simply exploring or playing with objects. Early actions with objects include mouthing, banging, throwing, and visually exploring. Later schemes include using objects or toys in conventional ways (stirring a spoon in a cup), and eventually using them in make-believe activities (putting a doll in a cradle, covering it with a blanket, and gently rocking the cradle). Such play behaviors are thought to be a nonverbal expression of a symbolic capacity just as language is the verbal expression of such a capacity.

Knowledge and Use of Language

There are two primary processes that reflect the child's knowledge of the language system: comprehension and production. In order to comprehend and produce oral language adequately, children must possess knowledge of the linguistic units and rules of phonology, semantics, and grammar. In addition, they must know how to use their linguistic knowledge to communicate with others. This knowledge of how to use language in context is referred to as *pragmatics* (Bates, 1976). In any language assessment, we will be concerned with children's comprehension and production of semantic forms and grammatical structures, their production of the phonemes of their language, and their pragmatic abilities. Each of these components—semantics, grammar, phonology, and pragmatics—has aspects which children need to master and which we, therefore, may want to assess.

Phonology. One aspect of assessing children's phonological systems is to obtain an inventory of the phonemes which they produce correctly and incorrectly. Phonemes are the smallest relevant sound unit in any language. They are considered relevant because they signal meaning differences among words; when you change a phoneme, you create a different word. For example, the words *bat, fat, cat, mat,* and *sat* differ only in the first sound, and yet they all mean something different. This example indicates that /b/, /f/, /k/, /m/, and /s/ are different phonemes in English. We must find out if children produce all of the phonemes which make up the sound system of their native language, and if they make errors in producing any of these phonemes.

Another component of the child's phonological system which we will want to explore is the sound contexts in which phonemes are produced correctly and incorrectly. For example, a child may produce the /k/ correctly in a word like *cake,* but may substitute a /t/ for the /k/ in *car.* It is important to determine if there are sound contexts in which a sound is produced correctly, indicating that the child's incorrect production is inconsistent.

A third aspect of our phonological assessment will be to analyze the child's error productions for *phonological process* (see Chapter 5). There are at least three major types of processes which have been described in normal and disordered children's speech:

1. Substitution processes in which one sound is substituted for another, often depending upon the sound's position in a word
2. Assimilation processes, in which two phonemes within a word become alike
3. Syllable structure changes in which the number or order of syllables in a word is reduced or changed

Examples of specific processes within each type are listed below (Edwards & Shriberg, 1983; Lund & Duchan, 1983):

A. Substitution Processes
   1. Stopping—substituting stops for fricatives (e.g., bu*t* for bu*s*)
   2. Fronting—substituting alveolars for velar and palatal consonants (e.g., *t*up for *c*up)
   3. Gliding—substituting glides for liquids (e.g., *w*adder for *l*adder)
B. Assimilation Processes
   1. Consonant harmony—consonants within a word become more alike in place or manner of articulation (e.g., [gɔgi] for doggy)
   2. Prevocalic voicing—consonants are affected by the following vowel and take on the voicing feature of the vowels (e.g., [dʌb] for tub)
C. Syllable Structure Processes
   1. Cluster reduction—one or more of the consonants within a cluster is deleted (e.g., [top] for stop)
   2. Deletion of final consonants—one or more of the consonants at the end of a word is deleted (e.g., [fi] for *fish*)
   3. Deletion of unstresed syllables—unstressed syllables are omitted (e.g., [nænə] for *banana*)
   4. Reduplication—a syllable, usually the stressed syllable, is repeated (e.g., [kækæ] for *cracker*

By analyzing children's sound production errors for these patterns, we can discover regularities in their speech deviations. The advantage to this approach is that all of the sound involved in a particular pattern can be worked on simultaneously in intervention.

Semantics. In assessing children's knowledge of the semantic component, we will be concerned with word meaning, sentence meaning, and nonliteral meaning. Word meaning can be assessed by determining the number and types of words that a child understands and produces. One way of categorizing words is on the basis of what they refer to. Some words, which we might consider concrete, refer to observable classes of entities, actions, and attributes. Other words, which might be considered abstract, refer to relationships among entities or events. These abstract words include dimensional, spatial, and temporal terms. For example, the word *dog* refers to an observable animal or class of animals, while the word *tomorrow* refers to a complex temporal relationship. Some children may comprehend and produce only concrete words, while other children's vocabularies include a number of relational words. Part of our semantic assessment will be to determine the types of words in the child's vocabulary.

Sentence meanings, which are compositional, depend on the relationships among words. Miller (1981) suggested that we look at meaning relations among, as well as within, sentences. Within sentence (intrasentence) relations include the semantic roles and relations expressed in children's early sentences. When young children say, "Doggie eat," they are identifying the agent of an action and naming the action. Complex intrasentence relations are evident in conjoined sentences such as "It broke when she hit it." We should obtain information about the child's comprehension and production of intrasentence relations.

Between-sentence (intersentence) relations are expressed through linguistic devices such as anaphoric and cataphoric reference, ellipsis, and lexical cohesion, all of which relate sentences to one another. These cohesion devices were defined in Chapter 5.

The inclusion of such discourse cohesion devices within the semantic component emphasizes the close relationship between semantics and pragmatics.

The last aspect of semantics to be assessed, particularly in older children, is nonliteral meaning. Nonliteral meanings are expressed in forms such as idioms ("She hit the roof,") metaphors ("He's as thin as a rail,") and proverbs ("Don't count your chickens before they're hatched"). In order to understand these nonliteral meanings, one must disregard the literal interpretation and rely on nonreferential, abstract, generalized concepts (Wiig & Semel, 1980). These nonliteral forms are not mastered until about 10 or 11 years of age; however, they are important in assessing older children's ability to deal with abstract meaning.

Grammar. The term "grammar" actually subsumes several levels of phonology, syntax, and semantics. However, for the purposes of our discussion, we will be concerned with only two aspects of grammar—morphology and syntax. Our assessment of morphology will focus on children's comprehension and production of grammatical morphemes. Grammatical morphemes are little words and inflectional endings that serve a grammatical function and carry subtle information about time, number, possession, etc. They include forms like noun plurals (dog*s*), past tense markers (push*ed*), and auxiliary verbs (*is* going). Brown (1973) has described them as those forms which "modulate," but do not change, the basic meaning within sentences. This description differentiates grammatical morphemes from lexical morphemes, which are content- or meaning-carrying forms.

Perhaps the distinction between grammatical and lexical morphemes is best illustrated in a telegram. If we retain lexical morphemes, we can omit many grammatical morphemes and still convey the basic message. For example, the telegram "Arrive 2:00 p.m. Saturday American flight 436. Expect you there" would undoubtedly be understood by most people. If you expand these telegraphic sentences, you can see that there are several grammatical morphemes absent (i.e., *I will* arrive *at* 2:00 p.m. *on* Saturday *on* American'*s* flight 436. *I will* expect you *to be* there.") Lexical morphemes are included in our analysis of the child's vocabulary under semantics.

Brown (1973) has described the early development of grammatical morphemes. He discussed 14 morphemes which children acquire at different rates, but with considerable similarity in the order of development. These 14 morphemes are presented in Chapter 5. Although there are other grammatical morphemes in English, their development has not received the systematic study of the 14 morphemes described by Brown. Other morphemes, such as modal and perfective verbs and adjectives, are included in the discussion of noun phrase and verb phrase analyses.

Syntax is the second aspect of grammar which should be assessed. The major areas of interest for syntactic assessment will include the child's knowledge of clause structure, of noun phrases and verb phrases within clauses, of rules for forming negatives and questions, and of rules for forming complex sentences through embedding and conjoining.

The first level in our syntactic analysis will be to assess the child's knowledge of basic clause structures. All clauses contain a subject and a verb or verb phrase (Crystal, Fletcher & Garman, 1976), although the subject may be omitted in imperative sentences or complex sentences. For every verb or verb phrase in an utterance, there is a

TABLE 6–1
Major Clause Structures

Clause Type	*Verb*	*Optional Elements*	*Structure*
Intransitive	Cannot take direct object	Adverbials (adverbs or prepositional phrases)	Subject + Verb ± Adverbial
Transitive	Takes direct object	Direct object and/or adverbials	Subject + Verb ± Direct object ± Adverbial
Equative	Copula and complement	Adverbials	Subject + BE + Complement ± Adverbial

separate clause. There are three major types of clauses in English, depending on the nature of the verb contained in the clause: intransitive, transitive, and equative.

Intransitive clauses contain an action or state verb which cannot take an object (e.g., "The dog barked"). However, intransitive clauses may contain one or more adverbials, which are adverbs or prepositional phrases (e.g., "The dog barked *loudly,*" "The dog barked *at the man,*" "The dog barked *loudly at the man every day*").

Transitive clauses contain an action or state verb which can take a direct object (e.g., "The girl ate the candy"). In addition, transitive clauses may contain an indirect object and adverbials (e.g., "The man gave *her* the candy," "The girl ate the candy *quickly,*" "The man gave *her* the candy *on the bus*").

Equative clauses contain a copula, or linking verb. Copulas are forms of the verb *be* (*am, is, are, was, were*) which are used as the main verb in the clause. They link the clause subject to some additional element which relates to the subject and is referred to as the *complement.* Other verbs, such as *seem, become, feel,* and *look,* may function as linking verbs and receive a complement. Complements can be nouns, adjectives, or adverbials (e.g., "He is *the boss,*" "The dog looks *big,*" "They are *in the house*"). Equative clauses also may contain other adverbials in addition to the complement (e.g., "They are in the house *today*").

Table 6–1 summarizes the types of clause structures found in simple sentences. By analyzing children's use of these clause structures, we will obtain information about their knowledge of the basic syntactic rules for forming sentences and their awareness of the optional elements, such as indirect objects and adverbials, associated with these clause structures.

The two major constituents of clauses are noun phrases and verb phrases. Thus, the next level in syntactic analysis will be to analyze the child's use of noun phrases and verb phrases.

Noun phrases always contain a main or head noun which is the central component of the phrase. In addition, noun phrases may contain several other optional elements which modify the head noun in some way. Crystal, Fletcher, and Garman (1976) discussed four such elements:

1. Initiators are the only element that can precede a determiner in a noun phrase. They frequently function to limit or to quantify a noun. Common initiators are *all, only, both, just, at least* (e.g., "*Only* that man is going").

2. Determiners include articles (*a, an, the*), possessive pronouns (*my, your, his, her, ours, their*), demonstratives (*that, this, these*), and qualifiers (*any, no, some, either, each*). They are always the first element in a noun phrase unless they are preceded by an initiator. An example of a sentence containing a determiner in both the subject and the object noun phrase would be "*Some* man stole *my* car."
3. Adjectivals are the largest class of elements that can modify nouns. Included in this class are adjectives (*little, blue, good*); ordinals (*first, next, final*); quantifiers (*two, many, few*); nouns used as descriptors (*party* hat, *cowboy* hat); and nouns marked for possession (*Mommy's* coat, *Billy's* dog).
4. Postmodifiers are modifiers which follow the head noun. They may include prepositional phrases (the man *in the picture*), clauses (the man *that came to visit*), and adjectives or adverbs (the boy *there*).

A noun phrase must contain a head noun: all of the other elements are optional. However, it is possible for a noun phrase to contain an initiator, a determiner, several adjectivals, and a postmodifier (e.g., "Only the last four strong, brave young women on the team . . ."). The rule for constructing a noun phrase would be as follows: NP = ± Initiator ± Determiner ± Adjectival + Head ± Postmodifier (Hubbell, 1981). In analyzing a child's use of noun phrases, we must determine first if the child is using nouns as sentence subjects and objects. Then we will look for evidence that the child is using early developing modifiers, such as determiners and adjectivals, and classify the types of determiners and adjectivals used. Finally, we will analyze for later developing noun modifiers such as initiators and postmodifiers.

Like the noun phrase constituent of the clause, the verb phrase contains one obligatory element and some optional elements. The obligatory element is the main or head verb. The optional elements within the verb phrase are as follows:

1. *Modals* include words such as *may, can, must, should, will,* which indicate mood or attitude.
2. Perfective constructions are used to specify certain types of action in the past. The perfective usually is symbolized by *have* + *-en* (e.g., *has seen, had done, have given*).
3. Progressive constructions indicate continuing or ongoing action. The progressive is represented by *be* + *-ing* (e.g., *is throwing, are eating, was running*).

The rule for constructing a verb phrase would be as follows: VP = ± Modal ± Perfective ± Progressive + Main Verb. In analyzing the child's use of verb phrases, we would first of all determine if the clause contains a main verb, and then we would look for the presence of the three optional verb constructions.

Tense markers and negation were not included in this discussion of verb phrases, even though some authors treat them as optional verb phrase elements (Dever, 1978; Hubbell, 1981). I have chosen to include tense markers in the analysis of grammatical morphemes and to discuss negatives as a separate type of simple sentence.

Our next level of analysis will focus on two major types of simple sentences—negatives and questions. In analyzing a child's negative sentences for knowledge of syntactic rules, we are looking for the negative morpheme *not,* either contracted or uncontracted, in conjunction with an auxiliary verb (e.g., *is not, don't, cannot, wasn't*). Although there are several lexical terms that express negation semantically (e.g., *no, nothing, gone, empty*), these are not considered syntactic forms of negation. Syntactic negatives negate affirmative propositions within sentences. We will be concerned with whether or not the child understands, as well as produces, sentences containing syntactic negatives.

Our assessment of children's knowledge of questions will involve analyzing their use and understanding of at least two major types of questions. One type includes questions that can be answered with either *yes* or *no.* Yes/No questions can be formed in several different ways:

1. By using a rising intonation with no change in word order ("See my new coat?")
2. By inverting the copula or auxiliary verb ("Is he going?")
3. By inserting the "dummy *do*" (so called because it adds no meaning to the verb) before the subject to act as an auxiliary ("Do you like ice cream?")
4. By adding a tag, consisting of a modal (with or without a negative) and a pronoun, onto a statement ("It's a nice day, isn't it?")

The second major type of question includes all questions beginning with words which specify the kind of information being requested. These are referred to as *Wh-* questions. Usually, the *Wh-* question word is the first word in the question followed by an auxiliary, copula, or "dummy *do*" and then the subject noun ("What is he doing?" "Who is that man?" "When did you go?") We will observe children's responses to various forms of Yes/No and *Wh-* questions and analyze the type and structure of whatever questions they produce.

The final level of syntactic analysis focuses on the child's knowledge of complex sentence structure. This level of analysis is especially important in assessing language in older school-age children, because complex sentence development in normal children continues well beyond the elementary school years (Haas & Wepman, 1974; Loban, 1968; chapter 5 in this book). Complex sentences contain two or more clauses, meaning that they contain two or more *main verbs.* Complex sentences can be formed by conjoining two clauses with a conjunction (*and, but, because*) to make a compound sentence, or by embedding one clause within another to make an embedded sentence. When two clauses are conjoined in compound sentences, each clause is independent and could stand as a separate sentence (e.g., "*He went to bed* because *he was tired*"). In embedded sentences, the subordinate clause is not independent, but is part of the structure of the main clause of the sentence (e.g., "*His father wanted him to go to bed early*"). In this example, the subordinate clause *him to go to bed early* served as the complement of the verb *wanted* in the main clause. Subordinate clauses can fulfill various grammatical roles within a sentence, including *subject, object, complement,* and *adjectival.* In our assessment, we will be concerned with the child's comprehension and production of various types of compound and embedded sentence structures.

Pragmatics. In assessing a child's pragmatic abilities, we are interested in how the child is using language to communicate. A detailed discussion of pragmatic assessment is beyond the scope of this chapter. However, there are at least two aspects of pragmatics that we will want to consider during our language assessment. One aspect is the child's use of language to express various communicative intentions. Language can be used for a variety of communicative functions, such as to request goods, services, or information; to express attitudes or feelings; to convey information; and to establish and maintain social interactions. Chapman (1981) described and discussed several of the taxonomies that have been developed to describe the communicative intentions expressed by children. Certainly, we will want to be aware of whether a child uses whatever language he has to express a variety of communicative intentions.

A second aspect of pragmatics with which we should be concerned is the child's conversational abilities. Being able to carry on a conversation involves several different skills. One basic component of conversations is turn-taking. In order to keep a conversation moving, we must be able to play the role of both speaker and listener, talking when it is our turn and allowing other people to talk during their turn. We use both verbal and nonverbal signals to indicate when we are ready to begin and end our turns as speaker and listener. Another component of conversations is that the participants maintain a common focus or topic. When one participant wants to change the topic, he indicates this in some way to the other participants. The new topic then becomes the focus of the conversation. Children seem to learn about turn-taking early, but the ability to maintain a topic is not well developed in young children. Bloom, Rocissano, and Hood (1976) found that children under three years old rarely maintained a topic for more than two turns.

Another important component of conversational interaction involves the ability to make accurate assumptions about shared information and cultural or social role expectations and to adjust what we say and how we say it on the basis of these assumptions. Such assumptions are called *presuppositions.* Presuppositions may be based on the speaker's information about the listener's background knowledge, the actual physical setting in which the conversation is taking place, and the role of the listener in relation to the speaker. For example, you would discuss children's language disorders differently with another speech-language pathology major than with a physics major who has little knowledge about language disorders. You modify conversation depending on whether the person you are talking with is in the same room or another room. You also adjust what you say and how you say it when you talk to a good friend versus a complete stranger. These kinds of changes in the content and form of what you say are based on presuppositions.

When we consider children's pragmatic abilities, we observe whether they use their language to serve various communicative functions, whether they take turns in conversations and maintain the topic, and whether they make accurate presuppositions and adjust their language accordingly. For a more detailed discussion of these pragmatic abilities, see Gallagher and Prutting (1983), Lund and Duchan (1983), and Rees (1978).

Table 6–2 outlines the major areas to consider in assessing a child's knowledge and use of the language system. It may not be necessary to do in-depth analyses of all areas for a particular child. The decision of which areas to focus on will be based on preliminary information about the child's level of functioning and particular strengths and weaknesses.

TABLE 6–2
Areas of Language to be Assessed

- I. Semantics
  - A. Word meaning
    1. Concrete words referring to observable objects, actions, attributes
    2. Relational words referring to dimensions, time, space
  - B. Sentence meaning
    1. Semantic rules and relations within simple sentences
    2. Abstract relational meanings within complex sentences
    3. Meaning relations among sentences
  - C. Nonliteral meaning
    1. Idioms
    2. Metaphors
    3. Proverbs
- II. Grammar
  - A. Grammatical morphemes
    1. Noun forms (plurals, possessive, prepositions, articles)
    2. Verb forms (progressive, past, third person singular, auxiliary, and copula)
    3. Adjective forms (comparative, superlative)
    4. Adverb forms (comparative, superlative)
  - B. Syntax
    1. Clause structures (intransitive, transitive, equative)
    2. Noun phrase constituent
    3. Verb phrase constituent
    4. Negatives and questions
    5. Complex sentences (compound and embedded)
- III. Pragmatics
  - A. Communicative intentions
    1. Requesting information/action
    2. Conveying information
    3. Expressing attitude/emotion
    4. Regulating social interactions
  - B. Conversational abilities
    1. Turn–taking
    2. Topic maintenance
    3. Presupposition

Now that we have established the dimensions of our assessment and know *what* kinds of knowledge and behaviors to focus on, we are ready to explore ways to obtain the necessary information about the child's knowledge and behaviors. In other words, we are ready to talk about *how* to assess language and communication.

GENERAL PLAN FOR ASSESSMENT

Before exploring specific methods of assessing children's language and communication abilities, we need to discuss the overall plan for assessment. Specific evaluation formats (the specific behaviors to be assessed and the procedures to be used) will vary, depending on the goal of the assessment and the characteristics of the particular child to be assessed. Therefore, we need a flexible assessment plan which will allow adapting the format to different goals and different children. Miller (1981) has proposed a general evaluation plan which meets this criterion. An adaptation of this plan is presented in Figure 6–1.

Figure 6–1. General Assessment Plan

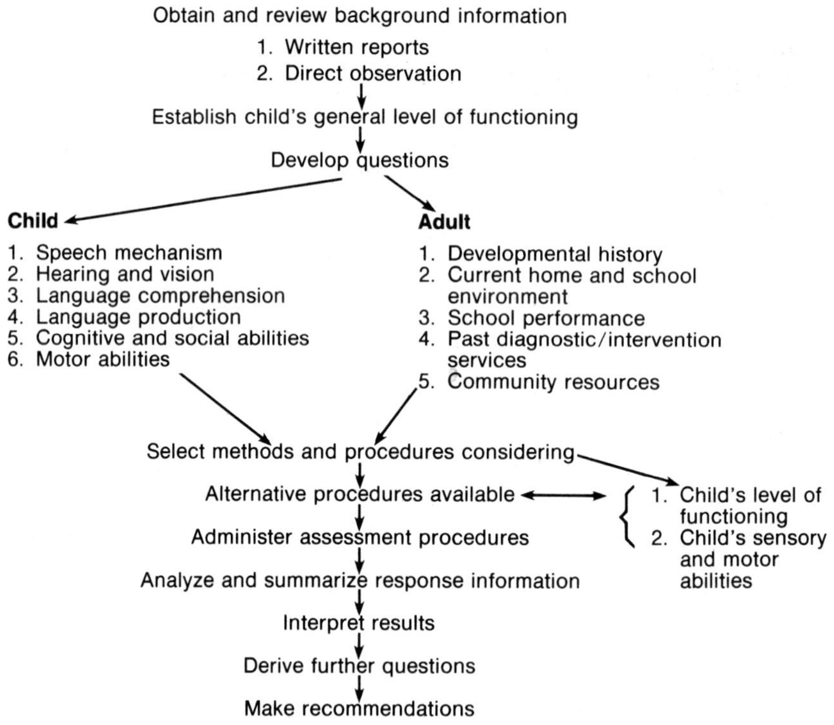

Note. From *Assessing Language Production of Children: Experimental Procedures* (p. 163) by J. F. Miller, 1981, Baltimore, MD: University Park Press. Copyright 1981 by University Park Press. Adapted by permission.

The first step in the plan is to gather and interpret background information regarding the child's level of functioning. This information may come from written reports of previous evaluations or from direct observations of the child prior to the formal evaluation. However it is obtained, it is used to draw some conclusions about the child's developmental level.

Once we have some idea of the child's developmental level, we can determine the kinds of information we want to obtain from the assessment. Miller (1981) suggested developing questions within various areas. (See Figure 6–1.) Some of the questions will focus on the child's knowledge and abilities, while others will be concerned with information about the child's past development and current environment. Information about the child's knowledge and abilities will be obtained from direct observation of the child as much as possible. The child's parents or other appropriate adults will provide answers to questions relating to history and environment. Extensive background information makes it possible to pose very specific questions such as "What optional elements does the child use in noun phrases?" However, there may be times when the background information will allow only general questions such as "What is the level of the child's language production?" The list of areas for questioning in Figure 6–1 is not exhaustive. Other important areas may be developed depending on the goals for assessment and the children.

The next step in this evaluation plan is to obtain information to answer the questions. We will need to select assessment procedures that will provide the relevant information and that are appropriate for the child's level of knowledge and abilities. Because a particular assessment procedure or task may not always be appropriate, we need to have alternative tasks or tests available.

Next, the tasks are presented and the child's responses are analyzed. Not only will the child's performance provide information about the particular area of knowledge or abilities being tested; the child's behaviors during the evaluation also can be analyzed for information about related areas such as social interaction skills and motor abilities. The results of the response analyses are then summarized and interpreted. Specific interpretation of the results will depend, to a large extent, on the purpose of the assessment. However, we will need to determine what the results tell us about the child's abilities and deficits in various areas. We also can develop further questions about specific aspects of behavior, either to clarify the results or to provide a more comprehensive picture of the child's abilities. Many of these questions probably are best answered once intervention has begun, and can serve as a framework for ongoing assessment within the intervention program.

Finally, we can make recommendations based on the assessment results. We will need to make a general recommendation about whether or not intervention is necessary. If it is needed, we will make specific suggestions about the content and structure of the intervention program.

This general plan for assessment allows considerable flexibility. The types of questions asked can be adapted to varying levels of background information, to individual children, and to different assessment goals. The particular methods and procedures chosen can be adapted to the type of information needed and to the characteristics of a particular child. Analyses and interpretations of the results can be adjusted to the purposes of assessment. In addition, the plan provides a framework for further or continuing evaluation.

METHODS OF ASSESSMENT

Developing a thorough description of a child's language and communication abilities requires obtaining information from all possible sources. As the general assessment plan indicates, the two major sources of information are adults who have contact with the child, such as parents, teachers, and other professionals, and our own observations of the child's performance.

Obtaining Information From Parents and Other Adults

Usually the adults who can give the most information about a child's past and current behaviors are the child's parents. It is important to let the parents know how valuable their information is so that their responses will be as accurate and complete as possible. One common method of obtaining information from parents is to have them fill out a questionnaire on the child's developmental history and current language functioning prior to the scheduled evaluation. A second method commonly used is to interview the parents either in a clinic setting or at home. It also can be helpful to observe the parents and child interacting in a clinic room or at home. A combination of all three of these methods—a questionnaire, an interview, and direct observation of parent-child interaction—provides the most complete and useful body of information about the child's past and present language functioning and about the nature of the parent-child relationship.

In addition to the child's parents, we may need to get information about the child from other professionals such as an audiologist, classroom teacher, resource room specialist, physician, and psychologist. This information can be obtained by requesting a written report or by interviewing the individual either on the telephone or in person.

Direct Observations of Child's Performance

The major source of information about a child's language knowledge and use will be direct observations of the child. These observations will serve as the basis for decisions about the need for and the nature of language intervention. Therefore, it is crucial that the samples of behaviors be as representative as possible of the child's actual language abilities and deficits. The issue of representativeness must be a major consideration in choosing assessment techniques and instruments.

Procedures for structuring our observations of the child's language behaviors can be divided into two basic categories: standardized and nonstandardized. We will discuss specific instruments or procedures that fall into each of these categories.

Standardized Tests of Language. Standardized tests provide a specific set of instructions and stimuli to elicit behaviors and a specific set of standards for scoring and interpreting the elicited behaviors. Usually the standards for interpretation are norms based upon a sample population's performance on the test stimuli. Test norms typically are reported as an average score plus some measure of variability, such as standard deviation. A child's performance on a test can be compared to the norms obtained from the standardization sample in one of two ways, yielding an age-equivalent score or a score of relative standing.

When a child's score is compared to the average scores for all the age groups in the standardization sample, an age-equivalent score is obtained; this score indicates to which age group the child's score is most similar. For example, a 5-year-old might score closest to the average score for 3 years, 6 months. Although it is convenient to be able to say that this 5-year-old is performing like a child at 3 years, 6 months it is difficult to determine what this statement means without some measure of variability. How many other 5-year-old children in the standardization sample had scores at the 3 years, 6 month level? Does an equal score indicate equal performance? A 5-year-old who achieved a score equal to the average score for 3 years, 6 months may in fact have performed very differently on this test than the children of that age. The specific items missed and the child's entire approach to the stimuli and tasks may be quite different. Age-equivalent scores should be viewed with some caution because of the difficulty in interpreting what they indicate about a child's language performance.

A second way of interpreting a child's score is to compare it to the performances of other children in the same age group. Comparisons of relative standing may be based on the concept of a "normal" distribution of scores. In a normal distribution, 68% of the scores will fall into a range $\pm$ 1 standard deviation from the average or mean score for that group, and 95% of the scores will be distributed within $\pm$ 2 standard deviations of the mean score. Standard deviation is simply a measure of how far away an individual's score is from the mean. Thus, if the mean score for a particular age group were 50, and the standard deviation was 5, we know that 95% of the group's scores would fall between 40 and 60 ($\pm$ 2 S.D.). Frequently, a score that falls more than 2 standard deviations below the mean is considered deviant.

A more sophisticated comparison of relative standing involves standard scores, which are derived by assigning an arbitrary number to the mean score and a constant value to the standard deviation. On many IQ tests, the arbitrary number for the mean is 100 and the standard deviation is 15. A child who obtained a score of 68 on such an IQ test would fall more than 2 standard deviations below the mean for her age group and, therefore, might be suspected of having a significant intellectual deficit.

A third type of relative standing comparison uses percentile ranks. Percentiles are derived by arranging all of the scores obtained from the sample age group and computing the percentage of children at and below each score. The 50th percentile corresponds to the median and is the score that divides the group into equal halves. A child who achieves a score at or below the 10th percentile performed more poorly than 90% of the standardization group. It should be kept in mind that the distance between points on a scale of percentile ranks is not constant. Siegel and Broen (1976) pointed out that a difference of only four items separates the 10th from the 90th percentile for the 7-year-old group on the Northwest Syntax Screening Test (Lee, 1971). Thus, "it is important to look at the total distribution and variation in scores and not simply at the child's score" (Siegel & Broen, 1976, p. 90) when using percentile ranks to interpret a child's performance.

The focus in most standardized tests is on a child's total or overall score. We compare the child's score to the norms to determine the child's level of functioning in the area(s) measured by the test. Generally, standardized tests are most useful in fulfilling the first purpose for assessment—identifying children with language disorders. Standardized tests can be very valuable during an initial assessment to determine whether or not children's language behaviors are age appropriate. However, they rarely provide the kind of comprehensive, in-depth information required for planning an intervention program. They may indicate that children are functioning below the level expected for their ages in areas such as vocabulary comprehension or grammatical production, but they will not reveal the specific aspects of vocabulary or grammar that need to be emphasized in therapy. The sampling of specific language forms and structures in most standardized tests simply is too limited to reveal children's strengths and weaknesses. These tests were not designed to yield that kind of information and we should not expect them to do so.

Table 6–3 contains a list of selected standardized tests that are used to assess language. The list indicates the abilities and components assessed, the age ranges specified, and the type of score derived. This list is by no means exhaustive, and it does not include tests of articulation. I have attempted to include some of the more recent and commonly used language tests which allow either age-equivalent or relative standing comparisons.

TABLE 6–3
Selected Language Tests by Type of Score, Age Range, and Dimensions Assessed

Test Name and Author	*Type of Score*			*Age Range*	*Production*		*Comprehension*	
	Standard	*Age Equivalent*	*Percentile*		*Grammar*	*Semantics*	*Grammar*	*Semantics*
Assessment of Children's Language Comprehension (Foster, Giddan, & Stark, 1973)		X		3:0 yr to 6:5 yr			X	
Bankson Language Screening Test (Bankson, 1977)			X	4:1 yr to 8:0 yr	X	X		
Boehm Test of Basic Concepts (Boehm, 1971)			X	Grades K to 2				X
Carrow Elicited Language Inventory (Carrow-Woolfolk, 1974)		X	X	3:0 yr to 7:11 yr	X			
Clinical Evaluation of Language Functioning (Semel & Wiig, 1980)		X		Grades K to 10	X	X	X	X
Developmental Sentence Analysis (Lee, 1974)		X	X	3:0 yr to 6:11 yr	X			
Illinois Test of Psycholinguistic Abilities (Kirk, McCarthy, & Kirk, 1968)	X	X		2:2 yr to 10:4 yr	X	X	X	X
Merrill Language Screening Test (Mumm, Secord, & Dykstra, 1980)			X	Grades K and 1	X	Pragmatics	X	X

Northwestern Syntax Screening Test (Lee, 1971)			X	3:0 yr to 7:11 yr	X		X	
Peabody Picture Vocabulary Test—Revised (Dunn & Dunn, 1981)	X	X	X	2:3 yr to 18:5 yr				X
Preschool Language Scale (Zimmerman, Steiner, & Evatt, 1969)		X		1:6 yr to 7:0 yr	X	X	X	X
Test for Auditory Comprehension of Language (Carrow, 1973)		X	X	3:0 yr to 6:11 yr			X	X
Test of Early Language Development (Hresko, Reid, & Hammill, 1981)	X	X	X	3:0 yr to 7:11 yr	X	X	X	X
Test of Language Development—Primary (Newcomer & Hammill, 1977)	X		X	4:0 yr to 8:11 yr	X	X	X	X
Test of Language Development—Intermed (Hammill & Newcomer, 1982)	X		X	8:6 yr to 12:11 yr	X	X	X	X
Test of Adolescent Language (Hammill, Brown, Larsen, & Wiederholt, 1980)	X		X	11:0 yr to 18:5 yr	X	X	X	X
The WORD Test (Jorgensen, Barrett, Huisingh, & Zachman, 1981)	X	X	X	7:0 yr to 11:1 yr		X		
Let's Talk Inventory for Adolescents (Wiig, 1983)						Pragmatics		

There are at least four limitations of this selected list of tests. One is that few of the tests listed allow children's scores to be converted to a standard score with a measure of how far the children deviate from the performance of their peers. Most of the tests allow only age-equivalent or percentile comparisons. This point is important because it suggests that many of the available standardized language tests yield scores which are difficult to interpret.

A second limitation is that there are no standardized tests available for assessing all the aspects of language about which we need to be concerned. All of the tests in Table 6–3, except two, assess some aspect of grammar or semantics only. The two tests designed to assess some aspect of pragmatics are the Let's Talk Inventory (Wiig, 1983) and the Merrill Language Screening Test (Mumm, et al., 1980). The Let's Talk Inventory is not norm-referenced and the MLST is a screening test, rather than an in-depth evaluation instrument. There are two major reasons for the lack of available tests of pragmatics. First and foremost, pragmatics involves language use in natural communicative situations. When we create standard stimuli to elicit responses, we may fail to obtain accurate information about a child's pragmatic abilities. Thus, standardized tests may not be the most valid or reliable techniques for assessing pragmatics. Secondly, pragmatics is a relatively new area of concern for professionals working with language-disordered children. We still are in the process of discovering and describing the kinds of abilities and behaviors that fall into the pragmatic domain. It is crucial that we know what the relevant behaviors are before we develop formal measures for assessing those behaviors. Again, we must be cautious about the validity of our procedures. Are we really assessing what we say we are?

A third limitation is the age range covered by many standardized tests. The majority of the available tests are not appropriate for children below 3 years or over 8 years of age. If the child to be assessed is not within this age range, the number of available tests will be limited.

A fourth area of concern that is not evident from the list in Table 6–3 relates to characteristics of the sample on which many language tests were normed. Frequently, the number of children sampled in each age group was small, even though the total sample may seem adequate in size. For example, the norms for the Test for Auditory Comprehension of Language (TACL) are based on a sample of only 50 children at each age level (200 total). Also, many of the language tests available were normed on middle- to upper-middle-class white children from a limited geographic area. Often minority groups and children with any identifiable handicap were excluded from the standardization sample. It is, therefore, very important to read about the standardization sample before administering any test. If the child to be tested is significantly different from the sample on which the test was normed, that test should not be used as a basis for determining the age-appropriateness of the child's language behaviors. This cautionary statement may seem quite obvious and unnecessary; however, it is too often ignored when assessment instruments are selected for an individual child.

The nature of the limitations or concerns raised about this selected list of standardized language tests suggests the need for alternative or additional ways of assessing language. Even when standardized language tests can be used to determine if a child has a language disorder, additional information to plan an intervention program is needed. Thus, to fulfill the second major assessment purpose, we must consider using some nonstandardized assessment procedures.

Nonstandardized Language Assessment Procedures. Nonstandardized procedures are not synonymous with informal or unstructured observations. Nonstandardized procedures differ from standardized procedures or tests in that they do not have a standard set of stimuli or instructions which must be adhered to, nor do they have well-established standards or norms for interpretation. They do have sufficient face validity to be used in assessing various aspects of language (Miller, 1978), and they include structured tasks as well as relatively unstructured observations. One of the primary assets of nonstandardized procedures is that they are flexible and can be adapted to fit the needs and characteristics of the child being evaluated. Because the assessor is not locked into a particular stimulus or method for eliciting information, a child's knowledge and abilities can be explored by varying the content, form, and presentation of the stimuli. For example, if a child gives an incorrect response to a *Wh-* question about a picture, a similar question about the immediate situation or about a familiar situation from the home or school environment can be asked. The child's incorrect response to the question about the picture might not reflect lack of comprehension of the *Wh-* question form. Rather, the child may lack the necessary information or vocabulary to answer the question referring to the pictured event. By asking the child the same *Wh-* question form in reference to familiar or immediate events, you can determine if he really doesn't understand the *Wh-* form or if the initial incorrect response was due to the stimulus situation. This kind of adaptation and probing is not possible with standardized tests.

Nonstandardized procedures include collection and analysis of spontaneous language samples, techniques for eliciting production of particular structures, and techniques for assessing comprehension. Some of the specific procedures within each of these general categories will be discussed.

Spontaneous Language Samples. The most common method for obtaining information about a child's language production is to analyze a sample of spontaneous conversation between the child and another person. Two major steps are involved in this assessment procedure: collecting and recording the sample, and analyzing the sample.

Collecting and recording the sample. The major concern in collecting a language sample is the accuracy of the sample. Is the recorded sample to be analyzed truly representative of the child's usual language? This issue, of course, is not unique to spontaneous language samples, but is a problem in any behavior sample. The language produced by a child during a natural conversation would seem to be more representative than language produced in highly structured test situations. However, several factors may influence the accuracy of the language sample and must be considered in collecting the sample. They include the conversation partner, the setting, and the stimuli or materials present.

Frequently, the conversation partner in an assessment situation is a clinician responsible for carrying out the assessment, and the setting is a diagnostic or therapy room within a school or clinic. Although there is evidence that an adequate and representative language sample can be obtained under these conditions (Olswang & Carpenter,

1978), children may produce longer utterances when the sample is collected at home by the mother than in the clinic by a clinician (Kramer, James, & Saxman, 1979). Experience in the Speech and Hearing Clinic at Syracuse University suggests that younger children (under 3 years) are more talkative when they interact with a familiar partner, such as the mother. Miller (1981) recommended recording both mother-child and clinician-child conversations during an evaluation to ensure a more representative sample and also to disclose whether the child adjusts his speech to different people.

Although a representative sample can be obtained in almost any setting, it is crucial to be aware of the potential constraints within a particular setting. For example, a child observed on the playground involved in strenuous motor activities at school may not talk much or may produce short simple sentences. Utterances produced during a small group activity in the classroom may consist mostly of responses to questions, which will affect the syntactic, semantic, and pragmatic aspects of language. Obviously, it is best to record a child's language in a variety of settings in order to obtain a representative sample.

The stimuli or materials used in collecting a language sample need to be considered carefully. Although pictures and picture books commonly are used in language sampling situations, there is evidence that pictures are less effective than toys or conversation without materials for eliciting adequate language samples (Bloom & Lahey, 1978; Lee, 1974; Longhurst & Grubb, 1974). James and Button (1978) found no differences in the length and complexity of the utterances produced by 5- to 9-year-old language-disordered children when toys were used as stimuli or when the conversation focused on no external materials. Stalnaker and Creaghead (1982) reported that preschool Head Start children produced their longest utterances when asked to retell a story using toys following the examiner's model; however, they produced the most utterances in a 15-minute period when the examiner asked them questions as they played with the toys. In general, toys with multiple pieces, such as the Fisher Price school, a barn and animals, or a dollhouse with furniture and people, are the best materials to use in collecting language samples from children under 5 or 6 years of age. With school-age children and adolescents, external materials are not necessary; the best topics of conversation for obtaining a good sample seem to be hobbies, friends, family, and school experiences. Miller (1981) and Lund and Duchan (1983) provided some excellent suggestions for engaging children in conversations.

The sample obtained must be long enough to include instances of the behaviors to be analyzed. A minimum of 50 to 100 different utterances is suggested as adequate for most analyses (Bloom & Lahey, 1978). In an assessment situation, it may be easier and more efficient to use a minimum time period rather than a minimum number of utterances as the criterion for a representative sample. Miller (1981) reported that children functioning at or above 24 months of age usually will produce 100 or more utterances in a 30-minute conversation. Lund and Duchan (1983) and Miller (1981) recommended observing children interacting with their caretakers for about 10 to 15 minutes and spending the rest of the 30 minutes in child-clinician interaction. The length of time required to get a representative sample will vary from child to child. Younger or more reticent children may require longer than 30 minutes to produce 50 to 100 utterances, while a very outgoing child may produce over 100 utterances in less than 30 minutes.

Language samples can be recorded in one of three ways: videotaping, audiotaping, and writing down the sample. Videotape recording, with a good audio microphone, yields the most complete and accurate record of the verbal and nonverbal aspects of the interaction. Video recording is strongly recommended when you wish to analyze certain aspects of semantics and pragmatics, such as semantic relations and communicative intentions. Whenever contextual information is crucial for an analysis, videotaping is the best method. Videotape recording equipment can be distracting and it is important to allow the child time to adapt to the presence of the camera and video recorder before you begin taping the interaction. Most children behave fairly naturally in front of the camera after a relatively brief warm-up period.

Audiotape recording, supplemented by notes on the situation and the child's nonverbal behaviors, will provide sufficient information for most analyses of the sample. Notes on the nonverbal context to carry out the desired analyses will be needed frequently and must be as complete and accurate as possible. Audiotapes should be transcribed as soon as possible after the taping in order to recall any helpful contextual information not included in the notes.

Writing down the conversation and nonverbal aspects of the interaction is not recommended as the usual recording method. However, in some situations it is impossible or impractical to audio record, such as in the child's classroom or on the playground. In such situations, the target child's utterances cannot be differentiated from utterances produced by other children. On-line transcription allows writing down only what the target child and the conversation partners say. It takes practice to do accurate on-line transcriptions, but they can provide needed information when other forms of recording are not possible.

Analyzing the Sample. Once the sample has been collected and transcribed, it can be analyzed. The types of analyses carried out will depend on the major purpose for the language assessment and on the child's general level of language abilities. At this point, the specific kinds of phonological, semantic, syntactic, and pragmatic analyses to be done will be decided.

Phonology. The child's language sample can be analyzed to determine those phonemes which are produced correctly and incorrectly in running speech. To facilitate in-depth analyses of the child's sound production errors, it is preferable to do a narrow transcription of a sample of the child's errors. Symbols used for narrow transcription can be found in Lund and Duchan (1983) and Shriberg and Kent (1982).

The sample also can be analyzed to determine the effects of different sound contexts on the child's correct and incorrect productions of problem sounds. Finally, the child's error production can be analyzed to determine which phonological processes she is using and with what frequency. Several systematic approaches for doing a phonological process analysis have been developed in recent years (Hodson, 1980; Ingram, 1981; Shriberg & Kwiatkowski, 1980; Weiner, 1979).

Semantics. One part of the semantic analysis of the child's language sample may describe the kinds of words the child is producing. Miller (1981) suggested creating a set of meaning categories in the transcript for words that the child uses. For example, nouns might be categorized as people, animals, clothing, and food, while verbs categories might include action (jump, hit), locative action (put, go), experience (want, love), notice (see, look), etc. Categories for modifiers might be shape, size, color, location, and time. This analysis would yield a description of the kinds of concrete and relational meanings expressed in the child's vocabulary. In addition, any instances of overextension of meaning (e.g., calling all cars and trucks "buses") or underextension of meaning (e.g., calling roses, but not tulips or carnations, "flowers") could be noted. We also would note instances when the child seemed to lack the word for a specific entity and used a nonspecific term to refer to it (e.g., calling an object "it" or "that thing").

The child's vocabulary diversity can be measured by computing a type-token ratio (TTR) for the language sample. To compute the TTR, the number of *different* words (type) is divided by the *total* number of words (token) produced in a 50-utterance sample. The resulting ratio is a measure of the diversity of the words used in the sample. Templin (1957), who developed the measure, reported that children between 3 and 8 years old achieve type-token ratios of about .45 to .50. A child whose TTR was considerably below .45 should be suspected of having a limited production vocabulary, indicating a need for more in-depth assessment of vocabulary production and comprehension.

We also can analyze a spontaneous language sample for information about the child's knowledge of intra- and intersentence relations. If the child is producing two- and three-word sentences, it would be appropriate to analyze the semantic relations expressed in these sentences. The usual method for doing such an analysis has been to place the child's utterances into predetermined categories of semantic relations, such as action, possession, location, nomination, recurrence, etc. (Bloom & Lahey, 1978; Miller, 1981; Prutting, 1979). An alternative clinical method for analyzing the meaning relations in children's early word combinations has been proposed by Leonard, Steckol, and Panther (1983). They referred to this method as the *interpretative approach.* Rather than using predetermined categories such as action, location, and recurrence, Leonard, et al. specified the meanings expressed through a careful analysis of a child's utterances and the situational context. One of the advantages of their analysis is that it seems to be a more accurate representation of the sentence meanings which are operative for an individual child, and it yields information about the relationship between regularities in word position and the meanings expressed. For example, one of the children observed by Leonard, et al. was noted to produce a number of word combinations identifying objects, people, and animals. These utterances contained the word *that* in first position (e.g., "that big ball"; "that Bobby"). Thus, *that* + "X" was determined to be a productive form expressing *identification* for that child. Although it is beyond the scope of this chapter to describe this interpretative approach in detail, it seems promising as a clinical tool for describing the meanings expressed in children's early sentences.

Intrasentence meaning relations also can be analyzed in complex sentences produced within the sample. Bloom, Lahey, Hood, Lifter, and Fiess (1980) found four meaning relations in children's conjoined sentences: additive, temporal, causal, and adversitive. These four types of conjoined sentences, which are discussed in Chapter 5, can serve as a framework for analyzing intrasentence relations.

Evidence of the child's ability to express intersentence relations would be found in the use of pronouns or demonstratives to refer to previously established referents (anaphoric reference) or to refer to upcoming referents (cataphoric reference), the use of synonyms to refer to previously noted referents (lexical cohesion), and in the omission of information which was stated in a preceding utterance (ellipsis). In addition to noting if the child uses these devices correctly, any instances in which such devices are used inappropriately should be noted. For example, some children use anaphoric references and ellipses in situations where the referent of information has not been established in a previous sentence. Such inappropriate use of these devices seems to indicate that the child does not fully understand the devices for relating sentences to one another in a conversation.

Information about a child's use of nonliteral meaning is more difficult to obtain from a language sample. However, older children's samples may include examples of jokes, riddles, or metaphors ("She's big as a horse"). The child's knowledge of nonliteral language may be elicited by asking the child to explain the meaning of idioms, proverbs, and metaphors.

Grammar. If the child is producing some word combinations (two or more words in an utterance), you can compute the mean length of utterance (MLU) for the sample. MLU is considered a gross, but reasonably accurate, index of grammatical development up to a ceiling of about four to five morphemes. It is a gross index because it provides no information about the form or structure of the child's utterances; it is considered a reasonably accurate index because as the child acquires grammatical structures, such as verb tense markers, modal verbs, and determiners, the length of the utterances, and therefore the MLU, increases.

To compute MLU, you add the number of morphemes for the entire sample and divide by the number of utterances in the sample. A minimum of 50 utterances is recommended for computing MLU (Darley & Moll, 1960). A child who produced 132 morphemes in 50 utterances would have an MLU of 2.64 morphemes (132/50 = 2.64). Detailed rules for counting morphemes can be found in James and Button (1978) and Miller (1981).

MLU has been used in several ways. Miller and Chapman (1981) have presented data on the relationship between chronological age and MLU and suggested that their data may be used, with certain cautions, to determine if a child's MLU is significantly below chronological age expectations. MLU also has been used to place children in one of Brown's (1973) five stages of linguistic development. The child's production of grammatical morphemes and sentence structures is then compared to what Brown (1973) described for that stage. Miller (1981) presented a detailed system, involving MLU, for analyzing children's grammatical production. The use of MLU as a predictive measure has been criticized by Lund and Duchan (1983). They argued that the variability across children and conditions is too great to allow accurate prediction of which forms or structures should appear in a given MLU stage. Although one may not want to use MLU as a basis for predicting what forms a child should produce, it can be useful as a general indicator of a child's level of grammatical production.

A general measure like MLU provides no information about the types of grammatical structure the child is or is not producing. In order to obtain this kind of information, the sample must be analyzed for those aspects of grammar including (*a*) the child's use of grammatical morphemes, (*b*) the types of clause structures used in the sample, (*c*) the elements contained in the child's noun phrases and verb phrases, (*d*) the structure of the child's negatives and questions, and (*e*) the use of complex sentences.

Grammatical morphemes. The best way to explore the child's use of all 14 grammatical morphemes in the sample is to analyze each utterance for the presence or absence of the morpheme in obligatory contexts. Obligatory contexts are those places within a sentence where an adult speaker would use the morpheme. In the following sentence, for example, there are obligatory contexts for the noun plural, the uncontractible auxiliary *were,* the present progressive, the preposition *on,* and the article *the:* "Two cat*s were* sitt*ing on the* chair." If a child said "two cats sitting on chair," the noun plural, the present progressive, and the preposition were used correctly, while the auxiliary and the article were absent. By noting the number of obligatory contexts for a morpheme and the number of times the morpheme was used correctly in those contexts, the percentage of correct use for the morpheme within that language sample can be calculated. Brown (1973) used 90% correct use as his criterion for acquisition of the 14 morphemes in normally developing children. It is useful clinically to consider a morpheme mastered when a child produces it correctly 80% of the time or more, while 40 to 80% correct use is considered evidence that the morpheme is emerging in the child's language.

In addition to analyzing the percentage of correct use of the 14 morphemes, these 14 morphemes and any other morphological endings such as the comparative (-er) and superlative (-est) endings that are added to adjectives and adverbs may be organized by word classes (Lund & Duchan, 1983). The morphemes associated with nouns would be the plural and possessive markers, prepositions, and articles; verb morphemes would include the present progressive, regular and irregular past tense, regular and irregular third person singular, and auxiliary and copula forms; adjectival and adverbial morphemes would be the comparative and the superlative endings. This organization helps determine if the child is having difficulty with those morphemes associated with a particular word class.

Clause Structures. In carrying out clause structure analysis of the sample, utterances which may not reflect the child's knowledge of basic clause structures should be excluded (Lund and Duchan, 1983). The utterances to be excluded are imitative responses; direct responses to questions, unless the response is a complete sentence; and stereotyped phrases such as greetings and rote sequences (e.g., nursery rhymes). Once all of the spontaneous utterances in the sample have been identified, the verbs in each utterance are circled (Lund & Duchan, 1983). All simple sentences (those with one main verb) will then be analyzed by clause type, while sentences with two or more main verbs will be analyzed as complex sentences.

Table 6–4 contains 25 utterances taken from the larger language sample of a language-disordered child named Scott. Although a sample of 25 utterances would not be considered adequate for a regular clinical analysis, it will be adequate to illustrate how to approach a syntactic analysis of a spontaneous sample. The verbs in each sentence have been circled. In order to begin looking at Scott's basic clause structures, we need to classify his simple sentences as intransitive, transitive, and equative. Table 6–5 presents a sample worksheet with the three types of clauses and the required (+) and optional (±) elements for each type. Scott's simple sentences have been classified into each clause type. Scott used all three clause types, and he produced all of the required elements for each. All of his intransitive clauses contained the optional adverbial ele-

TABLE 6–4
Selected Utterances from a Language Sample.

Name: Scott   Chronological Age: 5 years 6 months

V. missing
1. I be a pilot.
2. I saw a movie about them.
3. They were flying high.
4. Can you fly?
5. Pilots go everywhere.
6. I would fly to California.
7. Where you would fly?
8. I ride my Big Wheel.
9. I ride it all around.
10. Do you know what a Big Wheel is?
11. It's a small bike.
12. It isn't a tricycle.
13. It gots wheels and pedals, but it little. V. missing
14. I know how it goes.
15. It won't go in the grass.
16. You're too big for one.
17. We going to California.
18. My sister's there.
19. We went to Disneyland.
20. I like the big rides best.
21. My cousin rode one that went real fast.
22. She got scared and cried.
23. Why can't you go?
24. You can go with me.
25. I write you a letter. V. missing

TABLE 6–5
Clause Analysis

Intransitive Clauses

	+Subject	*+Verb*	*(±)Adverbial*
3.	They	were flying	high
4.	You	can fly	
5.	Pilots	go	
6.	I	would fly	everywhere
7.	you	would fly	to California
15.	It	won't go	Where
17.	We	going	in grass
19.	We	went	to California
23.	you	can't go	to Disneyland
24.	you	can go	Why
			with me

Transitive Clauses

	+Subject	*+Verb*	*(±)Indirect Object*	*+Direct Object*	*(±)Adverbial*
2.	I	saw		a movie	about them
8.	I	ride		my Big Wheel	
9.	I	ride		it	all around
20.	I	like		the big rides	best
25.	I	write	you	a letter	

Equative Clauses

	+Subject	*+BE*	*+Complement*	*(±)Adverbial*
1.	I	be	a pilot	
11.	It	's	a small bike	
12.	It	isn't	a tricycle	
16.	You	're	too big	for one
18.	My sister	's	there	

+ = Required element
± = Optional element

Note. From *Children's Language Disorders: An Integrated Approach* (pp. 168–169) by R.D. Hubbell, 1981, Englewood Cliffs, NJ: Prentice-Hall. Adapted by permission.

ment also; however, his transitive and equative clauses did not contain optional elements very often. In fact, he used an indirect object in only one of five transitive sentences and an adverbial in only one of six equative sentences.

After the basic clause structures have been analyzed, the next level of analysis focuses on the noun phrases and verb phrases within the clauses. Remember that noun phrases always contain a head noun and may contain at least four optional elements: initiators, determiners, adjectivals, and postmodifiers. Verb phrases have one required element, the main verb, and some optional elements, including modals, perfectives, and progressives. Table 6–6 presents a worksheet showing Scott's noun phrases and verb phrases. The required and the optional elements are listed for each type of phrase to show which elements Scott used and how frequently. The only noun phrases included from Scott's sample are those containing nouns, rather than pronouns, as head nouns. The first column, labeled subject or object, indicates whether the noun phrase

TABLE 6–6
Noun Phrase and Verb Phrase Analysis

	Noun Phrases *Subject or Object*	*Initiator*	*Determiner*	*Adjectival*	*Head*	*Post Modifier*
1.	o		a		pilot	
2.	o		a		movie	about them
8.	o		my		Big Wheel	
10.	o		a		Big Wheel	
11.	o		a	small	bike	
12.	o		a		tricycle	
18.	s		my		sister	
20.	o		the	big	rides	
21.	s		my		cousin	
21.	o				one	that went real fast
25.	o		a		letter	

	Verb Phrases *Modal*	*Perfective*	*Progressive*	*Main Verb*
1.	-(will)			be
2.				saw
3.			were + -ing	fly
4.	can			fly
5.				go
6.,7.	would			fly
8.,9.				ride
10.				know, is
11.				's
12.				isn't
13.				gots
14.				know, goes
15.	won't			go
16.				're
17.			-(are) + -ing	go
18.				's
19.				went
20.				like
21.				rode, went
22.				got, cried
23.	can			go
24.	can			go
25.	-(will)			write

Note. From *Children's Language Disorders: An Integrated Approach* (p. 184) by R.D. Hubbell, 1981, Englewood Cliffs, NJ: Prentice-Hall. Adapted by permission.

was in subject or object position. All but two of Scott's noun phrases were in the object position. He consistently used pronouns in the subject position. This pattern indicates that Scott expanded his object-noun phrases much more frequently than his subject-noun phrases. He used primarily two-word phrases. He used determiners frequently, but produced few adjectivals and postmodifiers, and no initiators. His single modifiers were always determiners, either articles or the possessive pronoun *my.* The only two adjectives produced were size terms.

Scott produced very few optional verb elements; most of his sentences contained the main verb only. In this limited sample, he used the modals *would* and *can;* he omitted *will* in two obligatory contexts (sentences 1 and 25), but included it in the negative *won't* (sentence 15). Use of the progressive element is questionable because he produced one correctly (sentence 3), but omitted the auxiliary verb from another (sentence 17). There were no examples of the perfective in this sample. Although tense markers would be analyzed with other grammatical morphemes, it can be noted here that Scott used irregular past tense consistently, and there was one example of a regular past tense.

The next analysis focuses on two types of sentences: negatives and questions. The analysis of negatives is fairly straightforward—all sentences which contain the word *not,* either contracted or uncontracted, in conjunction with an auxiliary verb are listed. Also note instances where the auxiliary verb is missing (e.g., "he not do it") and any sentences containing double negatives ("I don't never . . .). Scott produced the following negative sentences:

It isn't a tricycle.
It won't go in the grass.
Why can't you go?

He negated both the copula *is* and the modals *can* and *will* in this sample. Because he used the affirmative of both *is* and *can,* we can assume that they illustrate use of a productive negative rule. More information about *won't* is necessary because Scott omitted *will* in its two obligatory contexts.

Questions will be categorized by type and form for analysis. Table 6–7 contains a worksheet with Scott's questions listed by type and form. Based on this limited sample, Scott seems to be producing well-formed Yes/No questions with both auxiliary inver-

TABLE 6–7
Question Analysis

YES/NO QUESTIONS

Rising intonation

Inverse of copula/auxiliary
Can you fly?

Insertion of do
Do you know what a Big Wheel is?

Tag

Wh- QUESTIONS

No auxiliary/copula

Univerted auxiliary/copula
Where you would fly?

Well-formed
Why can't you go?

Note. From *Assessing Children's Language in Naturalistic Contexts* (p. 155) by N.J. Lund and J.F. Duchan, 1983, Englewood Cliffs, NJ: Prentice-Hall. Adapted by permission.

sion and insertion of the "dummy" *do*. It should be noted that his *do* insertion question is a complex sentence containing an embedded *Wh-* clause. Of the two *Wh-* questions in this sample, one is well formed with the auxiliary verb inverted. The other has an uninverted auxiliary.

The final syntactic analysis is to look at the complex sentence structures found in the sample. For some children, this level of analysis will be unnecessary because their sample will contain no complex sentences. Any sentences containing two or more main verbs in the initial clause analysis should be classified as compound or embedded. Compound sentences can be described further by the particular conjunction used and by whether the subjects and the verbs in the two clauses are the same or different. Embedded sentences can be classified by whether the grammatical role played by the subordinate is subject, object, complement, or adjectival. An alternative system for analyzing embedded clauses is presented by Paul in Miller (1981). She described nine types of embedded sentences including those with infinitive clauses, *Wh-* clauses, relative clauses, and gerund clauses. The sample from Scott contains two compound sentences: "It gots wheels and pedals, but it little", and "She got scared and cried." The first sentence actually contains two conjunctions; the object noun phrase of the first clause is conjoined with *and* ("wheels and pedals"), while the two clauses are combined with the contrastive conjunction *but*. The subject is the same for both coordinate clauses; the verbs would have been different, but the copula is omitted from the second clause. The other compound sentence conjoins two different verb phrases with *and;* the subject is the same for both verb phrases.

Scott produced three sentences with embedded clauses:

"Do you know what a Big Wheel is?"
"I know how it goes."
"My cousin rode one that went real fast."

The first sentence contains a *Wh-* clause embedded in a Yes/No question. The second sentence contains a *Wh-* question embedded in a declarative sentence. In both cases, the *Wh-* clause is the object of the verb. The third embedded sentence contains a relative clause beginning with the relative pronoun *that* which modifies the object noun (*one*).

Based on the limited sample of 25 utterances, the analysis of Scott's syntax could be summarized with the following brief description:

> Scott used all three basic clause structures in his simple sentences. He used the optional adverbials frequently in intransitive sentences which have only two required elements (S-V), but he rarely used optional elements in either transitive or equative sentences which both have three required elements (S-V-O and S-V-C respectively). Scott used primarily two-word noun phrases with determiners as the most frequent modifiers. His noun phrases were almost all in the object position; most of his sentence subjects consisted of pronouns. Scott's verb phrases were rarely elaborated, and modal verbs seemed to be his only productive optional verb element. He produced well-formed negatives. His Yes/No questions were well formed with both auxiliary verbs, but they were not inverted consistently. Scott formed complex sentences by conjoining two coor-

dinate clauses and by embedding one clause within another. He used two conjunctions, *and* and *but,* in his compound sentences. His embedded sentences contained *Wh*-clauses and a relative clause.

Based on this brief description, we might conclude that Scott needs help in learning to use optional elements in transitive and equative sentences and in expanding his noun phrases and verb phrases. These areas seem to be the weakest ones for him in the syntactic component.

Pragmatics. There are no clearly defined procedures for doing a pragmatic analysis of a child's language sample, and it is not necessary to do a formal analysis of pragmatics for every child. What is necessary is to observe the child's communicative interactions throughout the evaluation. Does the child's language serve different communicative intentions, such as requesting, informing, and expressing feelings? Does the child carry on conversations, taking turns, and maintaining the topic? Does the child seem to make appropriate assumptions? If any of these skills seems to be inadequate, a more in-depth analysis of that aspect of pragmatics is necessary.

Several taxonomies may be helpful for a detailed analysis of the child's communicative intentions. Halliday (1975) proposed a developmental sequence for the major functions of language based on longitudinal observations of his son. The proposed sequence was divided into three phases, with different functions and combinations of functions appearing in each phase. Six functions occurred during Phase I (approximately 10 to 18 months of age for Halliday's son):

1. Instrumental—language used to satisfy material needs and desires
2. Regulatory—language used to control or regulate the behavior of other people
3. Interactional—language used to establish interactions with other people
4. Personal—language used for the expression of personal feelings, attitudes, and interests
5. Heuristic—language used to explore and organize the environment
6. Imaginative—language used to create an imaginary environment

In the second phase of development, which extended from about 18 to 35 months for Halliday's son, the functions that emerged were combinations of the earlier developing functions. These functions include:

1. Pragmatic—language used to act on the environment. This is a combination of the earlier instrumental, regulatory, and interactional functions, and is represented in language used for requesting.
2. Mathetic—language used to learn about the environment. This function grows out of the earlier heuristic, personal, and interactional functions. It is represented in language use for commenting, recalling, and predicting.
3. Informative—language used to provide others with new information. This function appears well after the other previously mentioned functions and is represented in references to events that are remote in time or space.

The functions associated with Phase III (about 3 years of age for Halliday's son) mark entry into the adult linguistic system. There are three Phase III functions:

1. Ideational—language used to represent one's world. This function grows out of the Phase II mathetic function and is the representational, cognitive function of language. It allows speakers to talk about the world of observable objects and events.
2. Interpersonal—language used to participate in the world. This function grows out of the earlier pragmatic function and is represented by language used for social purposes.
3. Textual—language used to express meanings through verbal symbols. This function is part of all utterances. "It is meanings encoded into words or sentences" (Rees, 1978, p. 254).

Halliday's functional categories can be useful in establishing a framework for viewing children's use of language for different intentions. These categories should not be used to do an utterance-by-utterance analysis. Rather they should be the general functions of languages to look for when analyzing entire samples of interaction.

A detailed system for coding preschool-age children's conversational acts was developed by Dore, Gearhart, and Newman (1978). The categories in this system are based on the form, function, content, and conversational contingency of the utterances. Although the system was found to be reliable for coding the conversational acts of three-year-old children interacting with peers and the teacher, it is a fairly elaborate system for routine assessment purposes. It contains a large number of categories, and semantic content, as well as pragmatic function, must be considered in determining in which category an utterance belongs. However, it might be useful if a preliminary analysis has revealed that a child seems to be using language for limited intentions and a more detailed analysis is needed.

Regardless of what taxonomy or system is used to describe the child's use of language for different functions, the communicative contexts within the sample must be examined carefully. For example, was there any opportunity for the child to request an object, event, or information? Or were all needs anticipated and met, making requests unnecessary? Chapman (1981) referred to this situation as looking for "obligatory contexts" (p. 134) for communicative intentions.

In analyzing the child's language sample for conversational abilities, a quick glance through the transcript will determine if the child takes turns. If the child seems to produce monologues frequently, it must be determined if this behavior was appropriate within the context of the conversation. There are instances where narratives are quite appropriate within a conversation. Conversely, it must be determined if it were appropriate for the adult or other person in the conversations to produce a number of successive utterances with no intervening utterances from the child. Did the adult's monologue occur because the child did not take an expected turn? In this sort of analysis, it is helpful to view the videotape or listen to the audiotape for inappropriately long pauses. Such pauses frequently indicate that one of the conversation partners is not taking the expected turn. It is helpful to indicate long pauses on the written transcript.

A quick glance through the transcript can also indicate if the child's and the partner's utterances are semantically contingent, that is, related to the meaning of the previous utterances. This contingency is apparent when a person answers a *who* question by giving the name of a person. Young children frequently achieve semantic contingency by repeating part of their partner's preceding utterance. Semantic contingency is the basis of topic maintenance in conversations. If there are frequent topic shifts or the conversation seems fragmented or confused, topic maintenance should be examined in more depth.

Certain kinds of clues will help determine if the child has problems with presuppositions in conversations. Are there instances where the child fails to provide necessary background information for the listener? For example, does the child use pronouns to refer to people for whom no referent has been established. If so, he is not making appropriate presuppositions about and adjusting his language for the listener's knowledge. Does the child fail to relate another person's utterance to the situation? For example, a glass of juice is spilled and the adult says, "Oh, we'd better get a paper towel," and the child asks, "Why?" Is there evidence of the child's ability to make presuppositions about his relationship with the conversation partner? Does the child alter what he says and how he says it when talking to a family member versus an unfamiliar adult?

If any of these presuppositional skills appear to be problems within the language sample, the child should be observed in different situations interacting with different listeners. The setting (e.g., home, classroom, playground) and the listener (older, younger, peer; familiar, unfamiliar) should be varied to see if there are certain communicative situations or interactions that elicit adjustments in speech style.

Spontaneous language samples are the best source of information about the child's semantic, grammatical, and pragmatic production. However, it is necessary sometimes to set up situations to elicit structures that did not appear in the spontaneous sample or to see if the child *can* produce a particular form when it's required.

Elicited Production Procedures. There are at least two major methods of eliciting particular kinds of responses or forms from a child. One method is to provide a verbal stimulus designed to elicit particular responses. The second method is to provide a context or activity that is likely to elicit particular kinds of responses. Specific procedures falling within each of the major methods will be discussed.

Linguistic or verbal elicitation of responses. *Elicited imitation.* The most common procedure for eliciting particular responses to verbal stimuli is to have the child imitate what the examiner says. This procedure is used frequently in standardized language tests as a measure of syntactic production. Standardized tests using sentence imitation include the Carrow Elicited Language Inventory, the Clinical Evaluation of Language Functions, the Northwestern Syntax Screening Test, the Test of Early Language Development, and the Test of Language Development—Primary and Secondary. It also has been used in nonstandardized assessment tasks (Menyuk, 1968; Miller, 1981). The proponents of elicited imitation argue that it is a very efficient method for obtaining information about a child's ability to produce various kinds of linguistic structures. They assume that children's imitative responses reflect their linguistic knowledge, and that the errors found in the imitated utterances are similar to those they would make in spontaneous productions. The evidence, however, does not always support this assumption. Some investigators have reported that children's performance on elicited imitation tasks does not equal their spontaneous language performance (Bloom, Hood, & Lightbown, 1974; Connell & Myles-Zitzer, 1982; Prutting, Gallagher, & Mulac, 1975). However, there is evidence that children also may imitate forms that they do not use in their spontaneous speech (Kuczaj & Maratsos, 1975; Smith, 1970). Thus, the validity of elicited imitation as a measure of the child's language production abilities is questionable.

The most striking difference between spontaneous production and elicited imitation is the presence or absence of the intent to communicate (Hood & Lightbown, 1978). When children say something spontaneously, they usually intend to communicate with their listener. On an elicited imitation task, however, the only purpose for saying the model utterance is to carry out the examiner's instructions ("Say what I say"). Apparently, the intent to communicate plays a crucial role in the children's linguistic performance, and "the absence of communicative intent . . . may make sentence imitations a more complex matter than sentence formulation in the natural speaking situation" (Connell & Myles-Zitzer, 1982, p. 395).

Sentence imitation tasks should be used with considerable caution. Certainly, they should not serve as the only measure of children's language production abilities but as a supplement to information from a spontaneous sample when intelligibility is very poor or when the spontaneous sample is very limited.

Patterning. In this type of procedure, the examiner presents a set of linguistic stimuli as examples, and the child is to figure out and provide the appropriate type of response. An example of a patterning procedure is Bellugi's (1967) task for eliciting tag questions. The child is given instructions like the following:

> Sometimes I want to say something but I'm not sure if I'm right. So I might say, "That's a big dog" and then I might add, "Isn't it?" We're going to play a game like that. I'll say something and then you add the last part. Let's try it. I'll say "He can do it" and you say. . . .

This type of procedure can be used to elicit prepositions, auxiliaries, negatives, pronouns, and questions. Lund and Duchan (1983), Miller (1981), and Slobin (1967) presented various patterning procedures for eliciting a variety of forms.

Sentence completion. The examiner provides the first part of a sentence and the child fills in the end. Berko (1958) used this task to elicit morphological endings for nonsense words:

> "This is a wug. Now there are two of them. There are two ________."

The key to sentence completion tasks is to construct the first part of the sentence so that there are few possible correct responses for the fill-in. For example, a sentence like "The sun came out and the dog ________" has a large number of possible correct responses while "The sun came out and the snowman ________" has few correct responses. This kind of task can be used to elicit grammatical or conceptual knowledge.

Contextual elicitation of responses. One of the most common methods of creating a context to elicit particular forms or structures is role playing. Children's roles can require them to ask questions (e.g., teacher or interviewer), give commands (boss, parent), provide a lot of descriptive information (describing something for someone who cannot see).

Bringing a wrapped present or novel objects into an evaluation setting sets up a question-eliciting context. Hiding objects and having the child guess where they might be usually elicits Yes/No questions and various prepositions.

Creating contexts to elicit particular forms or structures is less structured than either imitation or verbal elicitation of responses. Various contexts within the spontaneous language situation increase the probability of obtaining a variety of grammatical, semantic, and pragmatic forms.

Thus far, I have focused on nonstandardized procedures for obtaining information about a child's language production abilities. We also need to consider ways of assessing language comprehension.

Language Comprehension. There are two basic types of comprehension of concern—linguistic comprehension and communicative comprehension. *Linguistic comprehension* refers to the ability to interpret a verbal stimulus using only linguistic cues and linguistic knowledge. An example of a task requiring linguistic comprehension is asking the child to act out a reversible active sentence such as "The girl chases the boy." In order to do this, the child needs to know the meaning of *girl, boy,* and *chase* and that the word order in the sentence (S-V-O) indicates that the girl is the agent and the boy is the object of the action. A child with this basic semantic and syntactic, or linguistic, knowledge could be expected to act out this sentence correctly.

I use *communicative comprehension* to refer to the ability to interpret a verbal stimulus using all of the information available in the communicative situation. For example, when someone tells a child to "Shut the door" and the child walks over to the only open door in the room and shuts it, we cannot assume that the child demonstrated linguistic comprehension of the command. If the speaker looked at or pointed at the door when giving the command, the child may have responded on the basis of that nonverbal cue and her own assessment of the situation. When someone points to an open door and says something, the most reasonable interpretation is that the door should be shut. In this case, the child would have needed no semantic or syntactic knowledge to respond correctly. However, she would have needed knowledge of the nonverbal cues and situational information on which to base an inference about the appropriate responses. The child also could have known the meaning of *door* and have responded correctly by simply inferring that the most reasonable thing to do with an open door is to close it.

It is important to be aware of these two types of comprehension in the assessment of the child's comprehension abilities. Standardized tests tap the child's linguistic comprehension, for the most part. The typical comprehension task on standardized tests requires the child to point to the picture, out of three or four choices, that best represents a word or sentence spoken by the examiner. These sentences are presented out of context, and, in order to choose the correct picture, the child must rely on the linguistic information in the verbal stimulus. In natural language situations, words and sentences are part of an ongoing verbal and nonverbal interaction that occurs within a specific setting or situation. The ongoing interaction and the setting or situation all provide important cues to aid the child in understanding what is being said. Most children are able to use these cues even when they lack full linguistic comprehension. Failure to use the various communicative cues is a real cause for concern.

Observation of children's communicative comprehension can be done during the collection of a spontaneous language sample. Note whether children respond to their mothers' and to the examiner's comments, commands, and questions. What kinds of cues, besides the verbal stimulus, were available? Children who have normal hearing, but frequently fail to respond appropriately to speech addressed to them, will need to be observed in other settings and with other people for evidence of communicative comprehension.

Assessment of children's ability to understand and use linguistic information will require more structured observations. In assessing children's linguistic understanding of words and sentences, we need to avoid asking them to do the expected or obvious thing. For example, if there are some blocks and a box, telling children to put a block in the box does not test their comprehension of the spatial relationship between the block and the box. Given an open box and a block, the expected action would be to put the block in the box and, in fact, the opposite is impossible. If you also told the children to put the block *on* and *under* and *beside* the box and they did all of these correctly (at least twice for each), then you might reasonably assume that the children comprehended *in* as well as the other prepositions. However, if they responded correctly only to "Put the block in the box," you could not conclude anything about their comprehension of *in*.

There are three major types of tasks that can be used in assessing comprehension of words and sentences: identification, acting out, and judgment (Leonard, Prutting, Perozzi, & Berkeley, 1978). In an identification task, children are asked to choose (e.g., point to) the object or picture that represents the word or sentence. An example of this type of task would be to place three or four objects in front of the child and tell him to "Show me ball."

Acting-out tasks require children to carry out an action or event described in the verbal stimulus. For example, a child may be given a group of toys and objects and told to "Make the boy chase the dog."

Judgment tasks require children to decide whether a verbal stimulus is acceptable. For example, a child might be asked if the sentence "The sisters was going" sounds okay. Or the child might be given two sentences, such as "The sisters was going" and "The sisters were going" and asked which one sounds better. Children also can be asked to explain why a sentence is acceptable or unacceptable to obtain additional information about their knowledge of the rules.

In assessing children's understanding or knowledge of connected sentences (discourse), it is necessary to go beyond tasks assessing understanding of single words or sentences. One way of tapping discourse comprehension is by reading or telling children a story and asking them to retell it. Johnston (1982) sugggested that children's narratives can be analyzed for evidence of various abilities. For example, they can be analyzed to determine if the children use underlying organizational rules in retelling the story, or to determine the ways in which their expectations about event sequencing influence their processing of the story. Chapter 5 contains a description of Johnston's model. The Merrill Language Screening Test (Mumm, Secord, & Dykstra, 1980) uses a story-telling format to provide some information about children's syntactic and pragmatics skills in discourse.

Early Cognitive and Communicative Behaviors. Many of the important social/communicative behaviors can be observed during child-caretaker interactions. Does the child establish and maintain eye contact with the caretaker and under what conditions? Will the child participate in social games, such as peek-a-boo and patty-cake, when the caretaker initiates them? Does the child vocalize in response to the caretaker's speech? Does the child only *respond* to the caretakers or does she also *initiate* interactions. If the child does initiate interactions, how does she do it—through sound production, gesture, or both? Does the child carry over any of the behaviors from the caretaker-child relationship to interactions with other adults, such as the examiner?

The sensorimotor concepts, such as mean-end relations and schemes for relating to objects, can be assessed through use of developmental scales such as Uzgiris and Hunt's (1975) Infant Psychological Developmental Scales. Nicholich (1977) and Westby (1980) have developed scales for assessing play (schemes for relating to objects) which allow more precise scoring than the Schemes for Relating to Objects Scale from Uzgiris and Hunt.

USING THE ASSESSMENT

The goal of assessment helps to determine the choice of assessment instruments. If the major purpose was simply identification of the child as either language-disordered or normal, then a standardized test would determine if the child's syntactic and semantic production and comprehension were similar to those of his peers. That information may be supplemented by information about pragmatics from observing the child in natural communicative interactions.

If the major purpose were to provide a comprehensive description of the child's language abilities and deficits, then a variety of nonstandardized procedures would provide the necessary information. Analyses of the child's spontaneous language sample provide information about phonological, semantic, syntactic, and pragmatic production abilities, as well as communicative comprehension. This information may be supplemented by results from elicited production tasks. The child's linguistic comprehension of various words and sentences can be assessed through nonstandardized identification, acting-out, or judgment tasks. Information on the child's discourse comprehension may be tested in a story-retelling task. At this point, there is a comprehensive picture of the child's strengths and weaknesses in language and communication. The next step is to interpret this information and to make recommendations.

Interpretation of Assessment Results

The way in which the assessment results are organized and interpreted depends, to a large extent, on the purpose of the assessment. If the purpose is identification of a child with a language disorder and standardized tests have been used in the assessment, interpretation of the results should be relatively simple. Children's performances on the tests will be compared to the norms to determine if they performed at the same level as their peers. If their level of performance was below that of their peers, then it must be determined if it is far enough below to indicate a language disorder. Some test makers suggest a point at which children should be recommended for therapy. For example, Lee (1974) suggested that children whose scores on the DSS place them at or below the 10th percentile should be seen for therapy. It is fairly common to consider scores that fall more than two deviations below the mean as indicative of a deficit or problem. However, there are no well-defined criteria for identifying children with a language disorder. Test scores are helpful in deciding whether there is a problem, but ultimately one will have to rely on informed judgment.

When the purpose for assessment is to develop an intervention program, organization and interpretation of results will be different than when the goal is identification. The concern is no longer with comparing the child's performance with that of his peers, but with identifying patterns that indicate problem areas. The differences between the nature and the interpretation of the information required for identification versus intervention can best be illustrated with a case profile.

CASE STUDY

Michele, age 4 years 2 months, was referred for an in-depth language assessment. She has been identified as language disordered by another agency. Following is a summary of the information obtained from that agency's evaluation of Michele at 4 years.

Language Production

Michele's MLU for a 50-utterance spontaneous sample was 3.3 morphemes. The predicted MLU for 48 months is 4.4 morphemes, with a $\pm$ 1 SD of 3.46 to 5.34 morphemes (Miller, 1981). Thus, Michele's MLU for this sample was below the lower limit of the predicted range for her age. In addition, Michele's sentences varied little in length and syntactic structure. About 95% of her sentences were simple active declarative sentences, three to four words long. She frequently omitted copula and auxiliary verbs from these simple sentences. The only questions produced were rising intonation Yes/No questions.

Michele willingly participated in conversations with the examiner about objects and events within the immediate environment. She took turns and was able to maintain topics for several conversational turns.

A few speech sound errors were noted in her quick speech, but these were primarily with later developing sounds like /ʃ/ and /θ/. Overall intelligibility was acceptable.

Michele's conversational skills and her speech sound production abilities seemed to be within normal limits. However, the low MLU and the lack of variation in sentence length and structure are not typical of the language of 48-month-old children.

Language Comprehension

During an unstructured play session with the examiner, Michele followed directions and gave appropriate answers to Yes/No and *Wh-* questions including *what, where, what do, who, how many,* and *why.* All of her responses were appropriate throughout this interaction.

Michele was given the Peabody Picture Vocabulary Test— Revised. Form L (Dunn & Dunn, 1981) to assess her receptive vocabulary. Her raw score of 46 is equivalent to a standard score of 104, placing her in the 60th percentile. The Test for Auditory Comprehension of Language (Carrow, 1973), which tests understanding of various grammatical structures, was administered also. Michele achieved a raw score of 67 which is equivalent to an age score of 4 years 1 month and places her in the 50th percentile for the age range from 4 to 4 years 5 months.

Michele's comprehension of language appears to be within normal limits. She demonstrated understanding of the language addressed to her in conversational context as well as age-appropriate vocabulary and grammatical comprehension on formal tests.

Other Impressions

No formal testing was done of Michele's social, cognitive, or motor abilities. However, informal observation of her interpersonal interactions, her approach to the assessment tasks, and her manipulation of objects suggests that she is developing normally in these areas.

Conclusions

Michele has a mild to moderate disorder of language production. The data from the initial evaluation were insufficient for designing an intervention program. A more detailed description of her language production was needed to indicate particular problem areas. The following summary provides the kind of information needed for establishing initial intervention goals. This summary is based on analysis of 120 utterances produced during a 30-minute unstructured play session between Michele and her mother.

A. Grammatical analysis
  1. MLU: 3.6 morphemes (range 1 to 6 morphemes)
  2. Grammatical morphemes
     a. 80% or more correct use: *in, on,* noun plural
     b. 40% to 80% correct use: progressive *-ing* (70%), noun possessive (60%), articles (60%), and uncontractible copula (42%)
     c. Less than 40% correct use: irregular and regular past tense; contractible copula; and contractible and uncontractible auxiliary
  3. Clause structure
     a. Produced intransitive, transitive, and equative clauses
        i. Intransitive clauses: 100% contained required elements (subject + verb) with a few optional adverbials
        ii. Transitive clauses: 100% contained the required elements (subject + verb + direct object) with some adverbials but no indirect objects
        iii. Equative clauses: 60% contained the required elements (subject + BE + complement); 40% lacked the copula (BE) verb
  4. Noun phrases
     a. Typically two words, with a few three-word phrases
     b. Single modifier always a determiner; her few three-word phrases contained a size modifier following the determiner
     c. Majority in the object position
  5. Verb phrases
     a. Typically contained only the main verb; used very few optional verb elements
     b. Optional elements included the progressive *-ing,* usually with the auxiliary omitted; and the modal verb *can*

6. Negatives
   a. Typically used *no* or *not* plus main verb; occasional use of *can't* and *don't*
   b. No other auxiliary or copula verbs used with negative markers
7. Questions
   a. Yes/No questions: typically signaled with rising intonation. There were some instances of correct copula/auxiliary inversion, although *do* was consistently omitted
   b. *Wh-* questions: *what, what-do, where,* and why were produced with the copula/auxiliary omitted
8. Complex sentences
   a. Two embedded sentences, both with simple infinitive clauses
   b. One compound sentence with duplicate subjects and verbs

B. Semantic analysis
   1. Type-token ratio: .47 (expected TTR for children between 3 and 8 years is about .50, according to Templin, 1957).
   2. Used words for location *(in, on, up, these),* size *(big, little),* quantity *(some, any, little bit),* and time *(last night, soon, now)*

C. Pragmatic analysis
   1. Used language to serve a variety of communicative intentions, including requesting, informing, expressing emotions, and establishing social interactions
   2. Took turns and maintained topic in conversations with her mother and with the examiner

D. Phonological analysis
   1. Produced all English phonemes
   2. Speech characterized by the following processes:
      a. cluster reduction (*pay* for *play*)
      b. deletion of unstressed syllables (*telphone* for *telephone*)
   3. Intelligibility when context is known was rated as good

Based on this information, the following conclusions and recommendations can be made:

1. Michele appears to have no major problems in semantic or pragmatic production and, therefore, these areas would not be a direct focus of intervention.
2. Although Michele uses some phonological processes in her speech, these do not seriously affect intelligibility. Therefore, phonology would not be a direct focus of intervention at this time.
3. Michele demonstrates a pattern of difficulty with the production of verbs. This pattern is reflected in various aspects of her grammatical use:
   a. inconsistent use of verb morphemes including uncontractible and contractible copula and auxiliary verbs and both the regular and irregular past tense
   b. omission of copula (BE) verbs from over one third of her single equative sentences
   c. restricted verb phrases expansion; most of her verb phrases contain only the main verb
   d. restricted use of auxiliary/copula verbs in negatives
   e. infrequent use of auxiliary/copula verbs in Yes/No questions and consistent omission of copula/auxiliary verbs in *Wh-* questions

4. The major focus of intervention should be on production of copula and auxiliary verbs within simple clauses, especially equative sentences, and then within negative sentences and questions. Other optional verb elements, beginning with modals, should be introduced to help Michele expand her verb phrases.

This case profile illustrates interpreting assessment information for two major purposes—identification and determining intervention goals. The third major purpose of assessment, monitoring change from intervention, requires interpreting current results in relation to results from previous assessments. In order to fulfill this purpose, it is crucial to have clearly defined intervention goals and to keep good records of the child's target behaviors. For example, one of the intervention goals for Michele would be to increase her production of the correct BE verb in equative clauses to 100%. In order to determine if therapy is helping Michele achieve this goal, the percentage of Michele's equative sentences containing copula verbs must be determined and then compared to the 60% reported in the previous evaluation. In addition, the forms of the BE verbs used most frequently, and the kinds of subjects (e.g., nouns, personal pronouns, demonstrative pronouns) most frequently followed by a BE verb. This kind of information would be important for determining the specific BE verbs to focus on and the kinds of sentence contexts which facilitate use of BE verbs.

In addition to determining if the child is acquiring the target language behaviors, it should be determined if the child is generalizing previously acquired skills and knowledge to new situations. Generalization of target behaviors is the ultimate test of any intervention program. In the case of Michele's use of BE verbs in equative sentences, we could observe her in a free play session with her mother, sibling, or peer, or observe her in another setting, such as nursery school, and record all of her equative sentences. Then we would analyze these sentences for presence of the BE verb, noting those particular contexts or situations in which it was used or omitted. The percentage of correct use of BE verbs in these nontherapy settings can be compared to the percentage of use in the therapy situation. The general goal is over 80% correct use in all situations.

SUMMARY

How assessment results are interpreted depends on the assessment goal or purpose. Interpretation when the goal is identification involves comparing children's language performance to the performance of their peers. When the purpose is designing a remediation program, interpretation of assessment information involves looking for patterns or regularities that indicate deficit areas. Finally, measuring change as a result of intervention requires interpreting assessment results in relation to previous assessment information.

Obtaining, organizing, and interpreting assessment information is no small undertaking. It requires curiosity, time, patience, and knowledge about language and communication. However, it is exciting and rewarding to uncover regularities in the child's language behaviors and to figure out what these patterns indicate about the child's abilities. This kind of information is necessary to fulfill the responsibility of designing and implementing effective language intervention programs.

STUDY QUESTIONS

1. What are the three major purposes for assessing children's language? What are the differences in the type and interpretation of the assessment information needed to fulfill each of these purposes?
2. What are some of the aspects of phonology, semantics, grammar, and pragmatics that may be assessed in a comprehensive language evaluation? What other aspects of behavior or development are important to consider?
3. What are the major sources of information about a child's development and current functioning? What kinds of information can be obtained from these sources?
4. Discuss the differences between the kinds of information obtained from standardized tests versus nonstandardized procedures. In what situation(s) would you recommend using each?
5. What are the two major types of comprehension? How would you go about assessing each type?

BIBLIOGRAPHY

Bates, E. (1976). *Language and context: The acquisition of pragmatics.* New York: Academic Press.

Bates, E. (1979). *The emergence of symbols.* New York: Academic Press.

Bankson, N. (1977). *Bankson language screening test.* Baltimore: University Park Press.

Bellugi, U. (1967). Bellugi's tag question test. In D. Slobin (Ed.), *A field manual for cross–cultural study of the acquisition of communicative competence.* Berkeley: University of California Press.

Berko, J. (1958). The child's learning of English morphology. *Word, 14,* 150–177.

Bloom, L., Hood, L., & Lightbown, P. (1974). Imitation in language development: If, when and why. *Cognitive Psychology, 6,* 380–420.

Bloom, L., & Lahey, M. (1978). *Language development and language disorders.* New York: Wiley.

Bloom, L., Rocissano, L., & Hood, L. (1976). Adult-child discourse: Developmental interaction between information processing and linguistic knowledge. *Cognitive Psychology, 8,* 521–552.

Boehm, A. (1971). *Boehm text of basic concepts.* New York: The Psychological Corporation.

Brown, R. (1973). *A first language: The early stages.* Cambridge, MA: Harvard University Press.

Bruner, J. (1975). The ontogenesis of speech acts. *Journal of Child Language, 2,* 1–19.

Carrow, E. (1974). A test using elicited imitations in assessing grammatical structure in children. *Journal of Speech and Hearing Disorders, 38,* 437–444.

Carrow, E. (1974). *Carrow elicited language inventory.* Austin, TX: Learning Concepts.

Carrow, E. (1973). *Test of auditory comprehension of language.* Austin, TX: Urban Research Group.

Chapman, R. (1981). Exploring children's communicative intents. In J. Miller, *Assessing language production in children,* pp. 111–136. Baltimore: University Park Press.

Connell, P., & Myles-Zitzer, C. (1982). An analysis of elicited imitation as a language evaluation procedure. *Journal of Speech and Hearing Disorders, 47,* 390–396.

Crystal, D., Fletcher, P., & Garman, M. (1976). *The grammatical analysis of language disability: A procedure for assessment and remediation.* London: Edward Arnold.

Darley, F. & Moll, K. (1960). Reliability of language measures and size of language sample. *Journal of Speech and Hearing Research, 3,* 166–173.

Dever, R. (1978). *TALK: Teaching the American language to kids.* Columbus, OH: Charles E. Merrill.

Dore, J., Gearhart, M., & Newman, D. (1978). The structures of nursery school conversation. In K. Nelson (Ed.), *Children's language,* Vol. 1, pp. 337–395. New York: Gardner Press.

Dunn, L., & Dunn, L. (1981). *Peabody picture vocabulary test—revised.* Circle Pines, MN: American Guidance Service.

Edwards, M., & Shriberg, L. (1983). *Phonology: Applications in communicative disorders.* San Diego: College Hill Press.

Foster, C., Giddan, J., & Stark, J. (1972). *ACLC: Assessment of children's language comprehension.* Palo Alto, CA: Consulting Psychologists Press.

Gallagher, T., & Prutting, C. (Eds.) (1983). *Pragmatic assessment and intervention issues in language.* San Diego, CA: College Hill Press.

Haas, W., & Wepman, J. (1974). Dimensions of individual difference in the spoken syntax of school children. *Journal of Speech and Hearing Research, 17,* 455–469.

Halliday, M.A.K. (1975). *Explorations in the functions of language.* London: Edward Arnold.

Hammill, D., Brown, V., Larsen, S., & Wiederholt, J. (1980). *Test of adolescent language.* Austin, TX: Pro-Ed.

Hammill, D., & Newcomer, P. (1982). *Test of language development—intermediate.* Austin, TX: Pro-Ed.

Hodson, B.W. (1980). *The assessment of phonological processes.* Danville, IL: Interstate.

Hood, L., & Lightbown, P. (1978). What children do when asked to "Say what I say": Does elicited imitation measure linguistic knowledge? In P. Connell (Ed.), *Comprehension and production of speech and language, Monograph I, Allied Health and Behavioral Sciences, 1,* 195–219.

Hresko, W., Reid, D., & Hammill, D. (1981). *The test of early language development.* Austin, TX: Pro-Ed.

Hubbell, R. (1981). *Children's language disorders: An intergrated approach.* Englewood Cliffs, NJ: Prentice-Hall.

Ingram, D. (1981). *Procedures for the phonological analysis of children's language.* Baltimore, MD: University Park Press.

James, S., & Button, M. (1978). Choosing stimulus materials for eliciting language samples from children with language disorders. *Language, Speech, and Hearing Services in Schools, 9,* 91–97.

Johnston, J. (1982). Narratives: A new look at communication problems in older language-disordered children. *Language, Speech, and Hearing Services in Schools, 13,* 144–155.

Jorgensen, C., Barrett, M., Huisingh, R., & Zachman, L. (1981). *The WORD test.* Moline, IL: Lingui-Systems.

Kirk, S., McCarthy, J., & Kirk, W. (1968). *Illinois test of psycholinguistic ability,* Revised Edition. Urbana, IL: University of Illinois Press.

Kramer, C., James, S., & Saxman, J. (1979). A comparison of language samples elicited at home and in the clinic. *Journal of Speech and Hearing Disorders, 44,* 321–330.

Kuczaj, S., & Maratos, M. (1975). What children *can* say before they *will. Merrill–Palmer Quarterly, 21,* 89–111.

Lee, L. (1974). *Developmental Sentence Analysis.* Evanston, IL: Northwestern University Press.

Lee, L. (1971). *Northwestern syntax screening test.* Evanston, IL: Northwestern University Press.

Leonard, L., Perozzi, J., Prutting, C., & Berkeley, R. (1978). Nonstandardized approaches to the assessment of language behaviors. *ASHA, 20,* 371–379.

Leonard, L. Steckol, K., & Panther, K. (1983). Returning meaning to semantic relations: Some clinical applications. *Journal of Speech and Hearing Disorders, 48,* 25–36.

Lewis, M. (1978). The infant and its caregiver. *Allied Health and Behavioral Sciences, 1,* 469–492.

Loban, W. (1968). *Language development during the school years.* Lawrence, KS: University of Kansas Publications.

Longhurst, T., & Grubb, S. (1974). A comparison of language samples collected in four situations. *Language, Speech, and Hearing Services in Schools, 5,* 71–78.

Lund, N., & Duchan, J. (1983). *Assessing children's language in naturalistic contexts.* Englewood Cliffs, NJ: Prentice-Hall.

Menyuk, P. (1968). Children's learning and reproduction of grammatical and nongrammatical phonological sequences. *Child Development, 39,* 849–959.

Miller, J. (1978). Assessing children's language behavior: A developmental process approach. In R. Schiefelbusch (Ed.), *Bases of language intervention* (pp. 269–318). Baltimore: University Park Press.

Miller, J. (1981). *Assessing language production in children: Experimental procedures.* Baltimore: University Park Press.

Miller, J., & Chapman, R. (1981). The relation between age and mean length of utterance in morphemes. *Journal of Speech and Hearing Research, 24,* 154–161.

Mumm, M., Secord, W., & Dykstra, K. (1980). *Merrill language screening test.* Columbus, OH: Charles E. Merrill.

Newcomer, P., & Hammill, D. (1977). *The test of language development.* Austin, TX: Pro-Ed.

Nicholich, L. (1977). Beyond sensorimotor intelligence: Assessment of symbolic maturity through analysis of pretend play. *Merrill Palmer Quarterly, 23,* 89–99.

Olswang, L., & Carpenter, R. (1978). Elicitor effects on the language obtained from language-impaired children. *Journal of Speech and Hearing Disorders, 43,* 76–88.

Piaget, J. (1952). *The origins of intelligence in children.* New York: International Universities Press.

Prutting, C. (1979). *Process* (/pra/,ses/n) The action of moving forward progressively from one point to another on the way to completion. *Journal of Speech and Hearing Disorders, 44,* 3–30.

Prutting, C., Gallagher, T., & Mulac, A. (1975). The expressive portion of the NSST compared to a spontaneous language sample. *Journal of Speech and Hearing Disorders, 40,* 40–68.

Rees, N. (1978). Pragmatics of language: Applications to normal and disordered language development. In R. Schiefelbusch (Ed.), *Bases of language intervention* (pp. 191–268). Baltimore: University Park Press.

Semel, E., & Wiig, E. (1980). *Clinical evaluation of language functions.* Columbus, OH: Charles E. Merrill.

Shriberg, L., & Kent, R. (1982). *Clinical phonetics.* New York: Wiley.

Shriberg, L., & Kwiatkowski, J. (1980). *Natural process analysis.* New York: Wiley.

Siegel, G., & Broen, P. (1976). Language assessment. In L. Lloyd (Ed.), *Communication, assessment and intervention strategies* (pp. 74–122). Baltimore: University Park Press.

Stalnaker, L., & Creaghead, N. (1982). An examination of samples obtained under three experimental conditions. *Language, Speech, and Hearing Services in Schools, 13,* 121–128.

Steckol, K., & Leonard, L. (1981). Sensorimotor development and the use of prelinguistic performances. *Journal of Speech and Hearing Research, 24,* 262–268.

Stern, D. (1977). *The first relationship: Infant and mother.* Cambridge, MA: Harvard University Press.

Templin, M. (1957). *Certain language skills in children: Their development and interrelationships.* Institute of Child Welfare Monograph No. 26. Minneapolis: University of Minnesota Press.

Uzgiris, I., & Hunt, J. McV. (1975). *Assessment in infancy: Scales of psychological development.* Chicago: University of Illinois Press.

Weiner, F.F. (1979). *Phonological process analysis.* Baltimore, MD: University Park Press.

Westby, C. (1980). Assessment of cognitive and language abilities through play. *Language, Speech and Hearing Services in Schools, 11,* 154–168.

Wiig, E. (1983). *Let's talk: Inventory for adolescents.* Columbus, OH: Charles E. Merrill.

Wiig, E., & Semel, E. (1980). *Language assessment and intervention for the learning disabled.* Columbus, OH: Charles E. Merrill.

Zimmerman, I., Steiner, V., & Evatt, R. (1969). *Preschool language scale.* Columbus, OH: Charles E. Merrill.

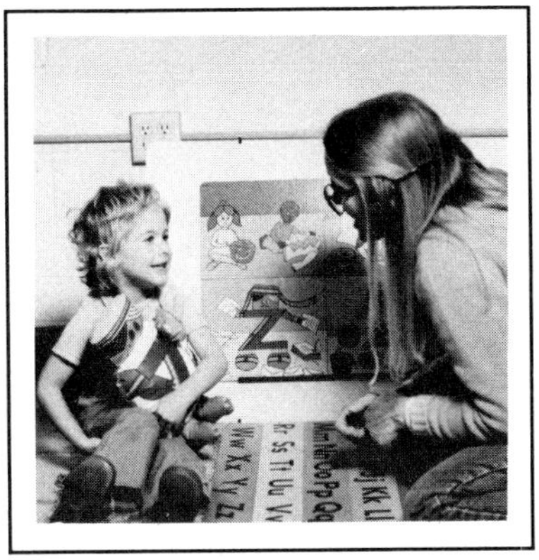

7

A Language-Communication Intervention Model

BASES FOR A THERAPY MODEL

The responsibility for designing and applying an intervention program for a child who has significant problems in communicating with other people is an awesome task. Communicative problems come in a wide variety of types and severities. Some children with significant language deficiencies may be the products of impoverished environments. Some may manifest intellectual deficiencies. Still others may carry the primary label of a specific and highly debilitating etiological category like brain injury or autism. A clinician faced with such variety in problem levels and client status must have some basic and pervasive organizing foundation from which to identify the intervention goals and procedures which will be applied in each case.

Professionals, by definition, have such foundations. They have a specific and comprehensive body of knowledge about their substantive areas. Their responsibility as professionals is to organize and apply this body of knowledge to the various clinical tasks that confront them. A body of knowledge organized in ways that allow it to be applied to varying types and levels of problems in a given area is a *model* for the activities of that professional. Because the requirements for a model in language intervention are so demanding, the process for developing that model is a crucial one. It is important in this chapter, therefore, to consider three basic questions:

1. What is an intervention model for language?
2. What does it need to contain?
3. How is it developed?

This chapter was written by Dr. James McLean, University of Kansas.

Finally, it becomes important to consider how such a model is to be applied to the specific problems of actual children.

Theory as a Basis for a Therapy Model

A therapy model is the design for practical application of a theory (or group of theories) about the behavioral domain in which the targeted problems exist. A theory model identifies the specific child behaviors that need to be trained, and determines the kinds of procedures which will be used to train these needed behaviors. A therapy model directs the overall course of training needed for children who begin such training at different levels and with different needs. Clinicians cannot design an individualized therapy plan for a child with a language deficit or disorder unless they have a well-developed theory about what human language is, what it does, and how it is acquired.

We often hear even experienced clinicians say, "I want something practical—not a lot of theory." What such clinicians seem not to recognize is that there is no formal therapy that is not based on some cogent and valid theoretical model of the behavioral domain being treated. Providing treatment without knowledge of the theoretical bases which generate it is the role of a technician—not a professional. Clinicians who do not have carefully organized and up-to-date knowledge from which to identify and select their therapy goals and procedures have little basis for individualizing their therapy offerings, revising their goals and procedures, or judging the overall progress made by their clients. Only clinicians who have this up-to-date knowledge base about what language is and what events and experiences affect its acquisition by both normal and handicapped children are truly prepared to assess, treat, and evaluate language disorders. Clinicians who do not have this theoretical base are dependent on the directions of others. Whether this outside direction is in the form of a prewritten program or is realized in the form of prescriptive orders of someone else, it should be clear that the clinician is not functioning as an independent professional. Considering the continuing struggle that is required to keep speech-language pathologists independent of the control of other disciplines, a clinician without a strong grounding in the theoretical bases of communication, speech, and language is indeed in jeopardy. So too is the client of such a technician.

Today's clinicians are fortunate because the current theories about human language are richer, and the research data supporting these theories are more robust than they have ever been. The content of this volume has been carefully thought out in order to emphasize these current theories. In this chapter, I will be offering some direction for the specific implications these theories have for a model which will identify the goals and procedures of language therapy.

Theories Underlying Current Therapy Models

At this point in your study, you have been exposed to the various theories and their supporting data that make up the current knowledge base in child language. Now, it is important to analyze these theories and discover what they tell about the targets a clinician must seek in therapy and the procedures which appear to be the most promising in attaining these targets.

Modern language theory holds that child language is a behavior that has one primary purpose—that of influencing the behaviors of other people. Language is used by children to request certain actions from other people, to direct the attention of other people to interesting objects or events, and to answer or reply to other people. Second, and importantly, this ability to intentionally influence other people's behavior begins in early infancy as babies interact with mothers and other family members who demonstrate that they are ready and willing to respond to any behaviors that indicate the infant's needs and desires (Bates, Camaioni, & Volterra, 1975; Bruner, 1975). The current theories of language also reflect the position that these abilities to affect the behaviors of other people to get help and attention and to carry on interesting activities are paralleled by growth in infants' abilities to act on the physical entities of their world, to solve problems, and to attain desired ends and effects in the physical environment, just as in the social environment. All of these parallel attainments in the physical dimension of the environment have been demonstrated in the theory and data on infant behaviors that are classed as developing in the sensorimotor period (Piaget, 1952).

The final important aspect of language development is that mothers and children work very hard at learning to communicate with and to have effects on one another. It is within these mother-child interactions that children learn the language skills that will enable them to communicate effectively with all of the other people in their environment. This ability begins with *action schemes* and gradually moves into *symbolic schemes.* That is, children move from reaching, pulling, and touching people and things to the point where they can gesture and, finally, *talk* about the action or attention they desire from others. In language acquisition, these behaviors do not just suddenly blossom; rather, they emerge gradually as a result of a child's experiences with people and things in the environment. You have seen some specific ways that mothers and caregivers facilitate the task of language learning when they interact with very young children.

A language clinician will work with children for whom this natural process has not been successful. Perhaps some of the children will be handicapped in ways that prevented them from learning some of the things taught by their caregivers. Perhaps, in some cases, the children's caregivers did not carry out the teaching process adequately or intensively enough to allow the children to move through all of the stages of language learning. For many children, both of these problems have occurred. When children have moderate to severe handicaps in any one of several areas, they often do not provide their caregivers with the reinforcement and feedback that these caregivers need to guide their teaching and facilitation. Thus, many handicapped children not only have problems associated with their primary handicaps, but they also have the problems which their deficient behaviors have *created* for those people who care for them, play with them, and teach them.

Therapy, then, becomes a matter of assessing children's language problems, evaluating the possible causes of these problems, and designing a program of activities which will enable the clients to acquire better communicative and language skills. The study of normal language has shown that learning language requires much work on the part of both the child and the teaching caregiver. Therapy requires activities in which both the clinician and the child work together to reach the language goals needed for that child. You will not be able to "pour" new knowledge and ability into children, but will be working to provide activities which allow children to *construct* the knowledge and behaviors that they need.

It is important that clinicians realize that therapy is not a one-way street; it is a partnership in which both the child and the therapist work to reach the goals identified as needed by the child. Therapy is not something that a clinician "gives" to the child. Therapy is a *process* of interaction between the therapist and the child in which both participants play important roles. The therapist must identify appropriate goal-behaviors, and design the activities and experiences which will allow the client to discover and acquire these needed skills and behaviors. The child, in turn, needs to work diligently to make these discoveries and acquisitions.

COMPONENTS OF A LANGUAGE THERAPY PROGRAM

A program of language therapy has three major components. First, such a program has *product goals;* that is, it specifies a set of behavioral products that are deemed appropriate and needed by a given client or group of clients. Second, it also has a *procedures* component; that is, it specifies exactly what activities and schedules will be used to facilitate a client's "discovery" or attainment of these content goals. Third, a therapy program has a *context;* that is, it has a milieu of physical, social, and activity elements in which therapy goals are sought. As we begin to identify the specific elements of these three components, we will be able to see how necessary a theoretical model of language is to the design of therapy.

Product Issues in Language Therapy

If we begin to think about the kinds of product goals we will identify for language therapy, we should find ourselves thinking about our theory of language. Thus, we should be considering that our therapy must be directed to all three of the dimensions of language that have been identified in our study to this point. Language has three dimensions:

1. *Content*—it must transmit a speaker's propositions and meanings
2. *Function*—it is used to attain certain desired effects on people in the environment
3. *Form*—only certain types and arrangements of communicative behavior or language structures will adequately carry the content and attain the goals of a language act

Therapy, then, must identify targets in all three domains for various children. Some children, for example, will need to learn how to *mean* certain things—how to talk about the events and entities in their environment in ways that others will understand. Do they want to direct attention? If so, they will need to be able to specify both the referent of interest and their communicative intent regarding that referent (e.g., "Look, cat"). Do they intend the function of their utterance to be that of specifically affecting their *mother's* attention? If so, they must add to the basic message ("Look cat, *mama*"). Although the preceding examples carry the appropriate content and function, the ideal goal would be to see that the content and function is carried in the *best language form* ("Look at the cat, mama").

The product goals for a child's language therapy program will not be simply a specific *linguistic form.* Rather, the target will be the appropriate *content, function,* and *form* for a desired communicative act (Bloom & Lahey, 1978; McLean & Snyder-McLean, 1978; Muma, 1978). In order to identify such multidimensional goals for language therapy, a clinician must know exactly what the content, functions, and forms of child language are. The therapy model, then, must contain all three elements. Figure 7–1 shows the three-dimensional model that is suggested by current language theory.

Figure 7–1 indicates that a child's utterance reflects the three dimensions of content, function, and form. Each of these three dimensions interacts with each of the others. A specific language *form* obviously must conform to the linguistic rules of a child's culture; but it is only fully appropriate if it carries the propositional *content* that a child desires and has the appropriate *function* (or effect) that a child intends it to have on the audience. The most important thing about the current therapy model is that it is a

Figure 7–1. A Transactional Model of Child Language

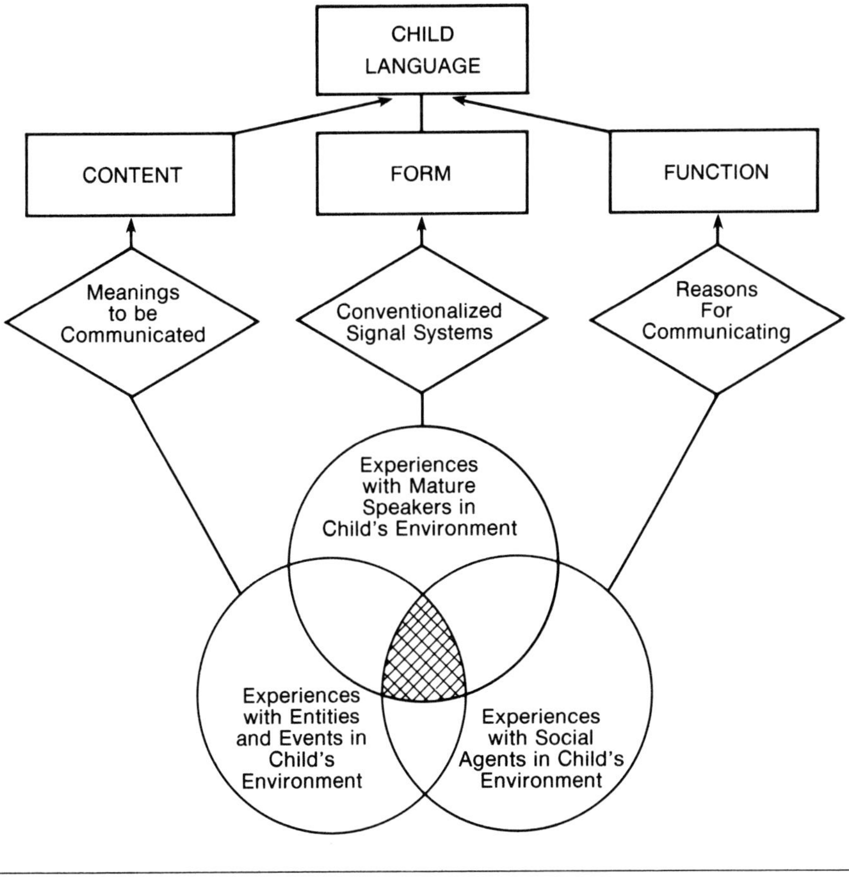

Source: J. E. McLean & L. K. Snyder-McLean (1978)
[a]See Table 7–1 for specification of priorities appropriate to each level.

communication model, as opposed to a strict linguistic model such as those followed in the past.

Procedural Issues in Language Therapy

The procedures for attaining such therapy goals are similarly multidimensional. We used to think that it was enough simply to present models of the desired language *forms* for children to imitate. However, such procedures are not at all adequate for many child clients. A language *form* that a child only imitates, but does not fully understand, is not likely to be used by a child in situations other than the clinical situation in which it is evoked. Thus, we have learned that children must:

1. Know what they wish to *mean*
2. Anticipate some desired effect on others
3. Know how such meaning can be encoded so that the listener will understand this meaning and will react appropriately to the intended function of the utterance

Current research and theory suggest that the attainment of such three-dimensional communicative behavior requires careful attention to therapy procedures. Because communication and language responses are controlled by many variables, therapy procedures cannot be one-dimensional. Current models emphasize language therapy procedures that reflect all of the dimensions that are critical to successful communication. The semantic *content* of a target utterance should be prominent in the knowledge base of the child and the context of the training. The *form* of the utterance should be modeled and evoked in a communicative context that supports both this semantic content and the communicative *intent* (or performative class) desired for the targeted response.

Context Issues in Language Therapy

Such a multidimensional procedural model calls for therapy *contexts* that are complex and *procedures* that are highly structured to assure that all of the needed dimensions are represented. In many cases, therapy for serious language problems is conducted in simulation of real communicative exchanges. For example, language therapy for preschool children or severely language-deficient mentally retarded children might be conducted within activity contexts which require the clinician and the children to interact with one another in complementary roles to attain the goals of the activity. If such activities are structured properly, targeted communication or language behaviors can be evoked, modeled, and reinforced in the same types of interactive contexts in which they will be needed in real life. Such procedures are called *interactive,* and they have become dominant in language therapy procedures for seriously language-delayed or -deficient children. There are many articles and published programs available which reflect this approach (Hart, 1981; Culatta & Horn, 1982; Hanna & Lippert, 1982; Waryas & Stremel-Campbell, 1982).

When interactive procedures and social contexts are combined and "milieu teaching models" (Hart & Rogers-Warren, 1978) are adopted, there is a great need to ensure that therapy procedures are carefully controlled and *systematic* in their application.

Goals must be specific; procedures must be carefully designed and applied; and, careful measurements must be made to assess the effects of the training program. Good language therapy is a demanding clinical process, and it requires a clinician who is knowledgeable and organized as well as effective in relating to and interacting with children.

PROGRAM CONTENT: THE GOALS OF LANGUAGE THERAPY

Considerations in Specifying Individual Therapy Goals

As we have discussed the kinds of general goals and procedures that are required in language therapy, we have described the fullest scope of such treatment. There are many children who will require this total approach to their communication problems. A clinician will also be treating children whose language needs are not as severe as the children who require such pervasive and intensive intervention. For example, some children may already have an adequate ability to express a full range of propositions and meanings in their language; they may demonstrate that they can use their language to achieve a full range of communicative effects on other people. Such children may need to learn only better language *forms* to express their known meanings and attain their desired functional effects on others. However, it remains important that children learn such forms in contexts that ensure that their content and function dimensions are salient. Thus, a truly communicative context remains important (Hart, 1981). Other children might not be communicating at all, and may need to acquire the most basic ability to affect others through gestural or other nonlinguistic communication systems. Still other children may be severely handicapped in their motor abilities and need to learn to produce language by using an electronic device attached to their wheelchair.

Therapy must be tailored to the various needs demonstrated by individual children. Only careful assessment of a child's abilities and deficits will tell a clinician what skills that child needs to attain in each of the major dimensions of language ability. Clinicians must use their own store of knowledge to design a therapy program appropriate for that child. A valid therapy model should guide a clinician in designing a program for any language-deficient child, regardless of the etiology of the child's problems.

A number of extremely important, related dimensions of therapy include assessment issues and the development of both long- and short-term goals for clients. Intervention for a serious communication or language deficiency often requires therapy over a period of many years. Overall or long-term goals for a client and reasonable short-term goals for a client's immediate therapy program are critical determinations. Many clinicians are frustrated by the failures that accrue when they let their desires to help a child push them to set goals that are two high for immediate achievement. It also happens that clinicians can fail a child by not expecting enough from the child. Many clinicians are caught in the trap of trying to be sure that their clients like them and "have fun," and thus fail to challenge a child to reach goals that require hard work and real commitment. However, a clinician can justify intensive efforts by a child only by knowing that such work is being directed toward goals that are both realistic and important to a child's attainment of improved communication.

Assessment and Therapy Planning

Intervention programs in speech and language are designed on the basis of a *deficit model.* That is, the critical elements of a communicative system that are deficient for a given client must be remediated through a therapy program. Such deficits can be identified only through a process of comparing the communicative repertoire that a child brings into therapy to the repertoire that might be expected of a child of comparable cognitive ability and social development. This means that a full inventory of the child's communicative repertoire must be made through a combination of assessment procedures which would include formal tests, language sampling procedures, and careful interviewing of a parent or teacher who knows the child well and can provide information about the communicative performance in environments other than the clinic. When the results of these various assessments are compared to the performances that might be expected from a child at similar developmental and ability levels, a clinician should have an inventory of the deficits that are apparent in a client's behavioral repertoire. These deficits, then, are analyzed to ascertain the appropriate course of intervention and an ordering of the goal behaviors that will be targeted in the therapy process.

Several aspects of these assessment procedures become critical in allowing a clinician to make appropriate decisions about an overall therapy plan. The first is to be sure that a major part of the assessment process is aimed at identifying communication and language deficits that will serve appropriately as therapy goals. For example, many of the so-called standardized tests measure representative developmental and skill levels that are simply milestones in normal child development. These standardized tests do not provide a *full* inventory of a child's current behavior, but sample a few behaviors for each of several domains at specific developmental levels. Thus, a general intelligence test might test young children's knowledge of spatial and combinatorial relationships by testing their ability to make a tower or a bridge out of blocks; or, it may measure whether or not they are able to understand certain vocabulary items. Although such tests are useful in making overall judgments about a child's relative intellectual level, they provide little basis for developing a fine-grained and functional communication therapy program.

In order to derive the specific information needed for planning a program of communication therapy, children must be assessed with instruments and procedures that will yield a detailed description and analysis of their communicative behavioral system. Does the child use speech, or is he communicating with a conventional gesture system augmented by intonated vocalization? If a child is talking, is he able to talk about those important semantic relationships which are available to children at comparable developmental levels? Is the form of a child's language reflective of both the complexity levels and specific grammar forms that are appropriate to his cognitive and social status? Is the client's phonological system adequate to carry his language intelligibly?

By assessing a child in the preceding communicative units, assessment can be made *prescriptive,* in that deficits identified in assessment can be directly translated into therapy goals. Thus, deficient semantic relations can be targeted, as can deficient communicative functions or performatives. Similarly, we can target grammar forms that are missing from a child's repertoire when their lack is significant in relation to the child's overall developmental level, and when he produces a number of utterances in which these forms would be obligatory. It is quite easy to use formal tests to document that a child is delayed or deviant in language development. However, it requires different types of assessment inventories to arrive at the specific kinds of communicative behaviors that a therapy program must teach or train. These inventories must reflect the content, function, and form elements which will be the basis for therapy designs. Thus, analyses of client language samples and other types of assessment data should allow comparisons with appropriate normal levels of development in the areas of semantics and semantic relationships (Bloom, 1970; Brown, 1973); pragmatic elements like performatives and presuppositions (Bates, 1976); grammar structures including grammatical morphemes (Brown, 1973); and syntactic forms and devices (Lee, 1974). Similarly, a phonological process analysis (Ingram, 1976) would indicate whether children's phonemic inventory and error patterns are atypical for their level of development.

The importance of having assessment instruments that measure the specific behaviors of speech and language cannot be overemphasized. These behaviors will be targeted in language intervention and must be inventoried so that deficits can be translated directly into clinical goals. The reason we assess is not simply to categorize a child and, thus, confirm that a handicapping condition exists. We assess and inventory children's behaviors in order to design and implement the most pertinent and appropriate treatment goals for each of them.

Setting Initial Goals

With a full and appropriate prescriptive assessment process completed, the clinician can begin to develop the therapy plan. Several components must be included in this plan. First, initial goals must be set. If assessment has been adequate, there should be some obvious indications of high priority needs for a child, and these should provide the basis for selection of initial therapy goals. Does a child have primarily language *form* needs, or does he demonstrate a need to expand the semantic relations needed to undergird the *content* component of language? Is the child appropriately social and communicative in all of the language *function* categories? That is, does a child understand that he can use language to direct the actions of other people and to direct attention to interesting entities or events? Does a child demonstrate the ability to request information of other people, and does he demonstrate the required communicative function for replying to communicative utterances directed to him? If such language performatives are not available in a child's repertoire, they will need to be targeted in therapy. Such analyses are basic to the identification of initial therapy goals.

In many cases, the clinician can discuss the indications of the formal assessment results with the child's parents or teacher to confirm that these initial goals also appear appropriate. Perhaps parents or teachers can identify some aspect of communicative performance that is particularly bothersome to them and, thus, important for immediate attention in therapy. The initial goals of therapy will need to be rather specific, but they should also be goals which are truly important to the child's overall communicative performance.

Occasionally, clinicians will not be able to determine from initial assessments exactly what type of training program a child needs or will benefit from. In these cases, clinicians will select the programming goals and procedures that they think are most appropriate and then take careful data to learn how a child is reacting to the therapy being offered. By making these observations, therapists will be able to learn more about the child's problems and needs. Perhaps the initial program will be too easy and thus below the child's need level. Perhaps it will be too difficult, and the clinician will find

Figure 7–2. Illustration of Decision–Making Process for Establishing Program Target Priorities for Children with Language Deficits

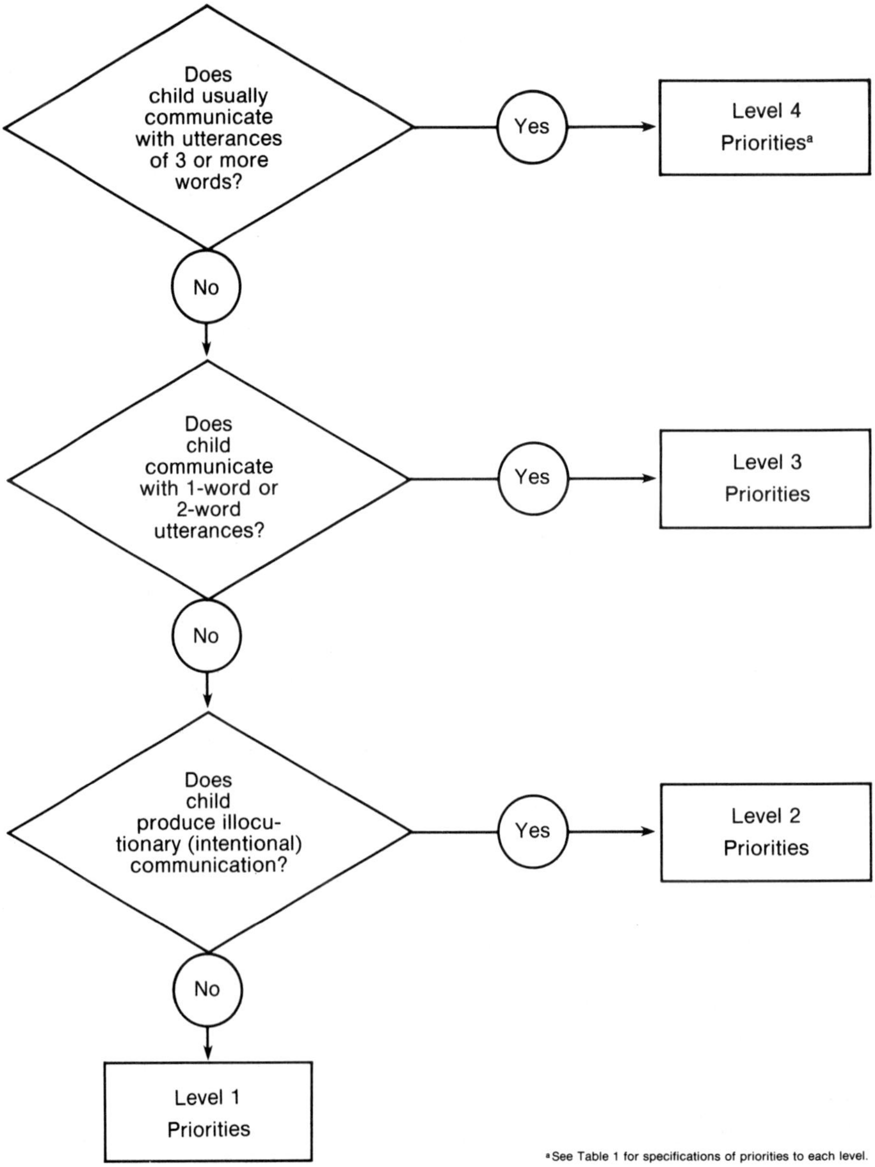

[a]See Table 1 for specifications of priorities to each level.

that the child is not yet ready to achieve the goals that have been targeted. Perhaps the procedures chosen will require the use of pictures, and the therapist finds that a child's vision problem prevents effective use of the size or types of pictures selected for therapy.

These examples demonstrate that a therapy program can be used to further assess a child's current status and needs. This process is known as *diagnostic therapy* and it is often the only way that one can fully determine the type of therapy program that is appropriate for a given child. There is little point in maintaining a therapy program that is too easy or too difficult. Such situations, however, can help the clinician design a program that is both appropriate and productive for a child.

When a clinician analyzes assessment data for identification of initial goals, it often helps to have developed a series of questions which will guide the process. Figure 7–2 illustrates this process in a flow-chart format. In this flow-chart, the major questions are arranged in the diamonds along the left side. As these questions are answered, the clinician is guided to either the next question or a set of therapy goals which will respond appropriately to the information gained. Table 7–1 shows examples of therapy reponses to the questions on the flow-chart in Figure 7–2.

Within each of the major levels indicated in Table 7–1, many additional questions and decision points need to be considered. Such processes ensure that every client's therapy programs are responsive to their specific needs.

Clients who have deficits at language levels higher than Level 4 may be assessed using currently available instruments that are specific to the *form* dimension of language or the *pragmatics* dimension. Thus, the standard tests available to assess grammar, vocabulary, and pragmatics style may be applied to identify therapy targets beyond those basic language problems covered in Levels 1 through 4. In these cases, the model remains the same as for more pervasive and basic problems. Targets are identified and the procedures for their modification are designed and applied. In cases of more advanced problems in grammar and pragmatics, the procedures may be much more tutorial than in severe language disorders. In advanced problems, clients are likely to be able to discuss language form and style in abstract terms. Such clients are said to be at a *metalinguistic* level in that they can talk about language and their problems with it. With such clients, therapy need not take on the *in situ* context needed for younger children or those with severe language deficiencies. Rather, language teaching is carried out using both written and spoken models of the desired behaviors; practice is carried out by the client; and, evaluation is given with appropriate rewards for good learning performances.

Long-Term Goals and Short-Term Objectives

The initial goals that are set according to the process described in Figure 7–2 and Table 7–1 generally take the form of *long-term* goals or objectives. Such long-term goals will not be targeted in their entirety; rather, they must be analyzed and broken down into a series of realistic component *short-term objectives* which, cumulatively, will lead to the attainment of major long-term goals. In the full process of implementing a series of sequenced short-term objectives, the long-term goals should be gradually accomplished. Clinicians must always guard against setting therapy goals that are too grand in scope for feasibility. By carefully analyzing the overall deficit patterns; asking

TABLE 7–1
Probable Program Target Priorities for Designing Treatment for Children at Different Levels of Communicative Functioning

Priority Levels	*Content Dimension*	*Function Dimension*	*Form Dimension*
Level 4 (For Children Using Multi-word Utterances	Identification of semantic needs for high-probability form and function targets Lexicon is appropriate and conventional	Full range of performatives served by child's utterance Demonstration of appropriate code-switching and polite forms in varying course contexts Appropriate presupposition and referencing for communicative effectiveness and efficiency	Consistent use of appropriate grammatical morphemes and syntax conventions where these are obligatory and expected at child's overall developmental level Consistent correct production of all phonemes in coarticulation contexts where these are expected at child's overall developmental level
Level 3 (For Children Using 1-word to 2-word Utterances	Full range of semantic notions and relations "mapped" in current 1- and 2-word utterances Adequate lexicon to "map" child's major meanings and referents	Full range of performatives served by child's current 1-word and 2-word utterances Available utterances used appropriately in discourse contexts	Increased length and complexity of utterance constructions used to convey existing meanings and intents (Potential use of nonspeech mode if warranted by assessment of speech intelligibility or receptive language competence)
Level 2 (For Children at Illocutionary Levels)	Broad range of knowledge of specific entities, events, and relationships that can be "mapped" or expressed as communicative content	Full range of internal communicative responses served by child's current nonlinguistic communicative abilities Appropriate attending and turn-filling-in communicative exchanges	Receptive language skills increased Stimulability in speech or augmentative mode sought Single words (in any mode) to map existing meanings and intents
Level 1 (For Children at Perlocutionary Levels)	Differential and appropriate responding to a variety of environmental entities and events Goal-directed (means-ends) responses	Illocutionary communicative responses in both the imperative and declarative functions Appropriate responding or turn-filling in dyadic interaction contexts	Production of a set of differential vocal and/or gestural responses that serve as communication signals

specific, detailed questions about the child's performance; and, following a complete theoretical model of language, reasonable and productive long-term goals and appropriate short-term objectives for achieving those goals can be chosen.

The determination of a long-term versus a short-term goal is a complex process. It is not simply a matter of time, (e.g., 6 months versus a year of therapy). Rather, such judgments should be made in terms of more qualitative aspects of the client's overall needs. For example, McLean, Snyder-McLean, Sack, and Decker (1982) considered two types of language therapy goals, *horizontal* and *vertical. Horizontal* goals are those which seek to increase the rate at which some *existing* level of communicative behavior occurs. For example, if a child is using two-word nongrammatical utterances to mark some semantic relations but using only one-word semantic notions to mark others, a hortizontal goal would be to increase the number of semantic relationships which are marked by two-word utterances.

On the other hand, a *vertical* goal is one in which an existing behavior is modified to achieve a qualitatively high level of behavior. For example, when a client begins to mark all relationships at a two-word level, a vertical goal would target the attainment of the appropriate *grammatical* multiword utterance to mark a few relationships. When this vertical move is accomplished on a few exemplars, the target again becomes horizontal in that an increase in an existing behavior is being sought.

In many types of therapy goals, this horizontal and vertical dichotomy will generate long-term versus short-term goals. In some cases, however, other criteria will be needed. The clinician must not allow too great a difference between long- and short-term goals. A short-term goal of sound imitation and a long-term goal of speaking in sentences leaves a great many in-between goals unspecified. However, setting imitation of five consonants and two vowels as a short-term goal, and the combining of these sounds into 20 word approximations as a long-term goal seems both reasonable and productive. The key to identifying therapy goals lies in one's knowledge about speech and language behaviors and the relationships that exist among their different types and levels. A good knowledge of speech and language acquisition in normal children suggests that the set of first goal statements is unrealistic and that the second set is both realistic and highly useful to the client.

In implementing such a goal-directed language therapy program, the effects of therapy toward both long- and short-term goals must be constantly evaluated. This evaluation process should alert clinicians to errors in setting goals and should direct them to goals and program revisions that match both children's needs and their ability and readiness to meet these needs. This overall process is *diagnostic therapy.* It suggests the need for clinicians to be always on the alert for indications that their current therapy goals are inappropriate so that revisions can be implemented.

PROCEDURES: IMPLEMENTING AN INDIVIDUALIZED PROGRAM OF THERAPY

Different therapy goals will require different therapy procedures. For example, therapy goals that include only improved language *forms* might well be accomplished by relatively simple modeling and reinforcement procedures. In the domains of both *content* and *function,* however, therapy procedures must reflect many more variables beyond the modeling of form. Meaning content must be made clear by arranging therapy contexts and materials in such ways that children can understand exactly what meaning a certain form encodes (MacNamara, 1972). Similarly, therapy contexts which include other people as *responders* to communicative utterances will allow a child to discover the effects certain utterances can have on the behaviors of other people. Children cannot discover these aspects related to meaning content and communicative functions just from learning the forms of language. They can discover the relationships between language forms and their meaning content and social functions only by having therapy contexts which allow them to use their language and experience the effects of such use. Such *transactional approaches* (McLean & Snyder-McLean, 1978); *milieu therapy* procedures (Hart & Rogers-Warren, 1978); or *interactive teaching* (Lee, Koenigsknecht, & Mulhern, 1975); are well represented in the literature and are reflected throughout this volume.

Contexts for Language Therapy

Language acquisition is a constructive process and language therapy is a set of interactive procedures that allow children to discover, acquire, and *use* new language behaviors. Obviously, this realization has important implications for clinicians, one of which is that many aspects of language learning must be carried out in the context of social activities that have some goal and some role for the participants. In this regard, I have discussed the dynamic processes associated with such contextual therapy and noted the literature which provides the details of these processes. I have also noted that there are many commercially available programs to aid the implementation of such a therapy model (e.g., Hanna & Lippert, 1983; Waryas & Stremel-Campbell, 1982). Certainly, many more programs of this *genre* will be appearing in the future.

The reason that this more dynamic, contextually based or *in situ* approach has become prominent in recent years is that older treatment models often failed to attain new reponses that children could carry from the clinical setting in which they were taught to the natural communicative contexts in which they were needed. One response to these generalization problems has been to incorporate more of the variables of natural communicative contexts and usage into therapy (Hart & Rogers-Warren, 1978). The overall rationale for such moves to larger therapy contexts is quite logical. If children are expected to use their language effectively and appropriately, they should first learn it as a means for communicating with others, rather than as a set of purely linguistic forms or structures.

McLean, Synder–McLean, Sack, and Decker (1982) have described the general characteristics of therapy contexts that are effective from the generalization standpoint:

1. A communicative therapy context most basically should allow and require some interaction between at least two people.
2. Further, these interactions should be so designed that they require the participants to transact some real *social commerce*—that is, each participant must negotiate referents and intents with the other, in order to achieve some common goal of their interaction.

3. Treatment contexts must allow and require multiple opportunities for clients to discover the properties and relationships which exist among entities and events in the world.
4. These environments must allow and require a *joint focus of attention* to be shared by the participants in an interaction.
5. Treatment must revolve around an activity in which participants have real roles, and in which a joint action is directed toward a common goal.
6. Finally, an ideal treatment context is one which will allow and require clients to participate in *consistent routines* and *roles* which they can learn and come to anticipate over a period of time.

Within the settings which reflect these characteristics, clinicians and significant others will *model* the desired communicative or linguistic responses appropriate to the situation. When clients respond with appropriate responses or utterances, they should be rewarded with the kinds of consequences which are obtained normally in such communicative contexts. Thus, if a request form is modeled and evoked from a client, the consequences should, quite logically, include an appropriate response to that request. Some past models of therapy concentrated only on the *form* of such responses. For example, clients who successfully imitated a model of a request like "I want drink" might be given an M&M as a reinforcement. The problem with such a procedure is that, although it may increase the rate of that response in that specific clinical situation, it provides the client with little experience with the way such an utterance functions in normal social contexts.

Many people are stressing the need to model, evoke, and reinforce language responses in ways that are more in line with the *natural* ways such events occur (Hart, 1981; Hart & Rogers-Warren, 1978). The rationale for moving to more natural teaching contexts emanates from evidence that, too often, new responses learned in contrived, clinical environments do not generalize to environments outside the clinic.

Such interactive therapy contexts require careful structuring and considerable planning. However, such contexts and the routines that they call for can be structured around a number of different activities that are basic and consistent in children's lives. Snack preparation in the preschool and simulated activities involving role-playing as firemen, policemen, and mothers and fathers can serve as ideal therapy contexts. With older, severely handicapped children, similar routines can be structured around prevocational tasks like assembling and sorting various kinds of materials; food preparation; self-help skills; and clothing care.

Involving the Significant Others in the Child's Environment

Other people who play significant roles in a child's environment are both necessary and useful in overall language therapy programs. If, for example, a child's mother can select an activity at home where her child is not communicating adequately, this context can be analyzed, goals can be selected, and treatment procedures can be designed to help that mother participate in her child's language and communication learning. With such an approach, the clinician is working on therapy goals that are important to both child and mother. In addition, the clinician is also educating the mother about general procedures that she can apply toward other language and communication goals for her child.

The same principles can be applied to involving a child's teacher in the therapy process. Specific language deficits that are interfering with the child's academic progress can be identified and systematically treated in the actual contexts in which they occur.

Historically, clinicians and teachers have not been committed too heavily to working with parents and other people of significance in a child's environment. Much of this historical neglect was the result of speech and language models which did not reflect our current, detailed understanding of how mothers and others facilitate children's language acquisition by playing out consistent routines (Bruner, 1975). With this new knowledge, however, it should be clear that language therapy targets should reflect goals which have been identified as important and useful to parents and other people. In addition, parents can provide important extensions and supplements to clinic-based therapy programs.

It should also be realized that some parents of language-deficient children may be contributing to their child's problem by interacting with them in ways that are not helping them learn and use language and communication behaviors. Parents and children often are mismatched in their styles of language teaching and learning. Some home environments reduce the opportunities that language-disordered children have to use what language they do have. Other home environments do not require language-deficient children to learn more and better ways to communicate; they adapt too well to their child's existing level of language. In these cases, clinicians not only have the child as a client, they have the parent or significant others as clients too. In fact, MacDonald (1982) maintained that this multiple constituency of child and significant others is *always* the case in severe language problems.

Clinicians must be able to use these significant others (MacDonald, 1982) in their overall therapy program. In order to do this, they must communicate to parents, teachers, grandmothers, and babysitters about the nature of human communication and language and the specific goals and procedures that are critical to a child's acquisition of these skills. Again, such responsibilities require that a clinician fully understand the many dimensions of human communication; the processes that allow children to acquire it; and, the specific content, function, and form products that therapy must attain. It also means that a clinician must have an overall therapy model that reflects these understandings.

Measuring Clinical Change

Finally, we must consider one more matter that demands the clinician's critical awareness; that is the need constantly to monitor and evaluate the effects of the therapy program being applied. Current federal and state laws call for accountability in the treatment of handicapped children, including communicatively deficient children. Clinicians and teachers are required to demonstrate that the treatment they are applying is producing positive effects on these children. Of course, ethical clinicians evaluate their therapy effects without the pressure of laws that direct them to do so. Whatever the specific motivation, therapy effects must be measured. Such measurements will document progress and will signal the clinician when a child's program should be changed.

A procedural plan for therapy, then, must not only specify the goals of therapy and the contexts and activities which will be used to attain these goals; but it must also contain a specific plan for measuring progress in therapy. These measures to evaluate therapy should be designed at the very beginning of therapy, and they should be used and responded to by the clinician. There is great security available to professionals who are specific and conscientious in the evaluation of their therapy. Not only are such clinicians rewarded by being able to document the progress of the client, but they are also able to demonstrate such progress to parents and supervisory personnel and thus establish the effectiveness of their services. It is surprising that many otherwise excellent clinicians do not maintain good evaluation plans and procedures. These clinicians deny themselves and their employers and consumers important data regarding both their own effectiveness and the effectiveness of their professional discipline. In many ways, the continued growth and value of speech and language services may depend on doing a better job of evaluating the services to children and adults with speech, language, and hearing disorders and deficiencies.

SUMMARY

There is a rich body of knowledge about human language currently available and well supported by research in child language. It requires and allows the designing of broad and highly detailed models for its application in therapy for children with language and communication deficiencies.

In the course of this chapter, I have suggested a general model for language therapy and demonstrated how it can be applied to the many dimensions of communication and language behavior. I have shown how the knowledge and model can be used to identify various goals and procedures for children with communication deficiencies of varying types, degrees of severity, and etiological origins. This model can facilitate a clinician's selection of therapy goals and procedures and can undergird a thorough evaluation process that will show the effectiveness of therapy and provide the clinician with data regarding the need to revise or alter therapy programs.

Finally, I have suggested that the procedures selected for therapy have important implications for communication and language learning, as well as for the generalization of that learning into the children's actual contexts, where they can use these abilities to have an effect on their environment of important people. I have also suggested that these other people can be extremely useful in helping them to attain desired communication and language behaviors.

In all of these considerations, I have made the point that communication therapy is *not* a set of simple procedures or techniques that are applied to a child. Communication therapy is an interactive process in which professionals constantly examine their knowledge in order to design therapy programs that meet individual needs. Successful communication and language therapy will allow children to acquire a most precious ability—the ability to affect the conditions of their existence with other human beings. It requires our best efforts.

STUDY QUESTIONS

1. What is the relationship between theory and therapy? What implications does this relationship have for the professional speech-language clinician?
2. Language has a number of basic social functions (performatives). What are some functions that would be typically in a list of these?
3. What are the three components of a therapy model? Characterize these components and provide specific examples of each.
4. How do etiological factors affect a basic therapy model?
5. Language assessment should be *prescriptive.* What does this mean and why is it important to a speech-language clinician?
6. Why is *diagnostic therapy* included as an assessment procedure?
7. Conceptualize a particular language-deficient child. Complete the questions from Figure 7–2 for this child and then select some specific goals appropriate for this child from those listed in Table 7–1.
8. Specify one *horizontal* and one *vertical* goal for the hypothetical child client from question 7.
9. Why are significant others important to language therapy?
10. Why is therapeutic accountability important to both clinician and client?

BIBLIOGRAPHY

Bates, E. (1976). *Language and context.* New York: Academic Press.

Bates, E., Camaioni, L., & Volterra, V. (1975). The acquisition of performatives prior to speech. *Merrill-Palmer Quarterly, 21,* 205–226.

Bloom, L. (1970). *Language development: Form and function in emerging grammars.* Cambridge, MA: M.I.T. Press.

Bloom, L., & Lahey, M. (1978). *Language development and language disorders.* New York: Wiley.

Brown, R. (1973). *A first language: The early stages.* Cambridge, MA: Harvard University Press.

Bruner, J. S. (1975). The ontogenesis of speech acts. *Journal of Child Language, 2,* 1–19.

Culatta, B., & Horn, D. (1982). A program for achieving generalization of grammatical rules to spontaneous discourse. *Journal of Speech and Hearing Disorders, 47,* 174–180.

Hanna, R. P., Lippert, E. A., & Harris, A. B. (1982). *Developmental communication curriculum.* Columbus, OH: Charles E. Merrill.

Hart, B. (1981). Pragmatics: How language is used. *Analysis and Intervention in Developmental Disabilities, 1,* 299–313.

Hart, B., & Rogers, W., A. (1978). The milieu approach to teaching language. In R. Schiefelbusch (Ed.), *Language intervention strategies.* Baltimore: University Park Press.

Ingram, D. (1976). *Phonological disability in children.* London: Edward Arnold.

Lee, L. L. (1974). Developmental sentence analysis. Evanston, IL: Northwestern University Press.

Lee, L. L., Koenigsknecht, R. A., & Mulhern, S. (1975). *Interactive language development teaching: The clinical presentation of grammatical structure.* Evanston, IL: Northwestern University Press.

MacDonald, J. D. (1982). Communication strategies for language intervention. In D. P. McClowry, A. M. Guilford, & S. O. Richardson (Eds.), *Infant communication: Development, assessment and intervention.* New York: Grune & Stratton.

MacNamara, J. (1972). Cognitive basis of language learning in infants. *Psychological Review, 79,* 1–13.

McLean, J. E., & Synder-McLean, L. K. (1978). *A transactional approach to early language training: Derivation of a model system.* Columbus, OH: Charles E. Merrill.

McLean, J. E., Snyder-McLean, L. K., Sack, S., & Decker, D. (1982). *A transactional approach to early language training: A mediated program for inservice professionals.* Columbus, OH: Charles E. Merrill.

Muma, J. R. (1978). *Language handbook: Concepts, assessment, and intervention.* Englewood Cliffs, NJ: Prentice-Hall.

Piaget, J. (1952). *The origins of intelligence in children.* New York: Norton.

Waryas, C. L., & Stremel-Campbell, K. (1982). *Communication training program.* Hingham, MA: Teaching Resources Corp.

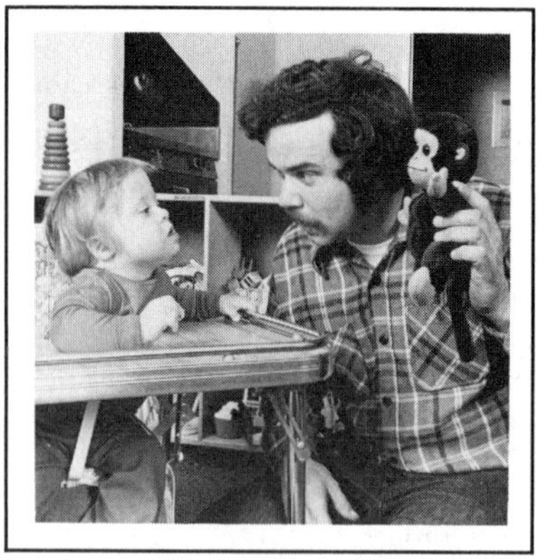

8

Mental Retardation: Difference or Delay?

> I wanted to make this book all about pop music, but my Dad says people will be more interested in my adventures. But I must write a bit about pop. (p. 89)

In *The World of Nigel Hunt,* Nigel Hunt expresses the interests of many other teenagers. This particular adolescent is mentally retarded. He was born with Down syndrome, a genetic disorder that is one of hundreds of identifiable causes of or factors related to mental retardation. Yet, Nigel is more like his nonretarded peers than he is unlike them.

It is difficult to characterize the mentally retarded population because of its diversity. This heterogeneous population includes individuals who are totally dependent and those who are nearly independent in their daily living. We can say, however, that they develop more slowly or at a more retarded rate than the nonmentally retarded population. This characteristic can be seen in several aspects of the development of mentally retarded individuals including language.

In this chapter, I shall explore a definition of mental retardation and discuss the implications for communication and language development. I will characterize the special language problems of this population and suggest intervention techniques and programs which might be helpful for the speech-language pathologist. More specifically, I shall address the following questions:

1. How can we characterize or define the mentally retarded population?
2. What are the cognitive and linguistic characteristics of the mentally retarded population? Do these characteristics reflect a difference or a delay?

This chapter was written by Dr. Robert Owens, State University of New York at Geneseo.

3. What is the developmental intervention approach, and how is it used?
4. What behaviors should be targeted, and what techniques should be used in intervention by the speech-language pathologist?

A DEFINITION OF MENTAL RETARDATION

The American Association on Mental Deficiency (AAMD), the primary organization for professionals working with the mentally retarded population, defines mental retardation as a "significantly subaverage general intellectual functioning existing concurrently with deficits in adaptive behavior and manifested during the developmental period" (Grossman, 1983, p. 1). In order to understand this definition fully, we must look at its various components.

Significantly subaverage is generally defined as an IQ of 70 or below, but this upper limit is not inflexible and may be extended upward, depending on the reliability of the testing that helped to establish the IQ. In the entire population, the mean or average IQ is 100, but the range of normality extends from 85 to 115. This range, which is considered to be one standard deviation from the norm, contains two-thirds of the population. An IQ of 70 is two standard deviations below 100, or significantly below average.

General intellectual functioning refers to the results of a standardized general intelligence test. The test should be pluralistic and culture-free and should be administered individually. The generally accepted measurement of intelligence is IQ, a ratio of mental age to chronological age. If the mental age is 10 years and the chronological age is 10 years, the relationship is 10/10 or 1, which is interpreted as an IQ of 100. In contrast, a mental age of 5 and a chronological age of 10 yields 5/10 or .5, which is an IQ of 50.

As stated previously, testing should be pluralistic and culture-free. A test based solely upon language abilities would be unfair to many second-language learners and to many learning-disabled children. Intelligence testing should also include nonlinguistic abilities, such as problem solving, sensorimotor development, and social skills. Likewise, culturally biased tests would be prejudicial to many minorities. The author knows of one recent Southeast Asian immigrant classified as mentally retarded based upon an English receptive vocabulary test.

Deficits in adaptive behavior are defined by Grossman (1983) as "significant limitations in an individual's effectiveness in meeting the standards of maturation, learning, personal independence, and/or social responsibility that are expected for . . . age level and cultural group" (p. 11). Adaptive skills vary for different ages. During infancy and preschool years, adaptive skills include sensorimotor, speech and language, self-help, and interactional development. In middle childhood and early adolescence, the emphasis shifts to academic and reasoning skill development and to group and interpersonal relationships. Late adolescent and adult adaptive skill development relates to vocational and social responsibility. Adaptive behavior frequently correlates very positively with intelligence but not always, especially for very low IQs (Grossman, 1983). One standardized measure of adaptive behavior is AAMD's Adaptive Behavior scale.

The *developmental period* generally denotes the span from conception to age 18. Development may be slow, arrested, or incomplete. The developmental rate decreases as all humans reach the late teens. Thus, profoundly retarded young adults may experience only moderate developmental change after age 18, although they function at a mental age of only 3 years.

The AAMD definition includes only those individuals who meet all the criteria. Learning-disabled children are not included because they possess normal intelligence; and elderly, aphasic patients do not qualify because their disorder did not manifest itself during the developmental period. Although individuals with both types of disorders might function within the retarded range on some tasks, they can not be classified as mentally retarded. Figure 8–1 illustrates the AAMD definition.

The definition does not specify causes or etiologies, but emphasizes the current functioning level of the individual. In other words, it is not assumed that Down syndrome is synonymous with mental retardation. In part, the definition reflects a bias that functioning levels can be modified or changed, that the mentally retarded individual is a developmental being.

Prevalence and Levels of Functioning

The number of mentally retarded individuals in the United States is unknown. Estimates vary from 1% to 3% of the population, or approximately 2.5 to 7 million individuals. Upper figures represent IQ score data solely. Mental retardation is 15 times more prevalent than blindness. Most of the approximately 125,000 retarded individuals born in the United States each year are only mildly retarded.

There are four categories of mental retardation based on IQ—mild, moderate, severe, and profound. The characteristics of each category are listed in Table 8–1.

The distribution of mental retardation within the population is not uniform. Although the distribution of the severely and profoundly involved reflect the general population,

Figure 8–1. AAMD Definition of Mental Retardation

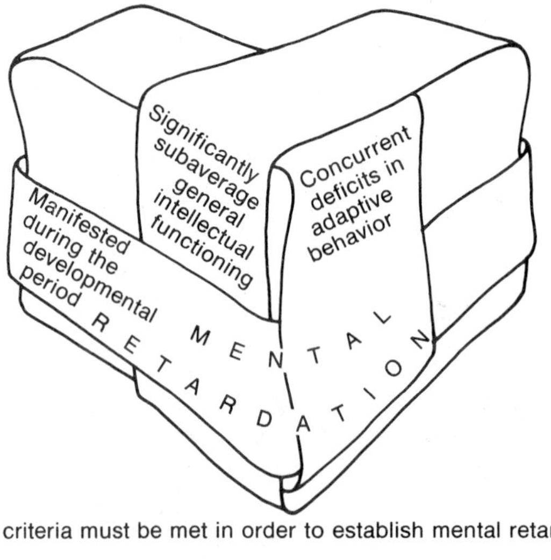

All criteria must be met in order to establish mental retardation.

Source: Adapted from H. Grossman (1983)

TABLE 8–1
Categories of Mental Retardation

Category	*IQ range*	*% of MR population*	*Characteristics*
Mild	52–68	89	Usually absorbed into the community where they work and live independently
Moderate	36–51	6	Capable of learning self-care skills and working within a sheltered environment. They live semi-independently, with relatives or in a community residence.
Severe	20–35	3½	Capable of learning some self-care skills and are not totally dependent. They often exhibit physical handicaps and deficits in speech and language.
Profound	below 20	1½	Capable of learning some basic living skills but require continual care and supervision. They often exhibit severe physical and/or sensory problems.

Source: Adapted from H. Grossman (1983)

the mildly and moderately retarded include a greater percentage of poor and minority populations, and of those with a family history of retardation (Birch, Richardson, Baird, Horobin, & Illsley, 1970). The disproportionately higher percentage among the poor may reflect the environmental effects of poverty or genetic influences. In the American culture, many minorities are also found in the lower socioeconomic levels because of discriminatory practices. Middle-class professionals are also more likely to classify lower-class or minority children as retarded. Lack of proper nutrition or poor health may contribute to delayed development among the poor. In addition, mildly mentally retarded parents are most likely to find themselves among the poor. These adults are more likely than nonretarded adults to produce offspring with depressed cognitive functioning. This factor does not occur with the severely and profoundly retarded because very few of these individuals produce offspring.

CAUSES OF MENTAL RETARDATION

According to Grossman (1983), biological factors account for only about 25% of the cases of mental retardation. Although social-environmental factors are related to a larger percentage of the cases of mental retardation, biological factors account for a greater proportion of the more severe forms of mental retardation. The correlation between intelligence level and biologic retardation is very strong.

Social-environmental factors are not as easy to identify as biological factors and involve many interactive factors. Poor housing and hygiene, as well as inadequate medical care and nutrition may contribute. Lack of prenatal care and of infant stimulation may affect the developing child more directly.

Known causes of mental retardation are listed in Table 8–2. In the majority of cases, the specific etiology is unknown.

TABLE 8–2
Known Causes of Mental Retardation

Type	*Examples*	*Characteristics*
Biologic		
Genetic and chromosonal	Down syndrome (Trisomy 21)	Broad head and characteristic facial features, small stature, mental retardation
	Klinefelter syndrome (sex-linked, XXY)	Feminine roundness to body, small testes, possible mental retardation
	Cri-du-chat syndrome	Cat-like cry, microcephaly, mental retardation
Infections processes	Maternal rubella	Cardiac defects, cataracts, hearing loss, microcephaly, possible mental retardation
	Congenital syphilis	Deafness, vision problems, possible epilepsy or cerebral palsy, mental retardation
Toxins & chemical agents	Fetal alcohol syndrome	Persistantly deficient growth, low brain weight, facial abnormalities, cardiac defects, mental retardation
	Lead poisoning	Central nervous system and kidney damage, hyperactivity
Nutrition and metabolism	Phenylketonuria (PKU)	Reduced pigmentation, motor coordination problems, convulsions, microcephaly, mental retardation
	Tay-Sachs disease	Progressive deterioration of nervous system and vision, mental retardation, death in preschool years
	Inadequate diet	Small stature, possible mental retardation

TABLE 8–2
Known Causes of Mental Retardation (Continued)

Type	*Examples*	*Characteristics*
Gestational disorders	Hydrocephalus	Enlarged head caused by increased volume of cerebral-spinal fluid, visual defects, epilepsy, mental retardation
	Cerebral malformation	Absence or underdevelopment of cerebral cortex and resultant mental retardation
	Craniofacial anomalies	Malformed skull and associated mental retardation
Complications of pregnancy and delivery	Extreme immaturity or preterm infant	Low birth weight, higher prevalence of central nervous system disorders
	Exceptionally large baby	Possible birth injury to central nervous system
	Maternal nutritional disorders	Low birth weight, higher prevalence of central nervous system disorders
Gross brain diseases	Tumors and Tuberous sclerosis	Tumors in heart, seizures, tuberous "bumps" on nose and cheeks, mental retardation
	Huntington disease	Degenerative neurological functioning evidenced in progressive dementia and cerebral palsy
Social-Environmental		
Psychosocial disadvantage	Subnormal intellectual functioning in immediate family and/or impoverished environment	Functional retardation
Sensory deprivation	Maternal deprivation Prolonged isolation	Functional retardation and failure to thrive

Source: H. Grossman, *Classification in mental retardation*. Washington, D.C.: American Association on Mental Deficiency, 1983.

Associated Disorders

There is a higher incidence of neurological disorders among the mentally retarded population, especially that segment which is severely and profoundly involved. Approximately one-third of the profoundly involved have at least two profoundly handicapping disorders (Cegelka & Prehm, 1982). Two disorder areas of note are neuromuscular disorders and emotional handicaps.

Neuromuscular Disorders. Cerebral palsy and/or epilepsy are found in a greater percentage of the mentally retarded population than in the nonretarded population. This difference is especially evident among the more severely retarded. This group frequently exhibits neuromuscular disorders as part of a complex of multiple handicaps.

Among the cerebral palsied population, approximately 50% demonstrate IQs below 70. Such scores may reflect a lack of sophistication by the tester or by the test. In other words, individuals with cerebral palsy may be difficult to test using standard procedures because of neuromuscular interference.

Epilepsy affects about one person in 160. The percentage increases with decreased intelligence, and in the profoundly retarded population, as high as 65% may exhibit seizure activity (Chaney, Eyman, & Miller, 1979). Frequent causes of epilepsy in young children are central nervous system (CNS) malformation, CNS injury from infection or accident, and CNS malfunction caused by a metabolic error.

Related neurological disorders further complicate the learning task for retarded persons. The increased occurrence with decreased intelligence may also indicate an underlying organic cause for the more severe forms of retardation.

Emotional Disorders. Mental retardation and mental illness are *not* the same although there is a high prevalence of emotional problems within the mentally retarded population (Phillips & Williams, 1975; Russell & Tanquay, 1981). Among children with schizophrenic disturbances, it has been estimated that one-third to one-half exhibit prolonged or permanent functioning within the mentally retarded range. Among retarded persons, behavioral disturbances are the second most frequent cause of institutionalization after intellectual deficiency (Russell & Tanquay, 1981). Emotional disorders may be of any type, and mentally retarded individuals may exhibit a full range of emotional and personality disturbances (Balthazar & Stevens, 1975; Syzmanski & Tanquay, 1980). Incidence figures may be higher than has been reported, according to Reiss, Levitan, and Szyszko (1982), because of "diagnostic overshadowing." In other words, the intellectual deficit may be such a salient feature that accompanying emotional disorders are overshadowed.

Very few depressive types of psychosis are reported for the mentally retarded population (Russell & Tanquay, 1981), however, many emotional diagnoses relate to bizarre behaviors, especially with institutionalized populations. Some institutionalized individuals have not been prevented from evolving behavioral repertoires which include self-injurious and self-stimulatory behaviors.

COGNITIVE FUNCTIONING: DIFFERENCE OR DELAY

Volumes of research have been published on the cognitive abilities of mentally retarded individuals. "Despite the number of articles in print," concluded Cegelka and Prehm (1982), "we have not significantly increased our understanding of retarded learning characteristics" (p. 166). There are a number of reasons for this conclusion. First, the complex nature of the cognitive process necessitates research which targets very limited aspects. Therefore, there are no definitive studies of the entire process of cognitive functioning among either the retarded or nonretarded population. Second, the cognitive functioning level of retarded subjects in many studies is poorly defined. This factor can be extremely important because there seems to be a very strong link between IQ and cognitive abilities. It is difficult to draw conclusions among studies when the functioning levels of the subjects differ greatly. Finally, it is difficult to extrapolate from a limited experimental setting to the daily environments of retarded individuals.

Researchers have interpreted their data in two general ways. One interpretation holds that there are discrepancies or differences in the cognitive processing abilities of the mentally retarded population that cannot be accounted for by mental age alone (Das, Kirby, & Jarman, 1975; Detterman, 1979; Greenspan, 1979; Spitz, 1979; Stephens & McLaughlin, 1974). Mentally retarded individuals do not perform in the same manner as nonretarded peers of the same mental age. Pointing to methodological problems in many of these studies, a second group of researchers considers the mentally retarded population to develop cognitively in the same manner as the nonretarded population, but at a slower rate (Balla & Zigler, 1971; Humphreys & Parsons, 1979; Kamhi, 1981).

In language intervention, the speech-language pathologist must understand underlying cognitive functioning. Our interest is in the learning processes and in memory. *Learning* is a change in behavior that results from rehearsal of the behavior to be learned. Cognitive abilities important for learning include attention, organization, transfer, and memory. The variables to which an individual attends and the organization of these variables is important for memory, which in turn, affects transfer or generalization to novel situations or problems. Figure 8–2 demonstrates this process schematically.

Attention. Attention includes awareness of a learning situation and active cognitive processing. As noted in Figure 8–2, we do not attend to all stimuli. Research on attention has examined the orienting, reacting, and discriminating abilities of mentally retarded individuals. Orientation is the ability to sustain attention over time. Karrer, Nelson, and Galbraith (1979) reported that mildly mentally retarded individuals have greater ability to sustain attention than their mental-age-matched (MA-matched) nonretarded peers. This finding may reflect the older age, and thus, longer attention span, of the retarded group. Other studies have found mildly retarded and nonretarded subjects to exhibit equal orienting abilities.

Reaction time refers to the amount of time that is required for an individual to respond to a stimulus. In Figure 8–2, the subject responds to stimulus F immediately. Baumeister and Kellas (1968) reported that mildly mentally retarded individuals react more slowly than chronological-age-match (CA-matched) peers. Studies with MA-matched peers are not as definitive, and the performance of the mildly mentally retarded is more individualistic (Krupski, 1977; Liebert & Baumeister, 1973). In part, reaction time is a function of the individual's ability to select the relevant dimensions of a task prior to responding. Mentally retarded individuals appear to be deficient in their abilities to scan and attend selectively.

Discrimination is the ability to identify differing stimuli from a field of similar stimuli. For example, a discrimination task might involve picking a different pitch tone from a series of pitch tones. In a more complicated task, a subject might be required to attend to several dimensions of a sample, such as color, shape, and size, at the same time. For example, in Figure 8–2, stimuli B and C are found to be similar to each other and to information already stored. In contrast, A and E are new information. In general, mentally retarded individuals exhibit difficulties identifying and maintaining attention to the relevant stimulus dimensions (Mercer & Snell, 1977; Zeaman & House, 1963, 1979). As a group, mildly and moderately retarded persons attend to fewer dimensions of a task than do the nonretarded, and these dimensions are not necessarily the salient or important ones. This deficiency reduces an individual's ability to compare new information with stored information from previous learning. In addition, it takes a longer time and more practice for mentally retarded persons to understand the dimensions of a task. Once a task is understood or learned, however, mentally retarded individuals can perform as well as their nonretarded MA-matched peers (Ross & Ross, 1979). Ellis and his colleagues (1982) found that as a group, higher functioning mentally retarded individuals could learn discrimination tasks more rapidly than their lower functioning CA-matched retarded peers. There were substantial individual differences among the

Figure 8–2. Schematic of Major Cognitive Functions

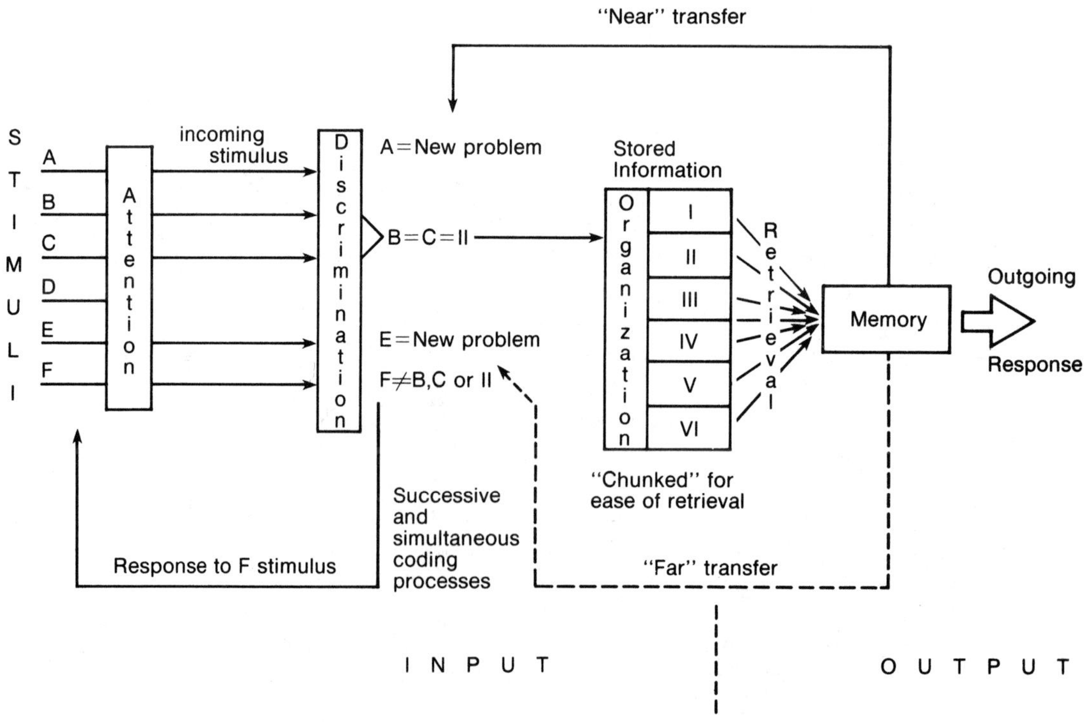

severely and profoundly retarded individuals, however, and some subjects learned the tasks as well as the mildly retarded.

In general, retarded persons seem able to attend as well as MA-matched nonretarded peers. There does seem to be some difference, however, in retarded persons' ability to select the relevant information from a field. Therefore, new or relevant material for a task needs to be more explicit.

Organization of Input Material. The organization of incoming sensory information is very important for later retrieval. This organization can be demonstrated when we try to recall the name of an object. Frequently, the names of related objects will also come to mind. Therefore, we may name the washing machine by "drier" or "refrigerator," but rarely "spoon" or "window". As in Figure 8–2, information is organized or "chunked" by category for easy retrieval. Stephens (1972) reported that mildly retarded and nonretarded persons exhibit similar developmental trends in the grouping of information. There is a shift with developmental level from grouping on the basis of physical similarities to grouping by function. Not all data can be classified in these manners. In general, mentally retarded individuals exhibit difficulty developing categorizing strategies for organizing new material into more easily remembered "chunks" (Herriot, 1972; Spitz, 1966). Any organizational deficit will hinder later recall and quickly overload memory capacity. It is much more difficult to remember unrelated bits of information. Every reader can recognize that it is easier to recall a ten-word sentence than ten unrelated words. Case (1978) has proposed that memory capacity is fixed. Therefore, more efficient processing requires increasingly better organization. In turn, better organization leaves more "room" for new input.

Teachers can aid learning by pregrouping information to facilitate organization and later recall. Organization strategies such as physical conceptual arrangement, grouping, and consistent ordering can also be taught (Burger, Blackman, Holmes, & Zetlin, 1978; Evans & Bilsky, 1979; Glidden, 1977; Taylor & Turnure, 1979).

Mildly and moderately retarded individuals do not seem to rely on mediation or associative learning strategies nor to use them efficiently as do the nonretarded. In mediating strategies, a word or symbol forms a link between two inputs. For example, a person's name might relate past experiences with feelings, life-styles, or opinions. In associative strategies, one word or symbol aids in recall of another. Common examples are "salt and ________," "black and ________," etc. Mildly retarded individuals can use associative strategies if the two symbols are easily associated and nonabstract.

In general, retarded persons are able to retain information better if it is organized first, and if the learning task is explained by the teacher. Mildly retarded individuals have better recall if material is grouped spatially rather than presented singly (Harris, 1982; MacMillan, 1972; Spitz, 1966). For example, a mildly retarded adult who is experiencing difficulty recalling four digits, such as 6-3-8-5, may do better if the digits are grouped in pairs to form 63 and 85. Such grouping does not seem to aid the recall of nonretarded individuals.

Das, Kirby, and Jarman (1979) have proposed four stages of information integration: input, sensory register, central processor, and output. The three components of the central processor are sequential or simultaneous synthesis, successive synthesis, and regulatory activities (Cummins, 1979; Cummins & Das, 1978; Luria, 1975). Simultaneous synthesis or coding, located in the occipital-parietal region of the brain, is related to higher thought. Separate elements are synthesized into groups so that all members of the group are accessible simultaneously for retrieval. For example, various examples of dog are coded for the "dog" category. Successive coding is related to language and located in the frontal-temporal region of the brain. Linguistic information is coded sequentially or successively. Both processes are used for coding input and for planning behavior. Obviously, these coding processes are influenced by sensory input, memory, and other intellectual processes.

Mildly retarded and nonretarded persons both exhibit simultaneous and successive coding (Jarman, 1978; Jarman & Das, 1977). There appears to be some difference in the use of this coding for the planning function however, and Das and his colleagues (1979) have concluded that the "two groups may *employ* the processes differently in solving more complex tasks" (p. 100). Down syndrome individuals may even possess different coding functions. As a group, Down syndrome persons perform more poorly than either brain-damaged individuals or other MA-matched retarded individuals on successive processing tasks. This deficiency may be an underlying cause for auditory memory and expressive language problems of the Down syndrome population (Burr & Rohr, 1978; Evans, 1977; Sommers & Starkey, 1977). More severely retarded persons may sustain some organic problems and, therefore, have qualitatively different neurological functioning also (Robinson & Robinson, 1976; Snart, O'Grady, & Das, 1982; Zigler, 1967).

In general, retarded individuals demonstrate some organizing difficulties and benefit from organized input. Organizational deficits can hinder recall and generalization, both essential for learning. Organizational skills have been taught with some success.

Transfer. Transfer or generalization is the ability to apply previously learned material in the solving of similar but novel problems. The greater the similarity between the learning situation and a subsequent task, the greater the transfer. Although mildly retarded persons can be taught cognitive processing strategies, attempts to generalize these strategies have been less successful (Brown, 1978; Campione & Brown, 1977; Evans & Bilsky, 1979). The learning of more severely retarded individuals is characterized by even weaker transfer (Bricker, Heal, Bricker, Hayes, & Larsen, 1969; Ellis, Deacon, Harris, Poor, Angers, Dirio, Watkins, Boyd, & Cavalier, 1982; Reid, 1980).

Burger, Blackman, Clark, and Reis (1982) developed a training program to facilitate generalization among mildly retarded individuals. Two types of generalization were assessed: near and far. *Near generalization* involves only minimal changes between the training and testing situations, while *far generalization* involves substantial changes. In Figure 8–2, stimulus A is considered to be similar enough to stored information to qualify for near generalization or transfer. Stimulus E is less similar and thus represents far generalization. As in other studies, the subjects in the Burger study demonstrated their ability to acquire learning strategies (Borkowski & Cavanaugh, 1979; Evans & Bilsky, 1979; Taylor & Turnure, 1979). Such learning enhanced performance but not generalization. Burger and her colleagues concluded that "reliable generalization effects for mentally retarded people may be found if all strategy components required are initially taught and the subjects are able to perceive the ready applicability of the trained strategy to the new task setting" (p. 412). Near and far generalization for retarded persons appear not to be a function of the similarity of tasks but of the level of awareness required by these persons to detect such similarity.

In a similar study, Burger, Blackman, and Clark (1981) studied the use of verbal abstraction strategies by mildly retarded persons in generalization. Other studies had reported some success in recall strategy generalization (Brown, Campione, & Barclay, 1979; Kendall, Borkowski, & Cavanaugh, 1980). Butterfield and Belmont (1977) hypothesized that generalization occurs only in the presence of analysis of the task and identification of the strategies required for the task. Thus, Burger and her colleagues (1981) trained their mildly retarded subjects to note the relevant attributes of a task and either to observe or to learn the task through self-instruction. All subjects were able to generalize their skills to novel situations better than those subjects who did not learn to analyze the task nor to identify strategies. Burger and her colleagues concluded that explicit training is not necessary for better generalization, because observation resulted in increased transfer also. Understanding of the task, however, is essential for transfer.

The generalization deficits of retarded individuals may reflect the selection and organization problems noted previously. Generalization can be facilitated, however, if the client is helped in analyzing the similarities between old and new tasks.

Memory. Necessary for transfer, recall or memory is the ability to retrieve needed information that was previously learned. Mildly and moderately retarded individuals seem to be able to retain information within long-term memory as well as nonretarded individuals (Belmont, 1967; Ellis, 1963). Organizational deficits, however, may result in an overreliance on rote memory by mildly retarded persons (Spitz, 1966). In contrast, profoundly retarded individuals, according to Ellis and his colleagues, exhibit significant forgetting of learned behavior within only a short interval.

Short-term memory deficiencies are more evident in the retarded population (Brown, 1974; Butterfield, Wambold, & Belmont, 1973; Ellis, 1970). In turn, such deficiencies may affect discrimination abilities (Lobb, 1974; Ullman, 1974). In general, short-term memory is very limited and even nonretarded individuals can hold fewer than ten entities only briefly. Information is retained and/or transferred to long-term memory through rehearsal or repetition. Yet, retarded persons do not seem to rehearse information spontaneously (Brown, 1974; Butterfield, Wambold, & Belmont, 1973; Ellis, 1970; Frank & Rabinovitch, 1974; Kellas, Ashcroft, & Johnson, 1973; Reid, 1980). Bray (1979) has called this lack a "rehearsal deficit." Mildly and moderately retarded individuals can improve their memory abilities, however, through the training of such rehearsal strategies (Brown, 1974; Burger, Blackman, & Tan, 1980; Engle & Nagle, 1979; Reid, 1980).

Lamberts (1981) examined the auditory memory of retarded school children and MA-matched nonretarded preschoolers. Each stimulus event has a sensory, or sign, impression which is inherent in the event and an abstract, or symbol, representation for that event (Dance, 1967; Whatmough, 1956). The sign is meaningful but nonlinguistic. For example, the sound of a horn may signal an automobile. In contrast, the abstract representation, or word, is linguistic in nature. Lamberts reasoned that auditory memory would be better for signs because internal representation is based originally on perception. In other words, our early meaning of "doggie" is based on the perceptual attributes of the examples of doggie that we have encountered. The name or word *doggie* is superimposed later. Our ability to infer an entity from an auditory sign is part of our early linguistic knowledge base (Ervin-Tripp, 1973; Macnamara, 1972). Lamberts found that retarded and nonretarded subjects had similar recall for signal information, but that the retarded subjects had significantly poorer recognition and recall of symbolic representations. There may be a link, therefore, between the reported language deficits and auditory memory deficits of the mentally retarded population (Brown, 1974; Ellis, 1970; Mittler, 1974; Reid & Kiernan, 1979).

Kintsch and van Dijk (1978) have stated that sentence recall involves reproduction of the memory episode and then editing of the text. Because retarded individuals make frequent word substitution errors, performance may break down in the second stage (Bilsky, Walker, & Sakales, 1983). Poor sentence recall by the retarded population may reflect poor editing skills.

Poor reading recall, on the other hand, may be related to failure to use important textual information for organization (Borkowski & Wanschura, 1974; Brown, Campione, & Murphy, 1974). Selective attention to important portions of reading passages can be taught, however, with resultant recall improvement (Luftig & Johnson, 1982).

Auditory memory deficits are particularly evident in the Down syndrome population. After study, Marcell and Armstrong (1982) concluded that "Down syndrome individuals have trouble remembering verbal-auditory material" (p. 92). This difficulty may be related to *echoic memory* which Watkins and Watkins (1980) defined as "the ability to hear a sound for some time after physical stimulation has ceased" (p. 252). In other words, echoic memory is the ability to remember what has been heard even when it is no longer present. Echoic memory is a passive retention strategy that is related to immediate recall of linguistic stimuli and seems to be most efficient with the fast rates found in conversation (Hockey, 1973). Among individuals with Down syndrome, however, this echo may decay more rapidly than in the nonretarded population or at a rate at which the slower processing of the retarded cannot access it. Marcell and Armstrong (1982) also theorized that Down syndrome individuals may not realize how to use such passive strategies effectively. Other studies have demonstrated the generally inefficient use of memory strategies by the retarded population (Engle & Nagle, 1979). As reported previously, Snart, O'Grady, and Das (1982) found moderately retarded Down syndrome individuals to have poorer successive cognitive processing than other retarded individuals and thus, poorer auditory sequential memory. This data would support the reportedly low language performance of those with Down syndrome in comparison to other retarded individuals (O'Connor & Hermelin, 1978).

In general, retarded persons demonstrate poorer recall than MA-matched nonretarded peers. Again, these skills can be taught with some success.

Conclusion. In general, the mentally retarded population develops cognitively in a manner very similar to the nonretarded but at a slower rate. According to Leahy, Balla, and Zigler (1982), experiential, not cognitive, factors may account for differences in personality and motivational functioning. Some cognitive processing differences exist, however, especially in organization and memory (Das, 1972; Das, Kirby, & Jarman, 1975; Semmel, Barritt, & Bennett, 1970; Stephens & McLaughlin, 1974). As the level of severity increases, wide individual differences become more apparent. With more severe retardation, cognitive functioning may be complicated by accompanying organic disorders. For mildly retarded persons, however, IQ alone is not a particularly powerful predictor of life adjustment (McCarver & Craig, 1974; Windle, 1962).

Kamhi (1981) investigated the overall difference-delay controversy by administering a number of tasks to retarded and nonretarded individuals of varying ages. MA-matched subjects performed similarly on five cognitive tasks: haptic (touch) recognition, conservation, classification, number conservation (relative quantity), and linear order. On a sixth task, mental displacement (matching), the retarded children actually performed better than the nonretarded normal children. The retarded children did perform slightly more poorly than the nonretarded on tasks involving symbolic skills. Symbolic skills are important for higher cognitive development and include, but are not limited to, language.

LANGUAGE AND COMMUNICATION SKILLS: DELAY OR DIFFERENCE?

The language behavior of the mentally retarded population is frequently the most seriously delayed or disordered area of adaptive behavior. In many early studies of the language of the retarded population, subjects were matched on the basis of chronological age. Naturally, these studies reported different behaviors for the retarded and nonretarded groups. In some studies, it was assumed that these differences represented disorders in the language of the retarded population. More recent studies, matching subjects for mental age or language level, have found more similarities between retarded and nonretarded persons. I shall examine these studies of language of the retarded population, threading through the mix of severity of retardation, subject matching, and level of development. The major characteristics of the language of the retarded population are listed in Table 8–3. This table is based on summarized data and on group data. Individuals or specific subgroups, especially the more severely impaired, may exhibit different behavior. Some profoundly retarded individuals will not use expressive language beyond single words.

Parameters of Language

Five parameters of language are generally recognized—syntax, morphology, phonology, semantics, and pragmatics. All five parameters have been examined in research studies of the language of retarded persons.

Syntax. In general, the overall sequence of development of syntactic structures is similar for the mildly retarded and the nonretarded population; however, the rate of development is slower (Ingram, 1972; Lackner, 1968; McLeavey, Toomey, & Dempsey, 1982; Naremore & Dever, 1975). Both sentence length and complexity increase

TABLE 8–3
Language Characteristics of Retarded Compared with Nonretarded Individuals

Syntactic	Same sequence of sentence development Shorter, less complex sentences Fewer subject elaborations or relative clauses Sentence word order has precedence over word relationships Reliance on more primitive forms
Morphologic	Same order of development
Phonologic	Higher incidence of articulation disorders Similar phonological rules but possibly serving different purposes
Semantic	Word meanings more concrete Less frequent uses of some semantic functions, particularly secondary and noun inflections
Pragmatic	Similar developmental patterns Less dominant conversational roles

with development (Graham & Graham, 1971; Lackner, 1968). The same sentence transformations appear and in the same order for both groups. There is a general trend of development of sentence types from simple declaratives through negatives, and then interrogatives to negative interrogatives (Lackner, 1968). Within interrogatives, the order of development is also similar (Ingram, 1972). For example, "what" and "where" types develop initially with "when," "why," and "how" being the last to appear.

Even at equivalent mental age levels, individuals with retardation appear to use shorter, less complex sentences than their nonretarded peers (McLeavey et al., 1982; Naremore & Dever, 1975). These characteristics are evident in the case study at the end of the chapter. Several studies have concluded that the syntactic development of retarded persons lags behind mental age (Bartel, Bryen, & Keehn, 1973; Lovell, 1968; McLeavey, Toomey, & Dempsey, 1982; Semmel, Barritt, & Bennett, 1970). Naremore and Dever (1975) reported that mildly retarded individuals use fewer complex structures, such as subject elaborations and relative clauses. These deficiencies may reflect the poorer linguistic rule generalization reported for retarded individuals. Poor rule generalization does not imply an inability to learn language rules, although Semmel (1967) concluded that retarded persons rely more on sequential placement than on grammatical rules. In other words, sentence word-order takes precedence over the relationships between different word classes. The result is less flexible linguistic structure. In contrast, McLeavey et al. (1982) concluded that "the types of deviations . . . suggest that mildly retarded children are rule-oriented in their approach to language" (p. 492). Graham and Graham (1971) reported that even individuals with severe retardation are capable of using linguistic rules. These seemingly contradictory findings may indicate that retarded persons learn and use linguistic rules but also rely more on primitive word rules than their language peers.

According to McLeavey and colleagues (1982), any syntactic lag noted among retarded persons may represent a dependence upon older syntactic forms for a longer time. Such reliance patterns have been suggested for the language learning skills of children with Down syndrome (Owens & MacDonald, 1982). McLeavey and colleagues concluded "the difference between nonretarded and mildly retarded children in syntactic development is quantitative rather than qualitative in nature" (p. 492). Advanced syntactic forms are learned but used less frequently.

Morphology. Several studies have assessed the morphological development of retarded individuals using the Test of Children's Learning of English Morphology (Berko, 1958). This test uses nonsense words to evaluate the child's morphological skills. In general, retarded children performed in a manner similar to MA-matched nonretarded peers, but with some minor differences (Bradbury & Lunzer, 1972; Dever & Gardner, 1970; Newfield & Schlanger, 1968). These results have been questioned because of the abstract nature of the testing task and the lack of relationship of rules for nonsense words to daily functioning (Dever & Gardner, 1970; Newfield & Schlanger, 1968).

In studies of a more developmental nature, differences were less pronounced. Newfield (1966) reported the same order of morphological development for both the retarded and nonretarded populations. Using Brown's (1973) morphological hierarchy from a study of the linguistic development of three nonretarded preschoolers, Johnston and Schery (1976) found the same developmental hierarchy for retarded children. Again the pattern of development seems to be delayed, even beyond what one might expect for mental age, but not to be significantly different.

Phonology. There have been a number of studies of the articulation deficiencies of the mentally retarded population (Bangs, 1961; Schiefelbusch, 1963; Spradlin, 1963; Wolfensberger, Mein, & O'Connor, 1963). In general, they demonstrate that a majority of institutionalized and/or severely retarded persons exhibit articulation disorders (Yoder & Miller, 1972). Articulation, or the production of speech sounds, is not the same as the rules for sound combinations, called phonology.

Prater (1982) reported that mentally retarded children exhibit some of the same phonological rules as younger nonretarded children, such as assimilation and reduplication. Consonant assimilation occurs when a consonant assumes a place of articulation similar to that of a second consonant. For example, dog becomes /dod/ or /gog/. The assimilated consonant is usually absent from the child's speech repertoire (Leonard, Miller, & Brown, 1980).

According to Prater (1982), however, retarded children assimilated consonants that they produced successfully in other words. Thus, consonant assimilation may serve different purposes (Vihman, 1978).

Similar behavior also exists for retarded and nonretarded children in the use of reduplication or syllable repetition. First, reduplication may aid monosyllabic children in production of multisyllabic words, such as "nana" for banana (Ingram, 1976; Leonard, Miller, & Brown, 1980). Reduplication also may aid the child in production of multisyllabic words in which one syllable contains consonants absent from the child's repertoire, such as "wawa" for water.

Semantics. Several studies have concluded that the word meanings of the retarded population are more concrete than those of the nonretarded (Semmel & Herzog, 1966). For example, *cold* may be defined in relation to temperature but not to the psychological aspects, such as a cold personality. Papania (1954) could find no difference in the quality of definition, however, as measured by the Stanford-Binet intelligence test.

Using Chafe's (1970) case grammar, Layton and Sharifi (1979) investigated the semantic functions of mildly retarded Down syndrome and MA-matched nonretarded subjects. According to Chafe, the verb is the central element of a sentence. There are four primary semantic features of the verb: state, process, action, and action-process. Secondary features such as locatives and temporals help to describe the scope of the basic feature. Finally, nouns also have semantic aspects that signal such features as possession or pronoun use. These features are illustrated in Table 8–4. Both the mildly retarded and the nonretarded subjects in Layton and Sharifi's study displayed all four basic features and the secondary features and noun inflections, but the Down's subjects used the secondary and noun features less frequently. Again, it appears that linguistic differences between retarded and nonretarded subjects are quantitative, not qualitative.

Pragmatics. The area of pragmatics or language use has generated considerable academic interest, especially in the field of retardation. McLean and Snyder-McLean (1978) have stated that many mentally retarded individuals "are seriously and basically deficient in this area of social . . . functions" (p. 190). Research studies have reached

TABLE 8–4
Simplified Version of Chafe's Generative Grammar

Primary semantic features of the verb: state, process, action, process-action.	
patient + state	The man is big.
patient + process	The toy broke.
agent + action	Tommy jumps.
agent + process-action + patient	Mother made the cake.
Additional secondary feature of scope	
Experiencer + experiential . . .	She likes . . . , she wants . . . , she knows . . .
Experiencer + experiential . . .	He feels . . . , he hears . . . , he sees . . .
Beneficiary + benefactive . . .	She has . . . , she owns . . . , she's got . . . , she takes . . .
Agent + completable . . .	He makes . . . , he plays . . . , he sings . . .
Patient + locative . . .	She is in (on, across)
Patient + directional . . .	The doll fell down.
Time + temporal . . .	Yesterday, . . .
Partive	All, most, some
Modal	Can, may, must
Semantic features of nouns	
Definite	The . . .
Indefinite	A . . .
Demonstrative	This, that, these, those . . .
Pronoun	You, me, he, she
Possessive pronoun	My, your, his, her

Source: Adapted from W. Chafe (1970)

varying conclusions, but there is little doubt that those retarded individuals residing in institutions demonstrate greater deficiencies in language use.

Pragmatic functions first become evident with the development of gestures. At this point, children begin to express primitive intentions, such as signalling notice, attracting attention, or making demands (Bates, 1976; Dore, 1974). Greenwald and Leonard (1979) reported that both mildly and moderately retarded Down syndrome and nonretarded children exhibited gestures at the same level of cognitive development, Piaget's sensorimotor stage V. Both groups of children used imperative gestures to enlist help or to gain an object and used declarative gestures to gain attention. Imperatives developed first, initially appearing in stage IV. These findings are supported by the findings of Lobato, Barrera, and Feldman (1981) who reported that gestures appeared by stage V for severely retarded children. These children used more sophisticated gestures for imperative than for declarative functions.

For both the retarded and nonretarded populations, language is strongly correlated with the cognitive functions of stage IV (Bates, 1976; Kahn, 1975; Lobato et al., 1981; Woodward & Stern, 1963). Woodward and Stern also stated that the speech of retarded children below stage IV is unintelligible, while their language is stereotypic, or irrelevant to context. In general, the language of retarded and nonretarded children fulfills the functions earlier expressed in gestures. The distribution of these functions is similar for both groups of children when matched for language development level (Owens & MacDonald, 1982). Both Down syndrome and nonretarded language-learning children are able to answer and to spontaneously ask questions, to reply to the comments of others, to make spontaneous declarations and demands, to name or label entities, and to imitate and spontaneously practice language.

At the single-word or early multiword stage, normally developing children begin to demonstrate "presuppositional" skills. They presuppose that their communication partners are aware of redundant or old information in a situation, and therefore, label only aspects of a situation that are undergoing change or are new information. For example, the child may not name the cup on the highchair each morning but may label with the word *cup* a new cup recently received from gram'ma. Leonard, Cole, and Steckol (1979) found that toddlers with mild retardation also exhibited this behavior.

Presuppositional skills may be a forerunner of several perspective-taking behaviors used in everyday communication. Ambron and Irwin (1975) cited three types of perspective-taking—perceptual, cognitive, and affective. Perceptual perspective-taking is the ability to assume the communication partner's perceptual viewpoint, as in interpretation of terms such as *here* and *there*. Cognitive perspective-taking concerns assessing the partner's knowledge; and, affective perspective-taking involves the partner's emotional state. Bender and Carlson (1982) found similar perspective-taking behaviors among mild-moderately retarded children and younger nonretarded 2nd-graders matched for cognitive abilities.

Other studies have reported that retarded individuals are delayed in role taking and in referential communication when compared with chronological and mental age-matched nonretarded children (Affleck, 1976; Chandler, Greenspan, Barenboim, 1974; Hoy & McKnight, 1977; Longhurst & Berry, 1975; Volpe, 1976). Blacher (1982) did not find these differences when subjects were matched for social maturity. "Results indicated that the social-cognitive skills of both retarded and nonretarded children were related to social age" (p. 473).

All of the preceding skills are interrelated in the conversational or discourse context. In a conversation, roles and topics change, and each partner must try to assess how much information his partner needs. The conversational role of retarded persons seems to be one of nondominance. Retarded children are more likely to keep greater interpersonal distance, a possible reflection of the child's perception of little personal control (Hayes & Koch, 1977). Likewise, Bedrosian and Prutting (1978) reported that retarded adults rarely exerted dominance in a conversation even when the communication partner was a child, although these adults possessed the communication skills to do so. This subservient conversational behavior is more pronounced in institutionalized populations (Prior, Minnes, Coyne, Golding, Hendy, & McGillivray, 1979) and can be noted in the case study at the end of the chapter.

Summary. Studies of the language of the mentally retarded population offer varying, sometimes conflicting, results. In general, however, the language abilities of retarded persons are similar to those of nonretarded mental-age-matched peers. Differences may be quantitative rather than qualitative. Although retarded persons have the ability to learn language relationships, these relationships appear less frequently in spontaneous use than they do among the nonretarded.

Any reported differences may reflect symbol processing deficiencies within the retarded population. Ashman (1982) has suggested for language intervention, therefore, that "it seems more defensible to teach individuals how to learn, and this implies the training of underlying processes" (p. 636).

Several studies have indicated that language abilities among retarded individuals are delayed beyond expectations based upon mental age alone, although the course of development is similar for retarded and nonretarded persons. This language delay is particularly evident in the Down syndrome population (Greenwald & Leonard, 1979; Ryan, 1975; Share, 1975; Snyder, 1978). Mahoney, Glover, and Finger (1981) concluded, "Down syndrome children are more delayed in their rate of language acquisition than might be predicted from general indices of their level of intellectual functioning" (p. 25).

Environmental Influences on the Language of MR Individuals

Retarded individuals are generally found in two types of environments: home-centered or residential. The different environmental influences upon learning have been well documented (Conroy, Efthimiou, & Lemanowicz, 1982). In general, institutionalized retarded individuals have fewer adaptive skills and are more dependent. Both language and communication are adaptive behaviors. Some aspects of language may be affected differently by institutionalization (McNutt & Leri, 1979; Montague, Hutchinson, & Matson, 1975). According to McNutt and Leri (1979), "The grammatical structure of language is apparently less affected by environment than are semantic or auditory elements" (p. 344). Phillips and Balthazar (1979) reported a deterioration of language abilities with extended institutionalization. The adult described at the end of this chapter exhibits few conversational initiations. Her verbal behavior is mostly responsive.

Parent-child Interaction. Is there some special feature of the language-learning home environment of retarded children that can account for the mental age-language age gap? One theory contends that if retarded infants behave differently from nonretarded infants, the mothers of each group must respond to their infants differently. The resultant alteration of mother-child interaction patterns adversely affects the child's language development.

The importance of early mother-child interaction has been increasingly recognized (Bruner, 1974/1975, 1977; Bullowa, 1979; Snow & Ferguson, 1977). Normally developing children have an established repertoire of communication skills prior to the appearance of their first words. These words usually fulfill the communicative functions already in place. The infant's communication skills develop within the interaction of mother and child (Owens, 1984).

The stress which accompanies birth of a handicapped infant alters the dynamics of family relations. There is an initial period of grief before a more normal relationship evolves. The sense of grief may be compounded by feelings of estrangement from an infant whose communication skills do not fulfill parental expectations (Fraiberg, 1979).

Because the interactional process is one of mutual adaptation by the two partners, some reseachers assume that a child with retardation will alter the mother's behavior differently than will a nonretarded infant. In addition, Down's infants may allow less time for maternal turn-taking and use less referential eye contact (Jones, 1977). "This reduction in the quality of the dialogue of emotional expression may result in parents being less effective with such children" (Trotter, 1983, p. 20). According to Eheart (1982), mothers of retarded children must contend with ambiguous parent-child social norms and with inconsistent child behaviors (Osofosky & O'Connell, 1972; Wolfensberger, 1967; Zigler, 1971). The situation is made more acute by a lack of information on and assistance with development (White, Watts, Barnett, Kaban, Marmor, & Shapiro, 1973), by feelings of grief and guilt (Klaus & Kennel, 1976), and by unknowns of the future (Kearsley, 1979). Several studies have attempted to assess the degree of modification in the interactions of mothers with their retarded children and the results of this modification.

Among children who are language delayed but who exhibit no other handicap, professionals have assumed that maternal or family language patterns are a contributing factor (Bee, Van Egeren, Streissguth, Nyman, & Leckie, 1969; Brophy, 1970; Emery & Ramey, 1976). For example, mothers of language-delayed children reportedly use more directives (Hess & Shipman, 1965), provide fewer opportunities for their children to use language (Jones, 1972), and are less verbally responsive (Wulbert, Inglis, Kreigsmann, & Mills, 1975). Although this maternal behavior is found in some language delay cases, it can not be assumed that this pattern represents general maternal interaction with language-delayed retarded children.

In general, more active and less irritable infants receive optimum maternal responsiveness (Rheingold & Eckerman, 1975; Stevenson & Lamb, 1979). Infants with Down syndrome or early medical disorders exhibit hypoactive behavior (Connor, Williamson, & Siepp, 1978; Field, 1979). Infants in intensive care nurseries are reported to have high irritability (DuHammel, Lin, Skelton, & Hantke, 1974). It might be expected, therefore, that mothers of these children would be less responsive than mothers of nondisordered infants. Lack of maternal responsiveness can result in the infant's withdrawal.

Predictable and responsive infants participate more in the parent-infant interactional environment (Goldberg, 1977). Affleck, Allen, McGrade, and McQueeney (1982) reported that at-risk infants are less predictable and less responsive. The resultant behavior was greater maternal restriction of the infant's activities and less maternal responsiveness.

In studies of the mothers of retarded children and CA-matched nonretarded children, the mothers of retarded children have been found to use more "primitive" forms of speech (Buium, Rynders, & Turnure, 1974; Kogan, Wimberger, & Bobbitt, 1969; Marshall, Hegrenes, & Goldstein, 1973). The unwarranted conclusion has been that these mothers are inhibiting their children's growth. We would expect children with retardation to function at a lower cognitive and language level than chronological peers. The real concern should be the appropriateness of this maternal input for the linguistic competence of the child.

Rondal (1976) studied 21 children with Down syndrome and 21 nonretarded children matched at three different language levels. He reported that the mothers of the Down's children altered their linguistic input appropriately for the language level of their children. There was no significant difference between the mothers of either group of children. This finding was substantiated by Buckhalt, Rutherford, and Goldberg (1978) who observed both verbal and nonverbal maternal behaviors. Both studies found that mothers used "motherese," a style of speaking that is characterized by short sentences, redundancy, long pauses, gesturing, and exaggerated intonation and stress patterns.

In a later study, Guttman and Rondal (1979) found mothers of Down syndrome and nonretarded children to use similar response classes (Skinner, 1957) with a few exceptions. Mothers of nonretarded children used more whole and partial repetitions, as did their children. In contrast, retarded children and their mothers used more comments and replies. In both groups, repetitions decreased and comments and replies increased with the children's increasing language abilities. In part, the more conversational style of the mothers with their retarded children may reflect the older age of these children compared to the nonretarded subjects.

Peterson and Sherrod (1982) reported other changes accompanying children's changing abilities. With retarded, language-delayed, and nonretarded children, mothers used language more prominently in interactions as their children's language progressed. Requests for nonverbal behavior decreased, while language-seeking utterances and verbal feedback increased. Language-seeking utterances consist of questions, requests for elaboration, labeling, and imitation. Buium (1975) had reported previously that mothers of 4-year-olds asked more questions and interpreted their children's gestures and vocalizations more than did mothers of 2-year-olds. Both negative and positive feedback increased within all three of the groups studied by Peterson and Sherrod. With their children's increasing language abilities, mothers became more discriminating and more demanding.

There were differences, however, and Peterson and Sherrod reported that mothers of language-delayed and of Down syndrome children demonstrated "a striking lack of rapport" (p. 396) with their children. One-third to one-half of the mother utterances were semantically unrelated to the children's activities. In a similar study with language-disordered children and their mothers, Millet and Newhoff (1978) concluded that the mothers incorporated fewer of their children's topics than did mothers of nondisordered children. According to Eheart (1982), mothers of retarded children dominated the parent-child interaction more than mothers of chronologically-matched nonretarded children. Mothers of retarded children were more directive and initiated interactions more frequently (Seitz & Riedell, 1974). For example, mothers of children with Down syndrome required their children to imitate more. Peterson and Sherrod (1982) concluded:

> It is difficult to determine whether such an emphasis on imitation would be helpful for these children who were functioning linguistically much like children of about 23 months who had no language delays. Interestingly, Nelson (1973) found that children's use of spontaneous imitation correlated negatively with some measures of language development. If a mother fosters a pattern of imitation beyond the time when it is most beneficial, the situation may eventually be deleterious to language acquisition. (p. 397)

Owens and MacDonald (1982) also noted the continued use of verbal imitation by children with Down syndrome long after such a language-learning strategy had ceased to be a viable learning technique.

Eheart (1982) reported that retarded children responded less frequently to their mothers' initiations. In addition, the children initiated only half as often as nonretarded children. In part, this behavior may reflect the larger ratio of adult to child utterances found within these dyads (Giattinno, Pollack, & Silliman, 1978).

Staff-client Interaction. Several studies have reported on the lack of appropriate verbal interactions within residential settings (Prior et al, 1979; Tizard, Cooperman, Joseph, & Tizard, 1973). Tizard and his colleagues found a large percentage of directives were used by the institutional staff. Such behavior is unlikely to elicit much verbal interchange. In fact, Prior and his colleagues reported that retarded clients were least responsive to staff directives, the most frequent staff verbal behavior. In contrast, the least frequent behavior, staff-initiated conversation, elicited the most client verbal responses. When clients did verbalize, staff personnel were equally likely to ignore the behavior as to respond with a verbal comment or reply. The most frequent staff behavior was a nonverbal agreement in the form of a head nod. Even though clients responded very little to staff instructions, such communication does provide language input. Yet, Prior et al. found that for most of the day, clients were left alone in unstructured settings. Prior and colleagues concluded that "there are features of the institutional environment which mitigate against the development of verbal communicative competence in mentally retarded persons" (p. 68).

Summary. The preceding studies indicate that in general, retarded individuals receive better linguistic input and more conversational opportunities within a home environment. The mother-child data are mixed, however, suggesting that while they adapt form and content to the linguistic competence of their retarded children, these same mothers provide primarily a responsive verbal environment. Thus, retarded children initiate less communication than their nonretarded peers. After examining maternal language use, Eheart (1982) concluded that "many of the maternal skills that are important for fostering the development of social adaptability in children are less frequently demonstrated by mothers of retarded children than by mothers of nonretarded children" (p. 24).

We can not assume, however, that differences indicate a cause for language delay. Bellinger (1980) summarized, "While many studies indicate that the language produced by mothers of language-delayed or impaired children differs from that of mothers whose children are progressing normally . . . , we cannot be sure that the atypicality of this speech is not a response to the children's language problems rather than their cause" (p. 485). Even if mothers of retarded and nonretarded children did provide similar linguistic form, content, and use styles, it might not be appropriate for the special language learning needs of retarded children.

LANGUAGE AND COMMUNICATION INTERVENTION

Many of the language and communication intervention techniques discussed with other language-disordered populations can also be used with retarded individuals. Some intervention methods, however, seem particularly germaine to the retarded population.

Most language intervention programs designed for the retarded population suggest a developmental or neodevelopmental approach (Bricker & Bricker, 1970, 1974; Guess, Sailor, & Baer, 1976; Horstmeier & MacDonald, 1978; Miller & Yoder, 1974; Owens, 1982). This approach generally is modified based upon a training rationale. Other language-disordered populations may also benefit from a developmental approach. In this section, I shall examine the developmental approach and discuss interaction with early, middle, and later language-learning retarded populations.

Language and Communication Intervention

Some language and communication intervention methods have particular application to retarded individuals because of the learning characteristics of this population. These methods are outlined in Table 8–5. In general, training goals should be explicit with

TABLE 8–5
Methodologies Particularly Applicable to the Retarded Population

1. Highlight new or relevant material
2. Preorganize information for easier learning and recall
3. Train the client to scan the task for relevant or similar stimuli to facilitate transfer
4. Train rehearsal strategies to facilitate cognitive organization and memory
5. Use similar situations and materials to facilitate transfer
6. Use concrete and/or familiar objects, persons, and situations for initial training
7. Change stimulus cues gradually and only one at a time over successive sessions
8. Use overlearning and repetition to facilitate later recall and transfer

the information organized for easy learning and recall. Hanley-Maxwell, Wilcox, and Heal (1982) found direct teaching of vocabulary words to be superior to more indirect training.

The clinician should consider the skills that the client brings to the task and those skills required for successful learning. To require too much in the form of new learning or transfer often hinders the client's ability to be successful. A question-probe technique can foster comprehension and help retarded individuals to assess the learning that they bring to a new situation (Zetlin & Gallimore, 1983).

Some structured training is usually necessary for initial learning, and repetition of initial procedures may aid further learning of the targeted skill. It may even facilitate learning if the material is presented in the same order until a certain criterion of performance is reached.

Transfer can be facilitated by keeping the training situation as close to the everyday environment as possible. The clever clinician will use objects, persons, and events from this environment for training.

The developmental model of language intervention also works well with the retarded population. Theoretically, the easiest structures are learned first by nonretarded children and, therefore, are targeted for the retarded client.

The Developmental Model

According to Haring and Bricker (1976), there are three tenets to a normative developmental model. First, development or change follows a developmental hierarchy. Children use single-word verbalizations prior to the use of short multiword utterances. Second, behavioral change goes from simple to complex. Short word-order rules appear prior to complex syntactic systems. Finally, complex behavior results from coordination or modification of simpler responses. Thus, localization to sound is presumed to result from a coordination of less complex visual and auditory skills. It is assumed that behaviors observed in normal development can serve as a basis for training with disordered populations, especially retarded individuals. Many training tools designed for the retarded population are based upon these tenets.

Professional caregivers or parents cannot teach all of the complex behaviors found among humans. Therefore, these individuals must determine which behaviors to target. Because development is rarely linear, educators must also determine the sequence of trained skills. Switsky, Rotatori, Miller, and Freagon (1979) concluded, "Since not all stages and sequences of normative development must be slavishly followed, two of the most important questions an educator must ask are which developmental behaviors and what sequences of mastery" (p. 169).

Selection of appropriate training targets is critical. "One cannot assume," stated Switzy and his colleagues (1979), "that behaviors that are clearly adaptive for a 'normal' child will be similarly adaptive for a biologically damaged severely/profoundly handicapped child" (p. 168). Selection of content for training should be based in part upon *ecological validity* and *ultimate functioning* (Brooks & Baumeister, 1977). Language training should reflect the expected functioning level and future use environment of the client.

Prutting (1979) has urged consideration of a stage approach of language intervention. At each stage, there are specific syntactic, morphological, phonological, semantic, and pragmatic targets to be trained. According to Switsky and his colleagues (1979), "While in infancy and early childhood developmentally significant behaviors seem so basic to the child's interaction with the environment they may serve as educational objectives—the face validity of this approach may decline with increasing chronological age" (p. 168). Therefore, Winitz (1983) concluded:

> Only perhaps in the very early stage of single-word development may children be operating within a clearly defined level. . . . Development stages, then, reflect age points at which mastery has been achieved, but do not indicate successive points in a learning sequence. . . . Children do not acquire language by accumulating stages of language achievement, as one would pile block upon block. (pp. 31–35)

Some professionals, such as Hogg (1975), have argued that normative development sequences cannot provide programming content, at least in a direct manner. For example, nonretarded children often use the regular past ending with irregular verbs. To teach such use to retarded children might confuse them when later they are required to learn irregular past tense. In contrast to Hogg, Bricker (1970) concluded that normative developmental behaviors can be used as educational objectives.

Winitz (1983) offered a compromise:

> Developmental language profiles should . . . serve as a guide for the "emphasis" of certain structures and, perhaps, the avoidance of others. However, these profiles should not be used as a fixed set of sequences from which the clinician cannot deviate. (p. 33)

The clinician should be free to adapt developmental guidelines to the particular learning characteristics of each child. According to Switzky and colleagues (1979), "Knowledge of the normative developmental sequences and integration of behaviors may be useful in drawing attention to some of the essential components of a skill" (p. 168). However, they cautioned that "additional non-normative behavioral sequences may have to be added to allow . . . children to acquire a skill" (p. 168). A developmental sequence might be modified based upon some sound educational rationale.

In the following sections, I shall discuss language intervention within a developmental framework. As suggested by Winitz, normal development shall serve as a guide.

Environmental Considerations and Generalization

For the retarded population, residential setting is an important variable affecting language development. The more immediate linguistic and nonlinguistic contexts are also determiners of linguistic behavior. Language development does not occur in a vacuum, devoid of purpose or use.

Although conceding that highly structured training may increase the rate of learning, especially for severely retarded individuals, Salzberg and Villani (1983) stated that such training "may well be limited to that context" (p. 403). Guess, Koegh, and Sailor (1978) concluded that "it appears easier to 'establish' a rudimentary language repertoire in language-deficient children than it is to teach the spontaneous use of skills in untrained situations" (p. 375). Highly structured settings offer a limited variety of communication situations. According to Spradlin and Siegel (1982), "The problem is how to incorporate procedures into the initial training that will actively induce generalization" (p. 3).

"Many teachers view language," stated Looney (1980), "as a 45-minute period or lesson . . . yet language is an integral part of any interpersonal communication and is best learned in the natural context of those daily interactions" (p. 31). We can expect little generalization with pictures or with objects not within the natural environment (Simic & Bucher, 1980; Welch & Pear, 1979). The typically limited stimuli used in the classroom or clinic often have little relation to the natural environment.

Language training is more functional if taught in the situations where there is actually a need for language to be used. The general result is more spontaneous usage which in turn, motivates the individual to learn more language (Rees, 1978). Wulz, Hall, and Klein (1983) concluded:

> One of the reasons so little spontaneity has been observed with this population is that the training has not been functional. Functional training employs stimuli, responses, and consequences which are similar to those in the target environment. (p. 3)

People within the natural environment should also be included in training. It is difficult to justify training that is limited to the training context only (Kozloff, 1977, 1979). According to Miller and Miller (1973), "The more parents are involved with the children's training, the more likely is the children's functioning to generalize to the home and other settings" (p. 84). Obviously, the present parent-child or caregiver-client interactional pattern is insufficient for training. These interactions can be systematically modified. "In our view," stated MacDonald, Blott, Gordon, Spiegal, and Hartmann (1974), "a major task in parent training is to demonstrate to parents that, since they are the children's major language teachers, they can become more effective by incorporating language training principles in their natural interactions with their children" (p. 411). Wulz et al. (1983) concluded that "systematically structuring these interactions to enhance the child's language behavior has been demonstrated to be effective (Culatta & Horn, 1981; Hart & Risley, 1980)" (p. 5). There is still no assurance that the new interactional patterns will be used in the home. Spradlin and Siegel (1982) offered several suggestions in Table 8–6 for facilitating language development in both clinical and more natural settings. Salzburg and Villani (1983) reported that "parents can readily acquire skills that allow them to be more effective educators of their handicapped children; however, effective parent training requires that parental skills be evident in circumstances beyond those in which they were initially acquired" (p. 412). There is often little or no generalization from the structured training mode to free-play situations in the home.

TABLE 8–6
Suggestions for Facilitating Language Generalization

In the natural environment:
1. Arrange environment to accomplish with language what cannot be accomplished easily in other ways
2. Delay reinforcement and provide cues when appropriate verbal response is obvious
3. Be responsive to communication attempts
4. Restructure environment to create opportunities for a particular response to occur

In the language training environment:
1. Teach language skills generalizable outside of the clinic
2. Vary the contexts, trainers, and training materials
3. Use consequences that are varied and related to language use being taught
4. Reduce density of reinforcement as performance improves

Source: Adapted from Spradlin and Siegel (1982)

Generalization doesn't just happen. The environment must be modified systematically to increase the likelihood of generalization. The skilled speech pathologist can train other language facilitators to use client content and developmental units in various settings and with various reinforcement conditions.

Initial Communication and Language Training

For many retarded individuals, training begins at a presymbolic or early symbolic level. Many young retarded children will participate in infant stimulation or preschool programs. Often nonspeaking, profoundly retarded adults can also be trained at this level.

Content. For best generalization, it is recommended that items and situations used for training come from the client's natural environment. These entities, including toys, clothing, utensils, and other people, can be used to train a variety of presymbolic or early symbolic skills. Skills essential to language acquisition form four categories: cognitive, perceptual, social, and communicative (McLean & Snyder-McLean, 1978; Owens, 1984). These categories and suggested presymbolic training levels are presented in Table 8–7.

In general, the client must possess certain cognitive or intellectual abilities in order to use symbols meaningfully. Several students have noted the relationship between language and cognitive development (Bloom, 1970, 1973; Bowerman, 1971; Brown, 1973; Mehrabian & Williams, 1971; Morehead, 1972; Schlesinger, 1971a, 1971b; Sinclair, 1970, 1971; Slobin, 1970). In addition, Bates, Benigni, Bretherton, Camaioni, and Volterra (1977) found a strong correlation between the cognitive stage of development and language use. More recent studies have questioned the exact relationship between cognition and language and have led Rice (1983) to conclude that the relationship "may vary as a function of age, linguistic abilities in question, and the type of cognition involved" (p. 354). In general, however, the cognitive "underpinnings" of symbol use have not been questioned.

Most studies with presymbolic children have focused on Piagetian sensorimotor substages of cognitive development. In general, these studies have concluded that children must attain or complete substage V cognitive functioning before they can

TABLE 8–7
Presymbolic Targets of Training

Behavior	*Cognitive*	*Perceptual*	*Social*	*Communicative*
Auditory notice—responding to sound		X		
Auditory search—looking for noise source	X	X		
Establishing eye contact—looking at people and objects		X	X	X
Localization—looking at noise source	X	X		X
Following a moving object—tracking visually	X	X		
Transferring eye gaze—focusing upon one entity, then another	X	X		
Physical imitation—imitating behaviors of others	X		X	
Imitation with objects—using extension of self for imitation	X			
Deferred imitation—retrieving a behavior for imitation	X			
Repetitive and sequential imitation—retrieving patterns	X	X		
Object permanence—retrieving object form from memory	X			

develop meaningful speech (Corrigan, 1978; Dihoff & Chapman, 1977; Ingram, 1975, 1978; James, 1980; Kahn, 1975; Woodward & Stern, 1963). Not all presymbolic skills are equally important. For example, object permanence skills do not seem to be good predictors of readiness for linguistic development (Bates, Benigni, Bretherton, Camaioni, & Volterra, 1977; James, 1980). Substage V means-ends and object relational skills are cognitive areas more closely related to developing language. The level of child play and language are also closely related (James, 1980). Several language intervention programs incorporate such a Piagetian or neo-Piagetian framework (Bricker & Bricker, 1974; Horstmeier & MacDonald, 1978; Mehrabian & Williams, 1971; Morehead, 1972; O'Regan-Kleinert, 1980; O'Regan-Kleinert, Rosenwinkel, & Robbins, 1979; Owens, 1982; Taenzer, Bass, & Kise, 1974).

Certain perceptual skills are also important, especially for decoding and self-monitoring. Nonhandicapped infants have well-developed auditory perceptual skills which enable them to discriminate auditory symbols and to retain them for processing. Auditory abilities are not essential for language, but the client must possess some input modality such as visual or tactile.

Presymbolic training might begin with attending and perceptual skills. Often, severely impaired individuals do not pay attention to relevant contextual cues nor do they

TABLE 8–7
Presymbolic Targets of Training
Continued

Behavior	*Cognitive*	*Perceptual*	*Social*	*Communicative*
Turn-taking—using motor imitation or eye contact in turn				X
Functional use—using objects for intended purpose in order to gain functional knowledge of meaning	X			
Means-ends—using one object or person to attain another	X		X	
Communicative gestures—displaying early intentions				X
Auditory memory—remembering sound patterns	X	X		
Word recognition—pairing names with entities				X
Vocal response—vocalizing in response to another person			X	X
Vocal turn-taking—vocalizing turns			X	X
Vocal imitation—shaping vocalizations to resemble a model		X		X
Sequencing vocal imitation—imitating vocal sequences		X		X

Source: R. Owens (1982)

integrate multisensory information efficiently (Zeaman & House, 1963). Several language programs for presymbolic populations target attending and/or perceptual skills (Bricker & Bricker, 1974; Horstmeier & MacDonald, 1978; McLean & Snyder-McLean, 1978; Owens, 1982; O'Regan-Kleinert, 1980).

Social behaviors are also important for the early use of language. The nonhandicapped infant is a very social being, an active participant in turn-taking activities and games. Even very young infants will focus upon the human face to the exclusion of all else. Eye contact and a social smile help establish early communication. Often, these behaviors need to be trained in the handicapped infant.

Finally, there are several communicative skills which seem essential to language development. Presymbolic children develop a repertoire of gestures that demonstrate their intentions, such as pointing, requesting, showing, and giving (Bates, 1976). Early words enhance the communication functions of these initial gestures. In fact, it is from the infant's general communication with the environment that language develops. Handicapped children and their caregivers may need to be trained in methods for establishing early communication skills. Sternberg, Pegnatore, and Hill (1983) have reported on a procedure for establishing communication awareness in profoundly retarded individuals. Basic awareness of others is often a first step in communication training.

Once the client possesses the necessary skills to use symbols, training can shift to the expression of single symbol units. These symbols may be words, pictures, or other visual images, signs or gestural systems, or a combination of these. These symbols can be used to fulfill a great variety of communication functions. For example, the semantic and illocutionary functions of early child language provide possible targets.

Bloom (1970, 1973), Brown (1973), and Schlesinger (1971a, 1971b) have described the underlying semantic organization of early child language. Bloom stated that she could find no evidence of a syntactic basis for single- and early multi-word utterances; and, Greenfield and Smith (1976) reported early prelinguistic and single-word semantic functions.

Halliday (1975) identified the general pragmatic functions of early child language, and Dore (1974) reported the more specific illocutionary acts found in early vocalizations and single-word utterances. He labeled these early illocutionary acts *Primitive Speech Acts,* or PSAs. McLean and Snyder-McLean (1978) recommended broadening early illocutionary targets in language initiation programs. They summarized the situation in this way:

> The lack of attention in current language programs to these pragmatic functions in language seems obvious and is demonstrated by the fact that so many current programs begin with almost exclusive targeting of the ability to "name" things. . . . It makes rather basic sense to concentrate on some basic reasons why we learn to "name" things. (p. 180)

McLean and Snyder-McLean concluded that although many programs are functional, in that they teach needs fulfillment, "such targets . . . do not represent an adequate representation of any one or all of the classes of language functions" (p. 181).

Once trained in imitation, the single word can be trained in a variety of semantic and illocutionary functions. As Miller and Yoder (1974) noted, "a single form may be used to express several functions and several forms can express a single function" (p. 523). Single words are typically trained in response to "What's this?", but this question-naming paradigm has only limited application. Possible semantic and illocutionary training targets appear in Table 8–8. Using this table, the clinician may pair behaviors in one column with those in the other. For example, a "location-answer" response might follow the cue "Where is baby?" A "nomination-question" might consist of "Cup?" or "What?" A "location-question" might also consist of "Cup?" if the client is trying to guess the location of some small object. Within these category combinations, longer utterances may also be earned. It has been demonstrated that children continue to use combinations of the semantic rules in utterances of up to four words. After this point, learning focuses upon internal sentence reorganization, and new structures are learned.

Some developmental guidelines exist for the semantic functions. Menyuk (1974) outlined the developmental sequence of single-word semantic functions. In general, the order is nomination, negation, action, objects, state or attribution, change in state or attribution, possession and location, experiencer of action, and agent. Bloom (1973) and Miller and Yoder (1974) reported that the first expansions are relational. Miller and

Yoder recommended that initial training with two-word utterances begin with the same type of expansions. Initial two-word functions include nomination ("that ______"), recurrence ("more ______"), and nonexistence ("no ______"). Next, separate semantic classes are combined to produce utterances to indicate agent + action ("Mommy eat"), possession ("baby cookie"), and location ("doggie bed").

Several programs target presymbolic and early symbolic skills (Guess, Sailor, & Baer, 1976; Hanna, Lippert, & Harris, 1982; MacDonald, 1978; 1982; Miller & Yoder, 1974; Musselwhite & St. Louis, 1982; Owens, 1982). Programs designed for less severely delayed clients, such as the Environmental Language Intervention Program (MacDonald, 1978), may contain fewer presymbolic skills than those presented in Table 8–7. Others, such as the Program for the Acquisition of Language with the Severely Impaired (PALS) (Owens, 1982), target more. Basic awareness skills may be taught using the methods outlined by Sternberg et al. (1983). Creative speech-language pathologists may select the training targets that they feel are essential for the client.

Guess, Sailor, and Baer (1976) targeted different language functions than those presented in Table 8–8. Of particular interest is their training of questions. In order to ask a question, the clients must realize that they do not know something and then formulate a question in order to gain that knowledge. Knowing when we don't know something is as important as knowing how to attain the answer. Often clients are trained to ask questions with obvious answers, thus negating the need for a question.

MacDonald and Gillette (1982) have produced some interesting clinical results using a conversational paradigm almost exclusively. By modifying the behaviors of significant others in the client's environment, the clinician can affect the communication behaviors of the language-delayed client. In a similar manner, the Facilitative Language Model of Blodgett and Miller (1981) builds conversationally upon the initial vocalizations of the client.

Evaluation. For presymbolic clients, it is essential that background data be integrated with observational and testing data to form an overall image of communication characteristics. Initial information can be gathered by observation and then supplemented through interviews with the client's caregivers. The speech-language pathologist should attempt to attain information on the following:

1. How does the client communicate primarily?
2. Does the client demonstrate any turn-taking behaviors?
3. What situations seem to be high-communication contexts?
4. What high-interest items does the client have?
5. Do caregivers provide enough time for the client to respond? How do caregivers cue the client to respond? How do they evaluate responses?
6. Which caregivers seem to elicit the most client responses? Why?
7. Does the client seem to enjoy making sounds? Give examples. How often does the client vocalize? Which situations elicit maximum vocalization? Imitated vocalizations?
8. Which daily situations result in the most client-caregiver interaction? Describe these interactions. When do these occur daily? Are the client's responses consistent?

TABLE 8–8
Semantic and Illocutionary Targets of Early Childhood

Functions	*Examples*
SEMANTIC	
Nomination—naming a person or object using a single- or multiword name or a demonstrative-plus as a name	Doggie, Choo-choo This horsie
Location—marking spatial relationships. Utterances may contain single location words or two-word utterances containing an agent, action, or object plus a location word. The function can be demonstrated in response to "where" questions.	Partner: Where's doggie? Client: Chair. Ball table, Doggie chair, Throw me, Throw here (X + locative)
Negation—marking of nonexistence, rejection, and denial using single negative words or a negative followed by another word (negative + X)	
Nonexistence generally develops first and marks the absence of a once-present object.	All gone (count as a single word), Away, No milk (client drank it), All gone car (the ride is over), No
Rejection marks an attempt to prevent or to stop an event	Partner: Time for bed. Client: No (or No bed) Stop it. No milk (pushes glass away)
Denial marks rejection of a proposition	Partner: See the bear? Client: No bear.
Modification	
Possession—appreciating that an object belongs to or is frequently associated with someone. Single-word utterances signal the owner's name. In two-word utterances, stress is usually on the initial word, the possessor.	Mine, My dollie, Johnnie bike (modifier + head) Dollie (client clutches doll)
Attribution—using descriptors for properties not inherently part of the object	Yukky, Big doggie, Little baby (modifier + head)
Recurrence—understanding that an object can reappear or an event can be reenacted	More, More milk, 'Nuther cookie (modifier + head)
Notice—signalling that an object has appeared, an event has happened, or an attempt to gain attention	Hi Mommy, Bye-bye, Look Jim
Action—marking an activity	
Action—single action words	Jump, Eat
Agent + Action—two-word signal that an animate initiated an activity	Mommy throw, Doggie eat, Baby sleep
Action + Object—two-word signal that an animate or inanimate object was the recipient of action	Eat cookie, Throw ball
ILLOCUTIONARY	
Answer—client responds to questions. The questioner's behaviors are a cue for the client's response; the response probably would not be produced without this cue. The client's responses are cognitively related to the question, although they may be incorrect.	Partner (holding doll): What's this? Client: Baby Partner: Is this a mirror? Client: No
Question—client asks for information or verification by addressing the other person verbally. The client's behavior is a stimulus or cue and indicates that he expects an answer. The client can ask himself questions when engaged in egocentric play.	Client (picks up toy telephone): Phone? Client: What this?

TABLE 8–8
Semantic and Illocutionary Targets of Early Childhood (Continued)

Functions	*Examples*
Reply—client makes meaningful response to the content of the other speaker's previous utterance, a verbal cue external to the client. The client may continue to build on the content and ignore the form of the utterance, such as responding to a word or thought in a question without answering the question. In many cases, the client will build on the content *and* respond with an appropriate form. This category does not include mere repetition.	Partner: Johnny, Bring me the scissors. (command) Client: No. Partner: May I have the keys? (request) Client: In a minute. Partner: This is a cute dog. (declaration) Client: My doggie.
Elicitation—client self-repeats in response to a request for repetition or clarification or in response to "Say x."	Client: Kitty go. (declaration) Partner: What? Client: Kitty go. Partner: Mary, say "ball." Client: Ball.
Continuant—client signals that he is listening and wants to continue the interchange, or that he missed what was said.	Uh-huh, Okay. I see, Yes What? Huh?
Declaration—client makes a statement that is situationally related and for communication but is not in response to another speaker. The utterance is more like a commentary. Cues are internal or situational but not verbal. This category also includes situationally related phonemic exclamations.	Client (playing game with mother and glances out): It raining out. Client (playing with car): Car go up. Partner: This is a cute doggie. Client: My doggie. (reply) He lives in a house. (declaration) Partner: This is a cute doggie. Client: My doggie. (reply) I have kitty, too. (declaration)
Practice—client repeats or imitates in whole or part what he or another person says with no change in intonation that would indicate a change of intent. In addition, internal replay without added new information is considered *practice.* This category also includes counting, singing, babbling, or rhyming behaviors in which the client seems to be experimenting or rehearsing. Perseverative responses, even if the other person interjects an utterance between them, are considered *practice* as long as they not mark discrete events or objects.	Partner: Ball. Client: Ball. Partner: See the red ball. Client: Red ball. Partner: See the red ball. Client: See ball. (practice) Ball, ball, ball. (practice)
Name—client labels an object or event that is present, but the label is not in response to a question. This verbal behavior is usually accomplished by pointing or nodding.	Client (picks up ball): Ball. Client (points to ball): That ball.
Suggestion, Command, Demand, Request—The primary function of the client's utterance is to influence another person's behavior by getting that person to do something or to give the client permission. The form may be imperative, declarative, or interrogative.	Client: Gimmie cookie. Client: Stop that. Client: Mommy. Client: Throw ball. (Parent throws ball) Throw ball. (Parent throws ball) Throw ball.

Note: From *Program for the Aquisition of Language with the Severely Impaired* by R. Owens, 1982, Columbus, OH: Charles E. Merrill. Copyright 1982 by Charles E. Merrill. Adapted by permission

9. Does the client ever initiate communication? How? In what situations?
10. Does the client
    Make wants known? How?
    Request help? How?
    Point to things, name them, or both? Does the client look at the object and/or partner while pointing or naming?
    Ask questions or seek information? How?
    Indicate emotions (pain, happiness, like/dislike)? How?
    Seek attention? How? What happens if attention doesn't follow?

This general information can be supplemented by specific questions related to the functioning level of the client. Several language intervention tools are available for this purpose. The Receptive-Expressive Emergent Language (REEL) Scale (Bzoch & League, 1971) probes both receptive and expressive language skills for individuals functioning below 36 months. At each level, respondents are asked three receptive and three expressive questions. In the Oliver (MacDonald, 1978) and the Caregiver Interview (Owens, 1982), questions relate more directly to specific levels of formal testing. The speech-language pathologist's goal is to attain an estimate of client functioning in order to provide a more thorough assessment. In addition, such probing familiarizes the caregiver with the behaviors to be tested and taught. This familiarization is vital if caregivers are to become fully participating members in the intervention process.

Formal testing should follow content similar to that mentioned in Tables 8–7 and 8–8. More valid results may be attained if caregivers attend with the client, and if the client uses familiar objects. The goal of formal assessment is to determine the functioning level at which to begin intervention. Westby (1980) has suggested a play format for assessing the development of early cognitive and language abilities. Her symbolic play scale describes ten stages of early development.

If the client uses symbols, the speech-language pathologist should attempt to gain a sample for analysis. Sampling may occur in a free-play situation or in a combination of free-play and structured sampling plus imitation (McDonald, 1978). Usually 50 utterances are adequate. The clinician should be interested in both the breadth and depth of semantic and illocutionary functions. Of particular interest are the nonexistence of certain functions, the low incidence of others, and the length of each function.

Leonard, Steckol, and Panther (1983) offered the following cautionary advice:

> To date, assessment has primarily taken the form of placing utterances produced by the child into semantic relation categories used in normal child language research. . . . Thus, for the language-disordered child the categories are predetermined, and may not adequately reflect his/her own semantic segmentations. (p. 25)

Leonard and his colleagues suggested that the speech-language pathologist look for patterns in early word combinations that suggest positional rules or combinations that serve as single-word utterances.

Because this chapter has recommended that caregivers act as language facilitators, it is necessary for the speech-language pathologist to attain a sample of the client-caregiver interaction. Owens (1982) suggested a 10-minute rated sample, while Wilcox and Campbell (1983) preferred a more descriptive analysis. Russo and Owens (1982) rated ten interactional behaviors, such as the caregiver behaviors of natural reinforcement, physical space, imitation, expansion, reply/extension, and content/child lexicon, and the client behaviors of attending, referencing, physical space, and naming/verbalization. In contrast, Wilcox and Campbell (1983) described the interaction in terms of engagement, termination, and reengagement activities, signalled by body posture and movement, and by vocalizations. MacDonald (1980) analyzed turn-taking and conversational strategies.

Once the initial evaluation is complete, the speech-language pathologist should know the client's interactional strategies, most frequent topics, communication partners, functioning level, and the quality of the client-caregiver interaction. Throughout the clinical intervention phase, the speech-language pathologist should continually test and probe in order to "fine-tune" training techniques.

Intervention. The first step in training is to decide what to teach, who will teach it, and under what circumstances. In the previous section, I suggested a number of training targets for early intervention. Who is involved and the circumstances are related and will significantly shape the intervention program.

It is essential in initial language programming that the natural environment of the retarded client be included. In establishing early communication, the speech-language pathologist must enlist the aid of the client's caregivers in the intervention process.

The effective use of parents as behavior change agents is well established (Baker, 1976; Heifetz, 1980). Several parent variables can affect the outcome. According to Clark, Baker, and Heifetz (1982), parent socioeconomic status, pretraining skills, and experience positively correlate with the short-term learning outcomes. This relationship may explain why parent training programs traditionally neglect low socioeconomic families (Hargis & Blechman, 1979). It is my experience, however, that lower-class mothers can make positive strides with their children, because prior to training, these mothers often overlook natural teaching situations used by middle- and upper-class mothers. Snell (1979) has reported successful use of higher functioning institutionalized individuals as language trainers for more severely retarded clients.

In a study with the parents of Down syndrome children, Stoneman, Brody, and Abbott (1983) reported that mothers assumed a manager or teacher role more often and were more responsive than fathers. Parents with some instruction were able to modify their speech to their retarded children in order to improve the children's expressive skills (Cheseldine & McConkey, 1979). Apparently, knowledge of the direction in which training should proceed is sufficient information to allow some parents spontaneously to adopt suitable teaching strategies.

The variables that control transfer of parental skills to natural settings are not fully understood (Forehand & Atkeson, 1977). Salzberg and Villani (1983) recognized two significant factors. First, transfer increases with the similarity of the tasks and of training structure to the natural environment (Mindell & Budd, 1977; Miller & Sloan, 1976). Second, feedback from the speech-language pathologist regarding the application of newly acquired training skills is also important (Polk, Schilmoeller, Embry, Holman, & Baer, 1976).

According to Salzburg and Villani (1983), successful use of parents as language facilitators depends upon three components. Parents must be asked to use their training skills at home, they must be specifically taught to adapt training techniques to these more informal situations, and they need to receive professional feedback.

Wulz, Hall, and Klein (1983) reported on successful use of their Instructional Communication Strategy. Within this model, the professional trains client responses, while the parents elicit these responses within the home. The components are environmental manipulation and teaching interaction. In environmental manipulation, parents restructure needs-meeting situations so that their children's needs are not anticipated but are dependent upon the children's communication behavior. Within the teaching phase, children are taught to respond to "need-to-communicate" situations. The purpose of the training is to expand the children's communication repertoire and to stimulate responding.

Home-based training should not be disruptive. According to Wulz et al. (1983), "Programs developed for the home should not add to the parent's existing responsibilities, but should restructure ongoing activities" (p. 6). Owens (1982) called this type of training "incidental teaching" and gave it primacy as an early communication training strategy. If, for example, the parent is training object permanence, nonfloating soap and toys can be incorporated into the bathing routine. Because almost any routine can be adapted for language training, there is no need to rely solely on formal, out-of-context training modes. With children, the modality for training may be play. Play is child-centered, and the child's activity can provide the focus of training.

MacDonald (1978) relied upon environmental rules to restructure client-caregiver interactions. Once the clients have learned a skill, they are required to perform that skill in order to attain desired entities or privileges. For example, if the client can sign "cookie," the sign is required in order to get a cookie. Previously accepted pointing or whining is unacceptable. Environmental rules affect both client and caregiver behaviors.

Language stimulation techniques can also be used in the natural environment (Cheseldine & McConkey, 1979; Owens, 1982). Ideally, such stimulation would precede slightly the client's actual level of functioning. Stimulation can take the form of "motherese" discussed earlier.

The importance of formal or structured training cannot be overlooked, but should be minimized when possible (MacDonald, 1978, 1982; Owens, 1982). Often this training can be adapted to a play modality (Manolson, 1982). Richmond and Lewallen (1983) reported that two trainers can facilitate client responding. One trainer cues the client while the second trainer models or prompts the appropriate response.

It is not always possible to train within the home. An alternative is the classroom (Brightman, Ambrose, & Baker, 1980). Within residential settings, aids, direct care staff, or foster grandparents may serve as language facilitators (Burke, Lepre, & Owens, in progress). Realon, Lewallen, and Wheeler (1983) reported that direct care staff teaching behaviors can be modified by simple praise or by feedback plus praise.

Augmentative Communication Aids

Some mentally retarded individuals, particularly the more severely impaired, experience great difficulty with speech and with the use of symbols. For these nonspeaking clients, an augmentative form of communication may be necessary. Augmentative forms increase or expand the symbolic communication capabilities of these nonspeaking individuals. Common forms of augmentative communication include manual communication, communication boards, and electronic or computer-based communication.

These augmentative communication forms will be discussed along with assessment and programming considerations.

Contrary to common misconception, use of augmentative communication systems does not deter further development of speech. Several studies have demonstrated that augmentative communication facilitates symbol learning (Bricker, 1972; Van Biervliet, 1977), increases verbalization of trained symbols (Burggraf, 1976), facilitates spontaneous verbal communication (Kahn, 1977; Konstantases, Oxman, & Webster, 1978; Reich, 1978), increases communication initiations (Harris-Vanderheiden, Brown, MacKenzie, Reinen, & Scheibel, 1975), and increases the range of meanings and communication partners (Harris, Lippert, Yoder, & Vanderheiden, 1979). Calculator and Luchko (1983) cautioned, however, that augmentative communication "will not, in itself, assure effective communication" (p. 185). According to Shane, Lipschultz, and Shane (1982),

> an augmentative communication system is not a panacea. It does not solve all of the communication problems of the non-speaking person. (p. 83)

Types of Augmentative Communication. There are three general modes of augmentative communication—manual, communication boards, and electronic. Manual communication includes signs, gestures, and fingerspelling. There are several types of sign systems from American Sign Language (AMESLAN), which is a language of its own, to Seeing Essential English (SEE_1) or Signing Exact English (SEE_2), which closely approximates English syntax. Signed English uses signs from both systems but does not adhere as closely to English morphological rules as SEE_1. American Indian sign language (Amer-Ind) has also been used successfully with retarded persons. One reason for these results may be the transparency of Amer-Ind. Transparency is the ease of understanding a sign once its origin is explained. Daniloff, Lloyd, and Fristoe (1983) found Amer-Ind to be significantly more transparent than AMESLAN.

Communication boards, the second type of augmentative system, come in many different shapes and varieties. In general, boards are easy to make, portable, and very adaptable. The visual symbols used may include, from least to most symbolic, models or miniatures, pictures, drawings, Rebus symbols, Blissymbols, or letters and words. Rebus symbols are pictographic representations of concepts. Blissymbols are generally less iconic than Rebus symbols but allow for more generative language use. Archer (1977) explained succinctly the origin and use of Blissymbols. These encoding forms are not exclusive and may be used in combination. In general, the more iconic or "guessable" the encoding system, the easier it is to learn (Clark, 1981). In turn, the less iconic systems are more flexible and generative, allowing more adult-like representation.

The final type of augmentative system is electronic or computer-based. The tremendous growth of computer technology is opening many new possibilities for the nonspeaking (Vanderheiden, 1982). Input systems may be similar to those used on communication boards, and output may include print, graphics, and/or prerecorded or synthesized speech. In general, there are three types of indicating methods used by clients—scanning, encoding, and direct selection. In the scanning method, the device continually scans the display of symbols. The retarded client stops the scan on the desired symbol. With encoding, a code such as numbers or digits is used to access the computer's memory. Finally, in direct selection, the client moves a cursor or pointer to the desired symbol or may, if possible, type the message.

According to Vanderheiden (1982), "The recent introduction . . . of portable and hand-held computers is opening up the potential for microcomputers to move out of the stationary writing-aid category and begin to address the categories of portable writing/note taking aids and conversational communication aids" (p. 138). Accessing these computers, however, may be the most difficult problem, particularly for severely motorically involved individuals. "The major barrier for using microcomputers as communication aids," cautioned Vanderheiden (1982), "is the need for custom interfacing to achieve optimum speech" (p. 139). The interface switch between the client and the microcomputer must often be modified or custom-designed to the motoric abilities of an individual client. The slowness of interface use may actually negate some of the speed advantages associated with microcomputers.

It may be advantageous for some retarded clients to have more than one type of augmentative system. Different systems may have application in different environments. In addition, the speech-language pathologist should continue to train speech.

Evaluation. Evaluative decisions on client use of an augmentative communication system are made by a team of professionals, usually consisting of a speech-language pathologist, psychologist, physical therapist, occupational therapist, special education teacher, a client advocate such as a parent, and the client. Assessment is a continuing process which, in this case, is essential to adapt the augmentative system to the client's changing needs and abilities.

The American Speech-Language-Hearing Association (ASHA) Ad Hoc Committee on Communication Processes and Non-Speaking Persons (1980) identified three components of the assessment for augmentative communication. First, the team must assess the appropriateness of an augmentative system. Not all nonspeaking individuals are candidates for augmentative communication. For example, the abilities needed for spontaneous symbol use apply to augmentative communication as well as to verbal language (Goossens, 1984; Owens & House, 1984; Shane & Bashir, 1980; Silverman, 1980). The environment also must be supportive of augmentative system use (Owens & House, 1984; Shane, Lipschultz, & Shane, 1982).

The second component of an evaluation is selection of the appropriate communication mode. The team must decide which type or types of augmentative systems will be appropriate for the nonspeaking individual. Of particular importance are the motoric abilities of the client (Shane & Wilbur, 1980; Silverman, 1980). "With the physically handicapped," cautioned Bottorf and DePape (1982), "interaction must be explored in the context of the body's total movement patterns" (p. 60). The evaluative team is interested in the range, speed, strength, and consistency of movement. Clients with good motor skills may be candidates for manual systems, while those with less ability may use communication boards or electronic systems. For electronic devices, Coleman, Cook, and Myers (1980) recommended a task analysis which includes the client's present skills and those behaviors needed in order to operate the communication aid.

Finally, the team must select the appropriate symbol system or systems. Questions of appropriateness relate to cognitive ability, visual accuity, and environmental receptivity (Chapman & Miller, 1980). For example, greater cognitive skills and visual discrimination abilities are needed for word use than for picture use. In addition, the use of a symbol system such as Blissymbols might hinder communication in a nonreceptive environment.

Several matrices have been developed to aid in the augmentative communication decision process (Owens & House, 1984; Shane & Bashir, 1980). These tools are guides and not rigid formulas. Clinical intuition and testing are very important.

Intervention. "Although the tool should be selected or created carefully and on an individual basis," Bottorf and DePape (1982) reminded, "the focus of intervention must always be centered on increasing successful interactions" (pp. 55–56). In general, communication interactions can be fostered by adapting the augmentative system to the individual client and to the communication environment.

The creative speech-language pathologist will attempt to establish an augmentative environment around the client. The augmentative system should be available at all times, and others should be encouraged to use the system. Signs are always available, but others may not use them when talking to the client. Their use may facilitate client comprehension and will help the client feel less an "odd-man-out." In addition, the daily routine of the client can foster augmentative communication use. "If an effective communication system is to be developed," explained Bottorf and DePape (1982), "intervention must take place within the context of day-to-day experiences unique to each individual" (p. 64).

The second principle, selection of individualized content, should reflect client routines, interests, and needs. The vocabulary selected will affect the types of interactions in which it is used (Bottorf & DePape, 1982). Fristoe and Lloyd (1980) proposed a guide to initial sign vocabulary based on ease of production and iconicity. They stressed, however, that their list is merely a guide, not a prescription. Initial vocabularies should be based upon each client's individual interests and routines, basic needs, and the recommendations of others within the environment. In addition, signs may be chosen on the basis of symmetry, taction, and iconicity. Kohl (1981) and Kohl, Karlan, and Heal (1979) reported that severely retarded individuals could learn signs more rapidly if the signs were symmetrical or contained identical hand movements, had some contact with the body (taction), and were iconic or highly representational.

Finally, the environment should be modified systematically to encourage augmentative communication. Nonspeaking mentally retarded clients must be given an opportunity to use their augmentative systems. Teachers and caregivers need to be cautioned not to dominate communication. Communication partners must be patient and await client responses. Clients should also be given a choice in their daily routine and among alternative activities in order to foster active system use.

Summary. Augmentative communication systems can be part of a nonspeaking individual's effective interaction system if continually evaluated and adapted to that client's communication needs. "As with speech," Shane et al. (1982) reminded, "an augmentative communication system can be used to express a variety of communication functions, but only if the environment provides opportunities for meaningful use" (p. 83).

Language Rule Training

Once the client begins to use symbols meaningfully, training targets become the rule systems used with these symbols. The speech-language pathologist should be knowledgeable in the rules used within the five generally recognized areas of language: syntax, morphology, phonology, semantics, and pragmatics.

Professionals frequently assume that only the adult forms of these rules are acceptable. A 2-year-old who says, "What mommy eating?" is not considered to be language disordered, but to be following an age-appropriate rule. Likewise, individuals with mental retardation follow rules that generally reflect their level of cognitive functioning. Luckily, these individuals have professionals to guide their language learning.

Not all child rules are appropriate for training. For example, nonretarded children develop a few irregular past tense verbs, such as "come" and "go", prior to learning the "-ed" rule for regular past. Once this rule is learned, however, forms such as "went" become "goed" or "wented". No one seriously proposes that we teach these forms to retarded individuals. On the other hand, it may be justifiable to teach "No eat peas" prior to "I no eat peas," followed by "I can't eat peas." Training in this sequence seems more logical than the previous example.

Evaluation. Initial evaluation should attempt to determine which rule systems the clients use expressively and which ones they comprehend. Assessment ideally would include both formal testing and informal evaluation.

There are very few formal tests designed for and normed on the retarded population. Most commercially available tests were developed and normed on nonretarded children. Careful consideration must be given to the appropriateness of such tests and materials with older retarded clients, particularly adults.

Owings and Guyette (1982) recommended the modification of existing materials and the development of new assessment tools. Many speech-language pathologists supplement formal tests with their own locally prepared instruments (Pickett & Flynn, 1983). This procedure is supported by a number of speech-language professionals (Mittler, 1976; Muma, 1978; Siegel, 1975).

Generally recognized formal tests are presented in Table 8–9. Each is identified by the specific areas tested. Such standardized measures may be employed in nonstandardized ways to gain knowledge of the client's functional level rather than a standardized score. In a survey, Rushakoff and Johnson (1979) found that four tests accounted for 54% of all language tests administered to the retarded the previous year. Pickett and Flynn (1983) reported that the language tests used most frequently with retarded adults are the Peabody Picture Vocabulary Test (Dunn & Dunn, 1981), the Test of Auditory Comprehension of Language (Carrow, 1973), the Utah Test of Language Development (Meacham, Merlin, & Jones, 1967), and the Illinois Test of Psycholinguistic Abilities (Kirk, McCarthy, & Winifred, 1968).

According to Dever (1978), "Attempts to assess the ability to use language on the basis of responses to items on a formal test are probably a waste of time and money" (p. 19). Informally collected language samples can be a valuable source of additional information. Samples can be analyzed in a number of ways. Initially, the speech-language pathologist should determine the mean length of utterance (MLU). Increasing MLU correlates with increasing complexity up to an MLU of 4.0 morphemes. Table 8–10 contains MLU values and equivalent ages.

Of the commercially available analysis methods, Miller's Assigning Structural Stage (1980) seems to be the most functional. Others, such as Developmental Sentence Scoring (Lee, 1974) result in a normative score but provide little direction for intervention. Using Miller's approach, the speech-language pathologist determines the correct percentage of use of Brown's (1973) 14 morphemes. This data, plus the MLU, suggest a developmental stage. Internal sentence analysis for noun phrase, verb phrase, and sentence type development results in assignment of the client to a stage or stages of language development. Because the instrument informs the speech-language pathologist of the characteristics of the next stage of development, programming is relatively straightforward. Similar analysis can be performed semantically and phonologically.

Intervention. Again, generalization is best assured by use of the natural environment for language training. Caregivers can be instructed in the use of evaluative feedback and in expansion techniques. For example, caregivers can provide corrective feedback in the form of modeling of the correct production. Incomplete or primitive responses can be expanded into a more adult-like form.

A training format similar to the one in Table 8–11 may be helpful for organizing training. In this table, sentence training targets are organized developmentally but modified for ease of training. Therefore, similar structures appear in proximity to facilitate carry over. As each new structure is added, all previously trained utterances which might contain that structure are retrained. New structures or uses represent an interplay of the different aspects of language.

When attempting to elicit full sentences, the speech-language pathologist should be very careful to use cues that make sense pragmatically and reflect general language use. For example, the cue "What do you want?" is most likely to elicit a single word or short phrase response, such as "Cookie." Demanding "I want cookie" as a response is inappropriate pragmatically.

In addition, speech-language pathologists should be aware of the special learning needs of the retarded population. Cognitive operations should be trained prior to linguistic skills that express those operations. For example, the client should understand reversibility of processes before learning linguistic concepts such as "before," "after," and "because."

Clients, such as Down syndrome individuals, may need help with successive processing skills. Simultaneous skills related to overall meaning may be employed to facilitate sequential operations.

Finally, some retarded populations, such as those with Down syndrome, will require additional input beyond auditory symbols. Visual and tactile input can enhance learning for these groups. The use of pictures or experiential activities might facilitate concept learning and elicit more client responses. Cook and Seymour (1980) reported that involvement in activity by the client resulted in more verbal responsiveness than involvement by the clinician or use of pictures. Likewise, Spiegel (1983) found active participation by the severely retarded client to become a cue for verbal behavior that was situationally appropriate.

Language Use: The Last Frontier

With higher functioning retarded adults or teenagers in prevocational or vocational training programs, the focus of training should shift from language form to language use. This proposal does not imply that language forms are unimportant, merely that they are not as critical to training. Naturally, a minimum of language structure is required.

Reiter and Levi (1980) reported that the main difference between occupationally and socially successful retarded adults and nonsuccessful ones was integration at work

TABLE 8–9
Language Test Content

	GRAMMATICAL																				
	Nouns				Verbs																
	Possessives	Plural (reg.)	Plural (irreg.)	Derivational Suffix	Present	Present Participle	Present Progressive	Past (reg.)	Past (irreg.)	Future	Present Perfect	Past Perfect	Past Progressive	Present Perfect Prog.	Passive	Modals	Copula	Auxiliary Verbs	Third Per. Sing (reg.)	Third Per. Sing (irreg.)	Infinitives/gerunds
ACLC						X															
Banksor.		X	X		X	X	X			X	X								X	X	
Berko	X	X		X			X	X	X										X		
CELI		X	X		X		X	X	X	X	X	X		X	X	X	X	X	X	X	X
ITPA	X	X	X	X			X	X	X						X						
Miller-Yoder	X	X			X		X	X		X					X			X	X		
NSST	X	X	X		X		X	X		X	X				X			X	X		
OLSIDI	X	X			X		X	X	X	X			X			X	X	X	X	X	X
OLSIST	X	X			X		X	X	X	X			X			X	X	X	X	X	X
PLST					X												X	X	X		
SICD		X	X		X	X		X		X							X	X	X		
TACL		X		X	X	X	X	X		X	X			X	X		X	X	X		
TSA				X	X		X	X	X	X	X				X	X	X	X	X	X	X
TSA-Screening				X			X	X	X	X					X		X		X		
Sampling Tools: Assign. Struc. Stage	X	X			X		X	X	X	X		X	X			X	X	X	X		
DSS					X	X	X	X	X	X	X	X	X	X	X	X	X	X	X		X
DST	X	X			X		X														
LSAT	X	X			X		X	X		X	X	X	X			X	X	X	X		X

and in society. Further results indicated that there was great need among the retarded population for attaining regular employment and for having nonretarded friends. One difference between the successful and unsuccessful group was found in the area of social skills including language. Therefore, more appropriate language use may become the training target.

Some language factors, such as following directions or asking questions, may be more important than others, particularly in the work setting. Malgady, Barcher,

TABLE 8–9
Language Test Content *(continued)*

	GRAMMATICAL																		OTHER						
	Pronouns					Adjectival							Clausal												
	Subject Pronouns	Object Pronouns	Possessive: Nom./Deter.	Indefinite Pronouns	Reflexive Pronouns	Adjectives	Demonstratives	Articles	Comparatives	Superlatives	Adverbs	Prepositions	Wh-Questions	Yes/No Questions	Embedding	Coordinated/Conjunction	Negatives	"Do" Insertions	Response to Commands	Quantity	Body Parts	Common Nouns	Color	Categorization	Miscellaneous
ACLC						X						X										X			
Banksor.	X	X	X			X			X	X		X					X		X	X	X	X	X	X	X
Berko						X			X	X															X
CELI	X	X	X	X	X	X	X	X	X		X	X	X	X	X	X	X	X				X	X		
ITPA			X		X	X			X	X		X										X			
Miller-Yoder	X	X			X	X						X					X						X		
NSST	X		X		X		X					X	X	X			X					X			
OLSIDI	X	X	X		X			X				X	X	X	X	X	X	X							
OLSIST	X	X	X					X				X	X	X	X	X	X	X							
PLST						X			X	X		X	X						X	X			X		X
SICD	X	X	X			X					X	X	X	X	X	X	X		X	X	X	X	X		
TACL	X	X	X			X	X		X	X	X	X	X		X		X			X		X	X		
TSA	X	X	X		X			X					X	X	X	X									
TSA-Screening	X	X	X		X			X					X	X	X	X	X								
Sampling Tools: Assign. Struc. Stage	X		X		O	X	X	X				X	X	X	O	O	X	X							O
DSS	X	X	X	X	X	X	X						X	X	X	X	X	X							
DST	X	X	X			X	X	X			X	X	X			X	X	X		X		X			
LSAT	X		X			X	X	X			X	X	X	X	X	X	X					X			X

Towner, and Davis (1979) compiled a list of maladaptive social behaviors observed by vocational training supervisors and used this list to rate mildly to severely retarded clients for employability. In general, language skills were rated as less important than acceptable verbal manners, such as not interrupting. Retarded adults are less likely to be employed if their languge use is inappropriate, such as being abusive, argumentative, vulgar, bossy, loud, interruptive, or irrelevant. Additional skills for training might also include conversational abilities and direction following.

TABLE 8–10
MLU and Approximate Age

MLU	*Predicted Chronological Age in Months*	*Predicted Age in Months ±1 S.D.*
1.5	23.0	18.5–27.5
2.0	26.9	21.5–32.3
2.5	30.8	23.9–37.7
3.0	34.8	28.0–41.6
3.5	38.7	30.8–46.6
4.0	42.6	36.7–48.5
4.5	46.6	40.3–52.9
5.0	50.5	42.1–58.9
5.5	54.4	46.0–62.8
6.0	58.3	49.9–66.7

Source: Adapted from J. Miller (1980)

These vocational-interpersonal skills can be modified through a combination of modeling, coaching, and behavior rehearsal (LaGreca, Stone, & Bell, 1983). Appropriate verbal behavior can be modeled while clients are trained in appropriate use. Rehearsal and role play in situations close to those of actual use can be beneficial. Social feedback in the form of praise, instruction, and reprimands has been more effective than reprimands and instruction in reducing inappropriate verbalizations (Dwinell & Connis, 1979).

Other conversational skills may also be taught. Mentally retarded teenagers may have particular difficulties communicating with their parents and expressing their feelings (Sheperd & Marshall, 1976). Rees and Wollner (1981) have constructed a taxonomy of pragmatic abilities for teaching the conversational use of language. These abilities relate to organizing and participating in a conversation, repairing conversational errors, establishing and varying conversational roles, and producing and comprehending speech acts. As conversational partners, mentally retarded individuals should observe the rules of turn-taking and be able to introduce, sustain, and contribute to the topic of conversation. In addition, they should be able to take their communication partner's perspective and to vary their own role and informational contribution accordingly.

Many mentally retarded individuals recognize the need for these conversational skills. In a "social" room in a day training program, the clients established the following rules:

Stay on topic
Be quiet when others are talking
Listen to what you hear
Don't interrupt others
Take turns—Give everyone a chance
Speak so others can hear you
Don't talk to yourself

TABLE 8–11
Possible Initial Integration of Language Training Targets

Basic Sentence Types	*New structure*
A. agent + action + locative [noun agent + verb + adverb (where)] (Boy jump up)	
B. agent + action + object [noun agent + verb + noun object] (Girl hit ball)	
C. action + modifier + object [verb + adjective + noun object] (Hit red ball)	
D. action + object + locative [verb + noun object + adverb or noun] (Throw ball here; Throw ball daddy)	
E. modifier + agent + action [adjective + noun agent + verb] (Big doggie jump.)	
F. modifier + X + locative [adjective + X + adverb or noun] (Big man chair)	
G. introducer + modifier + X (Hi big doggie)	
H. negative + agent + action (No daddy go)	
I. negative + action + object (No eat cookie; Not eat cookie)	
J. negative + agent + locative (No baby crib)	
K. negative + action + locative (Not eat table; No sleep bed)	
A. Experiencer + action + location [noun experiencer + verb + adverb] (Boy fall down: John want up)	Experiencer case
B. Experiencer + action + object noun experiencer + action + noun object (Mommy see dog; Daddy want car)	
A. agent + action [noun agent + verb(ing)] (Boy running)	Present Progressive -ing
B. action + object [verb(ing) + noun object] (Throwing ball)	
C. agent + action + locative [noun agent + verb(ing) + adverb] (Boy jumping up)	
D. agent + action + object [noun agent + verb(ing) + noun object] (Boy hitting ball)	
E. action + modifier + object [verb(ing) + adjective + noun object] (Hitting red ball)	

TABLE 8–11
Possible Initial Integration of Language Training Targets (Continued)

Basic Sentence Types	*New structure*
F. action + object + locative [verb(ing) + noun object + adverb] (Throwing ball daddy) G. modifier + agent + action [adjective + noun agent + verb(ing)] (Big doggie jumping) H. negative + agent + action [negative + noun agent + verb(ing)] (No daddy driving) I. negative + action + object [negative + verb(ing) + noun object] (No eating cookie) J. negative + action + locative [negative + verb(ing) + adverb or noun] (No throwing daddy)	
A. in/on + noun (object) (or here, there, that, this) (in box, in here, on table, on that) B. verb + in/on + noun (object) (put in box, jump in here, eat on table) C. verb (ing) + in/on + noun (object) (putting in box, eating on table) D. noun (agent) + in/on + noun (object) (boy in box, ball in here cup on table, cup in there) E. in/on + adjective + noun (object) (in red truck, on big wagon) F. noun (agent) + verb + in/on + noun (object) (Tom hide in box, Doggie sleep on chair) G. verb + in/on + adjective + noun (object) (sit in big chair, eat on little table) H. verb + noun (object) + in/on noun (object) (throw ball in box, sit dolly on floor, hide book in here) I. noun (experiencer) + verb + in/on + noun (object) (Boy fall in water)	Prepositions "in/on"
A. you (agent) + verb(ing) (you run, you running) B. you (agent) + verb(ing) + noun (object) (you, throw ball, you throwing ball) C. you (agent) + verb(ing) + adjective + noun (object) (you throwing big ball) D. you (agent) + verb + in/on + noun (object) (you sit on table, you sit in chair, you sit here) E. you (experiencer) + verb + noun (object) (You see kittie) F. You (experiencer) + verb + in/on + noun (object) (You fall in water)	Pronoun "you"

SUMMARY

Within this chapter, I have explored a definition of mental retardation which considers cognitive functioning and adaptive behavior. Overall, this definition reflects empirical findings that retarded individuals are developmental beings whose behavior is characterized by delay rather than by difference. Some differences do exist, but the overall developmental picture is one of delay. This finding is also true for the language development of the retarded population. Differences are quantitative rather than qualitative.

These characteristics suggest a developmental language intervention approach. The wise clinician will use nonretarded development as a guide for creative programming.

The language intervention targets will differ with the language skills of the client. Initial training should focus on cognitive, perceptual, social, and communicative skills and on the establishment of early communication. Early building blocks will be semantic and illocutionary. Once short multiword utterances are trained, the speech-language pathologist should target language rule systems. As the client becomes more capable in using language rules, language use becomes a tool for normalization training. Such training is particularly true of clients in vocational training programs.

As we began this chapter with a quote from Nigel Hunt:

> Thank you ever so much for letting me write this book. I am most delightful. (p. 124)

CASE STUDY

Catherine is a 33-year-old, severely retarded adult residing in a developmental center but attending a day training program in the community. She has been institutionalized since early childhood. The cause of retardation is unknown. Her mental age measured on the Wechsler Intelligence Scale is slightly above age 6, although her language performance is lower. She experiences seizures, primarily of the petit mal type. During seizure activity, Catherine usually stares and her expression is blank. Such episodes are usually a few seconds in duration, although, on a few occasions she has lost consciousness. Currently, her seizures are controlled through medication. At times, Catherine will become violent and strike other clients for no apparent reason. Her placement in a community residence is dependent upon control of this behavior. She has good self-help skills as evidenced on the AAMD Adaptive Behavior Scale.

Catherine's receptive vocabulary age is approximately 5 years as measured on the Peabody Picture Vocabulary Test. Although she can point to pictures named, she has difficulty explaining word meanings. Her equivalent receptive language age as measured by the Test of Auditory Comprehension of Language (TACL) is 4 years, 2 months. This score is corroborated by the Carrow Elicited Language Inventory. In this sentence imitation test, she received an age equivalent of 46 months. Her performance was characterized by sentence simplification, omission of articles, and difficulties with verb tensing and pronouns. On the TACL, she also made several errors in verb tensing and pronouns. A free sample analyzed using Miller's Assigning Structural Stage indicated that her language skills are primarily those found in Brown's stage IV. Her MLU is approximately 3.67. Language is primarily responsive and characterized by short sentences, a scarcity of complex or compound sentences, little use of pronouns beyond "you," "me," "he," "she," and "him," and absence of tensing markers. Some auxiliary verbs and modals are present, but there is some confusion with the verb "to be." Most sentences are simple declaratives or negatives.

In the vocational training program, Catherine's communication behavior is mostly responsive, although staff report that she also exhibits perseverative verbal behavior. While in vocational training, she will continually repeat instructions she has been given or statements made to her. This behavior is whispered but still annoys others around her. Staff report that it is difficult to stop this behavior.

Catherine is seen by the speech-language pathologist twice weekly for individual programming and once a week for group training. Within the individual sessions, the speech-language pathologist works primarily on verb tensing, focusing on the regular and irregular past and the future tense. Once a correct response is given, the speech-language pathologist attempts to gain a longer verbalization. Group work attempts to encourage initiation of conversation and use of longer utterances. In her vocational training program, Catherine is expected by the staff to provide longer responses in conversation. A questioning technique is used to elicit expansions of previous utterances. In addition, she is reinforced for short periods without perseverative whispering.

STUDY QUESTIONS

1. What is the AAMD definition of mental retardation? Explain each portion of this definition.
2. How does cognitive functioning of the retarded population differ from that of the nonretarded population? How might these differences relate to overall intervention considerations?
3. Compare all aspects of the language abilities of the retarded and nonretarded populations.
4. Explain the developmental model of intervention and its relation to language training with the retarded.
5. What are some of the targets for language intervention with the retarded population?

BIBLIOGRAPHY

Affleck, G. (1976). Role-taking ability and the interpersonal tactics of retarded children. *American Journal of Mental Deficiency, 80,* 667–670.

Affleck, G., Allen, D., McGrade, B., & McQueeney, M. (1982). Home environments of developmentally disabled infants as a function of parent and infant characteristics. *American Journal of Mental Deficiency, 86,* 445–452.

Ambron, S., & Irwin, D. (1975). Role-taking and moral judgement in 5- and 7-year olds. *Developmental Psychology, 11,* 102.

Archer, L. (1977). Blissymbolics—A nonverbal communication system. *Journal of Speech and Hearing Disorders, 42,* 568–579.

ASHA Ad Hoc Committee on Communication Processes and Nonspeaking Persons. (1980). Nonspeech communication: A position paper. *ASHA, 22,* 267–272.

Ashman, A. (1982). Coding, strategic behavior, and language performance of institutionalized mentally retarded young adults. *American Journal of Mental Deficiency, 86,* 627–636.

Baker, B. (1976). Parent involvement in programming for the developmentally disabled child. In L. Lloyd (Ed.), *Communication assessment and intervention.* Baltimore: University Park Press.

Balla, D., & Zigler, E. (1971). Luria's verbal deficiency theory of mental retardation and performance on sameness, symmetry and opposition tasks: A critique. *American Journal of Mental Deficiency, 75,* 400–413.

Balthazar, E., & Stevens, H. (1974). *The emotionally disturbed, mentally retarded: A historical and contemporary perspective.* Englewood Cliffs, NJ: Prentice-Hall.

Bangs, T. (1961). Evaluating children with language delay. *Journal of Speech and Hearing Disorders, 26,* 6–18.

Bartel, N., Bryen, D., & Keehn, S. (1973). Language comprehension in the moderately retarded child. *Exceptional Children, 40,* 375–382.

Bates, E., Benigni, L., Bretherton, I., Camaioni, L., & Volterra, V. (1977). From gesture to the first word: On cognitive and social prerequisites. In M. Lewis & L. Rosenblum (Eds.), *Interaction, conversation, and the development of language.* New York: Wiley.

Bates, E., Benigni, L., Bretherton, I., Camaioni, L., & Volterra, V. (1979). *The emergence of symbols: Cognition and communication in infancy.* New York: Academic Press.

Baumeister, A., & Kellas, G. (1968). Distribution of reaction times of retardates and normals. *American Journal of Mental Deficiency, 72,* 715–718.

Bedrosian, J., & Prutting, C. (1978). Communicative performance of mentally retarded adults in four conversational settings. *Journal of Speech and Hearing Research, 21,* 79–95.

Bee, H., Van Egeren, L., Streissguth, A., Nyman, B., & Leckie, M. (1969). Social class differences in maternal teaching strategies and speech patterns. *Developmental Psychology, 1,* 726–734.

Bellinger, D. (1980). Consistency in the pattern of change in mothers' speech: Some discriminant analysis. *Journal of Child Language, 7,* 469–487.

Belmont, J. (1967). Long-term memory in mental retardation. In N. Ellis (Ed.), *International review of research in mental retardation* (Vol. 1). New York: Academic Press.

Bender, N. & Carlson, J. (1982). Prosocial behavior and perspective-taking of mentally retarded and nonretarded children. *American Journal of Mental Deficiency, 86,* 361–366.

Berko, J. (1958). The child's learning of English morphology. *Word, 14,* 150–177.

Bilsky, L., Walker, N., & Sakales, S. (1983). Comprehension and recall of sentences by mentally retarded and nonretarded individuals. *American Journal of Mental Deficiency, 87,* 558–565.

Birch, H., Richardson, S., Baird, D., Horobin, G., & Illsley, R. (1970). *Mental subnormality in the community: A clinical and epidemiological study.* Baltimore: Williams & Wilkins.

Blacher, J. (1982). Assessing social cognition of young mentally retarded and nonretarded children. *American Journal of Mental Deficiency, 86,* 473–484.

Blodgett, E., & Miller, V. (1981). The facilitative language model. Paper presented at the American Speech-Language-Hearing Association Annual Convention, Los Angeles.

Bloom, L. (1970). *Language development: Form and function of emerging grammars.* Cambridge: MIT Press.

Bloom, L. (1973). *One word at a time: The use of single-word utterances before syntax.* The Hague: Mouton.

Borkowski, J., & Cavanaugh, J. (1979). Maintenance and generalization of skills and strategies by the retarded. In N. Ellis (Ed.), *Handbook of mental deficiency: Psychological theory and research.* Hillsdale, NJ: Lawrence Erlbaum.

Borkowski, J., & Wanschura, P. (1974). Mediational processes in the retarded. In N.R. Ellis (Ed.), *International review of research in mental retardation* (Vol. 7). New York: Academic Press.

Bottorf, L., & DePape, D. (1982). Initiating communication systems for severely speech-impaired persons. *Topics in Language Disorders, 2,* 55–72.

Bowerman, M. (1973). Structural relationships in children's utterances: Syntactic or semantic? In T. Moore (Ed.), *Cognitive development and the acquisition of language.* New York: Academic Press.

Bradbury, B., & Lunzer, E. (1972). The learning of grammatical inflections in normal and subnormal children. *Journal of Child Psychology and Psychiatry, 13,* 239–248.

Bray, N. (1979). Strategy production in the retarded. In N. Ellis (Ed.), *Handbook of mental deficiency: Psychological theory and research.* Hillsdale, NJ, Lawrence Erlbaum.

Bricker, W. (1970). Identifying and modifying deficits. *American Journal of Mental Deficiency, 75,* 16–21.

Bricker, D. (1972). Imitative sign training as a facilitator of word-object association with low-functioning children. *American Journal of Mental Deficiency, 76,* 509–516.

Bricker, W., & Bricker, D. (1970). A program of language training for the severely handicapped child. *Exceptional Children, 37,* 101–111.

Bricker, W., & Bricker, D. (1974). An early language training strategy. In R. Schiefelbusch & L. Lloyd (Eds.), *Language perspectives: Acquisition, retardation, and intervention.* Baltimore: University Park Press.

Bricker, W., Heal, L., Bricker, D., Hayes, W., & Larsen, L. (1969). Discrimination learning and learning set with institutionalized retarded children, *American Journal of Mental Deficiency, 74,* 242–248.

Brightman, R., Ambrose, S., & Baker, B. (1980). Parent training: A school-based model for enhancing teaching performance. *Child Behavior Therapy, 2,* 35–47.

Brooks, P., & Baumeister, A. (1977). A plea for consideration of ecological validity in the experimental psychology of mental retardation: A guest editorial. *American Journal of Mental Deficiency, 81,* 407–416.

Brophy, J. (1970). Mothers as teachers of their own preschool children: The influence of socioeconomic status and task structure on teaching specificity. *Child Development, 41,* 79–94.

Brown, A. (1974). The role of strategic behavior in retardate memory. In N. Ellis (Ed.), *International Review of Research in Mental Retardation* (Vol. 7). New York: Academic Press.

Brown, A. (1978). Knowing when, where, and how to remember: A problem in meta cognition. In R. Glaser (Ed.), *Advances in instructional psychology.* Hillsdale, NJ: Lawrence Erlbaum.

Brown, A., Campione, J., & Barclay, C. (1979). Training self-checking routines for estimating test readiness: Generalization from list learning to prose recall, *Child Development, 50,* 501–512.

Brown, A., Campione, J., & Murphy, M. (1974). Keeping track of changing variables: Long-term retention of a trained rehearsal strategy by retarded adolescents. *American Journal of Mental Deficiency, 78,* 446–453.

Brown, R. (1973). *First language: The early stages.* Cambridge: Harvard University Press.

Bruner, J. (1974/1975). From communication to language—A psychological perspective. *Cognition, 3,* 255–287.

Bruner, J. (1977). Early social interaction and language acquisition. In R. Schaffer (Ed.), *Studies in mother-infant interaction.* New York: Academic Press.

Bryan, T. (1977). LD children's comprehension of nonverbal communication. *Journal of Learning Disabilities, 10,* 501–507.

Buckhalt, J., Rutherford, R., & Goldberg, K. (1978). Verbal and nonverbal interaction of mothers with their Down's syndrome and nonretarded infants. *American Journal of Mental Deficiency, 82,* 337–343.

Buium, N. (1975). Interrogative types in parental speech to language-learning children: A linguistic universal? *Journal of Psycholinguistic Research, 5,* 135–142.

Buium, N., Rynders, J., & Turnure, J. (1974). Early maternal linguistic environment of normal and Down's syndrome language-learning children. *American Journal of Mental Deficiency, 79,* 52–58.

Bullowa, M. (Ed.) (1979). *Before speech: The beginning of interpersonal communication.* New York: Cambridge University Press.

Burger, A., Blackman, L., & Clark, H. (1981). Generalization of verbal abstraction strategies by EMR children and adolescents. *American Journal of Mental Deficiency, 85,* 611–618.

Burger, A., Blackman, L., Clark, H., & Reis, E. (1982). Effects of hypothesis testing and variable format training on generalization of a verbal abstraction strategy by EMR learners. *American Journal of Mental Deficiency, 86,* 405–413.

Burger, A., Blackman, L., Holmes, M., & Zetlin, A. (1978). Use of active sorting and retrieval strategies as a facilitator of recall, clustering, and sorting by EMR and nonretarded children. *American Journal of Mental Deficiency, 83,* 253–261.

Burger, A, Blackman, L., & Tan, N. (1980). Maintenance and generalization of a sorting and retrieval strategy by EMR and nonretarded individuals. *American Journal of Mental Deficiency, 84,* 373–380.

Burggraf, A. (1972). *Sign language as a verbal facilitator with mentally retarded children.* Master's thesis, Ohio State University, Columbus.

Burke, L., Lepre, C., & Owens, R. The use of language facilitators with residential retarded populations. (Study in progress).

Burr, D., & Rohr, A. (1978). Patterns of psycholinguistic development in the severely mentally retarded: A hypothesis. *Social Biology, 25,* 15–22.

Butterfield, E., & Belmont, J. (1978). Assessing and improving the cognitive functions of mentally retarded people. In I. Bialer & M. Sternlicht (Eds.), *The psychology of mental retardation: Issues and approaches.* New York: Psychological Dimensions.

Butterfield, E., Wambold, C., & Belmont, J. (1973). On the theory and practice of improving short-term memory. *American Journal of Mental Deficiency, 77,* 654–669.

Byers, P., & Byers, H. (1972). Nonverbal communication and the education of children. In C. Cazden, J. Hymes, & D. Hymes (Eds.), *Functions of language in the classroom.* New York: Teachers College Press.

Bzoch, K., and League, R. (1971). *Assessing language skills in infancy.* Baltimore: University Park Press.

Bzoch, K., & League, R. (1970). *The receptive-expressive emergent language scale.* Gainesville, FL: Tree of Life Press.

Calculator, S., & Luchko, C. (1983). Evaluating the effectiveness of a communication board training program. *Journal of Speech and Hearing Disorders, 48,* 185–191.

Campione, J., & Brown, A. (1977). Memory and metamemory development in educable retarded children. In R. Kail & J. Hagen (Eds.), *Perspectives on the development of memory and cognition.* Hillsdale, NJ: Lawrence Erlbaum.

Carrow, E. (1973). *Test for auditory comprehension of language.* Austin, TX: Urban Research Group.

Case, R. (1978). Intellectual development from birth to adulthood: A neo-Piagetian interpretation. In R. Siegler (Ed.), *Children's thinking: What develops?* Hillsdale, NJ: Lawrence Erlbaum.

Cegelka, P., & Prehm, H. (1982). *Mental retardation: From categories to people.* Columbus, OH: Charles E. Merrill.

Chafe, W. (1970). *Meaning and the structure of language.* Chicago: University of Chicago Press.

Chandler, M., Greenspan, S., & Barenboim, C. (1974). Assessment and training of role-taking and referential communication skills in institutionalized emotionally disturbed children. *Developmental Psychology, 10,* 546–553.

Chaney, R., Eyman, R., & Miller, C. (1979). Comparison of respiratory mortality in the profoundly mentally retarded and the less retarded. *Journal of Mental Deficiency Research, 23,* 107.

Chapman, R., & Miller, J. (1980). Analyzing language and communication in the child. In R. Schiefelbusch (Ed.), *Nonspeech language and communication: Analysis and intervention.* Baltimore: University Park Press.

Cheseldine, S., & McConkey, R. (1979). Parental speech to young Down's syndrome children: An intervention study. *American Journal of Mental Deficiency, 83,* 612–620.

Church, J. (1971). Methods for the study of early cognitive functioning. In R. Huxley & E. Ingram (Eds.), *Language acquisition: Models and methods.* New York: Academic Press.

Clark, C. (1981). Learning words using traditional orthography and the symbols of Rebus, Bliss, and Carrier. *Journal of Speech and Hearing Disorders, 46,* 191–196.

Clark, D., Baker, B., & Heifetz, L. (1982). Behavioral training for parents of mentally retarded children: Prediction of outcome. *American Journal of Mental Deficiency, 87,* 14–19.

Coleman, C., Cook, A., & Myers, L. (1980). Assessng non-oral clients for assistive communication devices. *Journal of Speech and Hearing Disorders, 45,* 515–526.

Connor, F., Williamson, G., & Siepp, J. (1978). *Program guide for infants and toddlers with neuromotor and other developmental disabilities.* New York: Teachers College Press.

Conroy, J., Efthimiou, J., & Lemanowicz, J. (1982). A matched comparison of the developmental growth of institutionalized and deinstitutionalized mentally retarded clients. *American Journal of Mental Deficiency, 86,* 581–587.

Cook, D., & Seymour, H. (1980). A comparison among three language elicitation procedures. Paper presented at the American Speech-Language-Hearing Association Convention, Detroit.

Corrigan, R. (1978). Language development as related to stage 6 object permanence development. *Journal of Child Language, 5,* 173–189.

Culatta, B., & Horn, D. (1981). Systematic modification of parental input to train language symbols. *Language, Speech, and Hearing Services in the Schools, 12,* 4–12.

Cummins, J. (1979). Language functions and cognitive processing. In J. Das, J. Kirby, & R. Jarman (Eds.), *Simultaneous and successive cognitive processes.* New York: Academic Press.

Cummins, J., & Das, J. (1978). Simultaneous and successive synthesis and linguistic processes. *International Journal of Psychology, 13,* 129–138.

Dance, F. (1967). Toward a theory of human communication. In F. Dance (Ed.), *Human communication theory: Original essays.* New York: Holt, Rinehart, & Winston.

Daniloff, J., Lloyd, L., & Fristoe, M. (1983). Amer-Ind transparency. *Journal of Speech and Hearing Disorders, 48,* 103–110.

Das, J. (1972). Patterns of cognitive ability in nonretarded and retarded children. *American Journal of Mental Deficiency, 77,* 6–12.

Das, J., Kirby, J., & Jarman, R. (1979). *Simultaneous and successive cognitive processes.* New York: Academic Press.

Das, J., Kirby, J., & Jarman, R. (1975). Simultaneous and successive synthesis: An alternative model for cognitive abilities. *Psychological Bulletin, 80,* 97–113.

Detterman, D. (1979). Memory in the mentally retarded. In N. Ellis (Ed.), *Handbook of mental deficiency: Psychological theory and research.* Hillsdale, NJ: Lawrence Erlbaum.

Dever, R. (1978). *TALK—Teaching the American language to kids.* Columbus, OH: Charles E. Merrill.

Dever, R., & Gardner, W. (1970). Performance of normal and retarded boys on Berko's test of morphology. *Language and Speech, 13,* 162–181.

Dihoff, R., & Chapman, R. (1977). First words: Their origin in action. *Papers and Reports in Child Language Development, 13,* 1–7.

Doll, E. (1965). *Vineland Social Maturity Scale.* Circle Pines, Minnesota: American Guidance Service.

Dore, J. (1974). A pragmatic description of early language development. *Journal of Psycholinguistic Research, 3,* 343–350.

Duhammel, T., Lin, S., Skelton, A., & Hantke, L. (1974). Early parental perceptions and the high risk neonate. *Clinical Pediatrics, 13,* 1052–1056.

Dunn, L., & Dunn, L.M. (1981). *Peabody picture vocabulary test.* MN: American Guidance Service.

Dwinell, M., & Connis, R. (1979). Reducing inappropriate verbalizations of a retarded adult. *American Journal of Mental Deficiency, 84,* 87–92.

Eheart, B. (1982). Mother-child interactions with nonretarded and mentally retarded preschoolers. *American Journal of Mental Deficiency, 87,* 20–25.

Ellis, N. (1963). Stimulus trace and behavioral inadequacy. In N. Ellis (Ed.), *Handbook of mental deficiency.* New York: McGraw-Hill.

Ellis, N. (1970). Memory processes in retardates and normals. In N. Ellis (Ed.), *International review of research in mental retardation* (Vol. 4). New York: Academic Press.

Ellis, N., Deacon, J., Harris, L., Poor, A., Angers, D., Diorio, M., Watkins, R., Boyd, B., & Cavalier, A. (1982). Learning, memory, and transfer in profoundly, severely, and moderately mentally retarded persons. *American Journal of Mental Deficiency, 87,* 186–196.

Emery, G., & Ramey, C. (1976). Maternal teaching styles as a function of mothers' level of education. Paper presented at fourth biennial Southeastern Conference on Human Development.

Engle, R., & Nagle, R. (1979). Strategy training and semantic encoding in mildly retarded children. *Intelligence, 3,* 17–30.

Ervin-Tripp, S. (1973). Some strategies for the first two years. In T. Moore (Ed.), *Cognitive development and the acquisition of language.* New York: Academic Press.

Evans, D. (1977). The development of language abilities in Mongols: A correlational study. *Journal of Mental Deficiency Research, 21,* 103–117.

Evans, R., & Bilsky, L. (1979). Clustering and categorical list retention in the mentally retarded. In N. Ellis (Ed.), *Handbook of mental deficiency: Psychological theory and research.* Hillsdale, NJ: Lawrence Erlbaum.

Field, T. (Ed.) (1979). *Infants born at risk: Behavior and development.* New York: Spectrum.

Fisher, M., and Zeaman, D. (1970). Growth and decline of retardate intelligence. In N. Ellis (Ed.), *International Review of Research in Mental Retardation, Vol. IV.* New York: Academic Press.

Fisher, M., and Zeaman, D. (1973). An attention-retention theory of retardate discrimination learning. In N. Ellis (Ed.), *International Review of Research in Mental Retardation, Vol. VI.* New York: Academic Press.

Forehand, R., & Atkeson, B. (1977). Generality of treatment effects with parents as therapists: A review of assessment and implementation procedures. *Behavior Therapy, 8,* 575–593.

Fraiberg, S. (1979). Blind infants and their mothers: An examination of the sign system. In M. Bullowa (Ed.), *Before speech.* New York: Cambridge University Press.

Frank, H., & Rabinovitch, M. (1974). Auditory short-term memory: Developmental changes in rehearsal. *Child Development, 45,* 397–407.

Fristoe, M., & Lloyd, L. (1980). Planning an initial expressive sign lexicon for persons with severe communication impairment. *Journal of Speech and Hearing Disorders, 45,* 170–180.

Giattinno, J., Pollack, E., & Silliman, E. (1978). Adult input in language impaired children. Paper presented at the American Speech and Hearing Association Annual Convention, San Francisco.

Glidden, L. (1977). Stimulus relations, blocking, and sorting in the free recall and organization of EMR adolescents. *American Journal of Mental Deficiency, 82,* 250–258.

Goldberg, S. (1977). Social competence in infancy: A model of parent-infant interaction. *Merrill-Palmer Quarterly, 23,* 163–177.

Goossens, C. (1984). Assessment for nonspeech. Paper presented at the annual conference of American Association on Mental Deficiency, Minneapolis, MN.

Graham, J., & Graham, L. (1971). Language behavior of the mentally retarded: Syntactic characteristics. *American Journal of Mental Deficiency, 73,* 623–629.

Greenfield, P., & Smith, J. (1976). *The structure of communication in early language development.* New York: Academic Press.

Greenspan, S. (1979). Social intelligence in the retarded. In N. Ellis (Ed.), *Handbook of mental deficiency: Psychological theory and research.* Hillsdale, NJ: Lawrence Erlbaum.

Greenwald, C., & Leonard, L. (1979). Communicative and sensorimotor development of Down's syndrome children. *American Journal of Mental Deficiency, 84,* 296–303.

Grossman, H. (1983). *Classification in mental retardation.* Washington, DC: American Association on Mental Deficiency.

Guess, D., Koegh, W., & Sailor, W. (1978). Generalization of speech and language behavior: Measurement and training tactics. In R. Schiefelbusch (Ed.), *Bases of language intervention.* Baltimore: University Park Press.

Guess, D., Sailor, W., & Baer, D. (1976). *Functional speech and language training for the severely handicapped.* Lawrence, KS: H and H Enterprises.

Gutmann, A., & Rondal, J. (1979). Verbal operants in mothers' speech to nonretarded and Down's syndrome children matched for linguistic level. *American Journal of Mental Deficiency, 83,* 446–452.

Halliday, M. (1975). *Learning how to mean: Explorations in the development of language.* New York: Edward Arnold.

Hanley-Maxwell, C., Wilcox, B., & Heal, L. (1982). A comparison of vocabulary learning by moderately retarded students under direct instruction and incidental presentation. *Education and Training of Mentally Retarded, 3,* 214–221.

Hanna, R., Lippert, E., & Harris, A. (1982). *Developmental communication curriculum.* Columbus, OH: Charles E. Merrill.

Hargis, K., & Blechman, E. (1979). Social class and training of parents as behavior change agents. *Child Behavior Therapy, 1,* 69–74.

Haring, N., & Bricker, D. (1976). Overview of comprehensive services for the severely/profoundly handicapped. In N. Haring & L. Brown (Eds.), *Teaching the severely handicapped.* New York: Grune & Stratton.

Harris, D. (1982). Communicative interaction processes involving nonvocal physically handicapped children. *Topics in Language Disorders, 2,* 21–38.

Harris-Vanderheiden, D., Brown, W., MacKenzie, P., Reinen, S., & Scheibel, C. (1975). Symbol communication for the mentally handicapped. *Mental Retardation, 13,* 34–37.

Hayes, C., & Koch, R. (1972). Interpersonal distance behavior of mentally retarded and nonretarded children. *American Journal of Mental Deficiency, 82,* 207–209.

Heifetz, L. (1980). From consumer to middleman: Emerging roles for parents in the network of services for retarded children. In R. Abidin (Ed.), *Parent education and intervention handbook.* Springfield, IL: Charles Thomas.

Hess, R., & Shipman, V. (1965). Early experience and the socialization of cognitive modes in children. *Child Development, 36,* 886–896.

Hockey, R. (1973). Rate of presentation in running memory and direct manipulation of input processing strategies. *Quarterly Journal of Experimental Psychology, 25,* 104–111.

Hogg, J. (1975). Normative development and educational program plannng for severely educationally subnormal children. In C. Kiennan & F. Woodford (Eds.), *Behavior modification with the severely retarded.* Amsterdam, The Netherlands: Associated Scientific Publishers.

Horstmeier, D., & MacDonald, J. (1978). *Ready, set, go—talk to me.* Columbus, OH: Charles E. Merrill.

Hoy, E., & McKnight, J. (1977). Communication style and effectiveness in homogeneous and heterogeneous dyads of retarded children. *American Journal of Mental Deficiency, 81,* 587–598.

Humphreys, L., & Parsons, C. (1979). Piagetian tasks measure intelligence and intelligence tests assess cognitive development: A reanalysis. *Intelligence, 3,* 369–382.

Hunt, N. (1967). *The world of Nigel Hunt: The diary of a mongoloid youth.* New York: Garret.

Ingram, D. (1972). Transivity in child language. *Language, 47,* 888–910.

Ingram, D. (1975). The acquisition of fricatives and affricatives in normal and linguistically deviant children. In A. Carramazza & E. Zuriff (Eds.), *The acquisition and breakdown of language.* Baltimore: Johns Hopkins University Press.

Ingram, D. (1976). *Phonological Disability in Children.* London: Edward Arnold.

James, S. (1980). Language and sensorimotor cognitive development in the young child. Paper presented at the New York Speech-Language-Hearing Association convention.

Jarman, R. (1978). Patterns of cognitive ability in retarded children: A reexamination. *American Journal of Mental Deficiency, 82,* 344–348.

Jarman, R., & Das, J. (1977). Simultaneous and successive synthesis and intelligence. *Intelligence, 1,* 151–169.

Johnston, J., & Schery, T. (1976). The use of grammatical morphemes by children with communication disorders. In D. Morehead & A. Morehead (Eds.), *Normal and deficient child language.* Baltimore: University Park Press.

Jones, O. (1977). Mother-child communication with prelinguistic Down's syndrome and normal infants. In H. Schaffer (Eds.), *Studies in mother-infant interaction.* New York: Academic Press.

Jones, P. (1972). Home environment and the development of verbal ability. *Child Development, 43,* 1081–1086.

Kahn, J. (1975). Relationship of Piaget's sensorimotor period to language acquisition of profoundly retarded children. *American Journal of Mental Deficiency, 79,* 640–643.

Kahn, J. (1977). A comparison of manual and oral language training. *Mental Retardation, 15,* 21–23.

Kamhi, A. (1981). Developmental vs. different theories of mental retardation: A new look. *American Journal of Mental Deficiency, 86,* 1–7.

Karrer, R., Nelson, M., & Galbraith, G. (1979). Psychophysiological research with the mentally retarded. In N. Ellis (Ed.), *International Review of Research in Mental Retardation* (Vol. 7). New York: Academic Press.

Kearsley, R. (1979). Iatrogenic retardation: A syndrome of learned incompetence. In R. Kearsley & I. Sigel (Eds.), *Infants at risk: Assessment of cognitive functioning.* Hillsdale, NJ: Lawrence Erlbaum.

Kellas, G., Ashcroft, M., & Johnson, N. (1973). Rehearsal processes in the short-term memory performance of mildly retarded adolescents. *American Journal of Mental Deficiency, 77,* 670–679.

Kendall, C., Barkowski, J., & Cavanaugh, J. (1980). Maintenance and generalization of an interrogative strategy by EMR children. *Intelligence, 4,* 255–270.

Kintsch, W., & van Dijk, T. (1978). Toward a model of text comprehension and productions. *Psychological Review, 85,* 363–394.

Kirk, S., McCarthy, J., & Winifred, K. (1968). *Illinois test of psycholinguistic abilities.* Urbana: University of Illinois Press.

Klaus, M., & Kennell, J. (1976). *Maternal-infant bonding.* St. Louis: Mosby.

Kogan, K., Wimberger, H., & Bobbitt, R. (1969). Analysis of mother-child interaction in young mental retardates. *Child Development, 40,* 799–812.

Kohl, F. (1981). Effects of motoric requirements on the acquisition of manual sign responses by severely handicapped students. *American Journal of Mental Deficiency, 85,* 396–403.

Kohl, F., Karlan, G., & Heal, L. (1979). Effects of pairing manual signs with verbal cues upon the acquisition of instruction-following behaviors and the generalization to expressive language with severely handicapped students. *AAESPH Review, 4,* 291–300.

Konstantases, M., Oxman, J., & Webster, C. (1977). Simultaneous communication with autistic and other severely dysfunctional nonverbal children. *Journal of Communication Disorders, 10,* 267–282.

Kozloff, M. (1977). A comprehensive training program for parents of autistic children. In D. Upper (Ed.), *Perspectives in behavior therapy.* Kalamazoo, MI: Behaviordelia.

Kozloff, M. (1979). *A program for families of children with learning and behavior problems.* New York: Wiley.

Krupski, A. (1977). Role of attention in the reaction-time performance of mentally retarded adolescents. *American Journal of Mental Deficiency, 82,* 79–83.

Lackner, J. (1968). A developmental study of language behavior in retarded children. *Neuropsychologia, 6,* 301–320.

LaGreca, A., Stone, W., & Bell, C. (1983). Facilitating the vocational-interpersonal skills of mentally retarded individuals. *American Journal of Mental Deficiency, 88,* 270–278.

Lamberts, F. (1981). Sign and symbol in children's processing of familiar auditory stimuli. *American Journal of Mental Deficiency, 86,* 300–308.

Layton, T., & Sharifi, H. (1979). Meaning and structure of Down's syndrome and nonretarded children's spontaneous speech, *American Journal of Mental Deficiency, 83,* 439–445.

Leahy, R., Balla, D. & Zigler, E. (1982). Role-taking, self-image, and imitativeness of mentally retarded and nonretarded individuals. *American Journal of Mental Deficiency, 86,* 372–379.

Lee, L. (1974). *Developmental sentence analysis.* Evanston, IL: Northwestern University Press.

Leonard, L., Cole, B., & Steckol, K. (1979). Lexical usage of retarded children: An examination of informativeness. *American Journal of Mental Deficiency, 84,* 49–54.

Leonard, L., Miller, J., & Brown, H. (1980). Consonant and syllable harmony in the speech of language-disordered children. *Journal of Speech and Hearing Disorders, 45,* 336–345.

Leonard, L., Steckol, K., & Panther, K. (1983). Returning meaning to semantic relations: Some clinical applications. *Journal of Speech and Hearing Disorders, 48,* 25–35.

Letlin, A., & Gallimore, R. (1983). The development of comprehension strategies through the regulatory function of teacher questions. *Education and Training of Mentally Retarded, 18,* 176–183.

Liebert, A., & Baumeister, A. (1973). Behavioral variability among retardates, children, and college students. *The Journal of Psychology, 83,* 57–65.

Lobato, D., Berrera, R., & Feldman, R. (1981). Sensorimotor functioning and prelinguistic communication of severely and profoundly mentally retarded individuals. *American Journal of Mental Deficiency, 85,* 489–496.

Lobb, H. (1974). Effects of verbal rehearsal on discrimination learning in moderately retarded nursery-school children. *American Journal of Mental Deficiency, 79,* 449–454.

Longhurst, T., & Berry, G. (1975). Communication in retarded adolescents: Response to listener feedback. *American Journal of Mental Deficiency, 80,* 158–164.

Looney, P. (1980). Instructional intervention with language-disordered learners, *Directive Teacher, 2,* 30–31.

Lovell, K. (1968). Some recent studies in cognitive and language development, *Merrill-Palmer Quarterly, 14,* 123–138.

Luftig, R., & Johnson, R. (1982). Identification and recall of structurally important units in prose of mentally retarded learners. *American Journal of Mental Deficiency, 86,* 495–502.

Luria, A. (1975). Basic problems of language in the light of psychology and neurolinguistics. In E. Lenneberg & E. Lenneberg (Eds.), *Foundations of language development: A multidisciplinary approach.* New York: Academic Press.

MacDonald, J. (1978). *Environmental language intervention program.* Columbus, OH: Charles E. Merrill.

MacDonald, J., Blott, J., Gordon, K., Spiegal, B., & Hartmann, M. (1974). An experimental parent-assisted treatment program for preschool language-delayed children. *Journal of Speech and Hearing Disorders, 39,* 295–415.

MacDonald, J., & Gillette, Y. (1982). *ECO, ecological communication system: A clinical handbook for parents and teachers.* Columbus, OH: Nisonger Center.

MacMillan, D. (1972). Paired-associate learning as a function of explicitness of mediational set by EMR and nonretarded children. *American Journal of Mental Deficiency, 76,* 686–691.

Macnamara, J. (1972). Cognitive basis of language learning in infants. *Psychological Review, 79,* 1–13.

Mahoney, G., Glover, A., & Finger, I. (1981). Relationship between language and sensorimotor development of Down syndrome and nonretarded children. *American Journal of Mental Deficiency, 86,* 21–27.

Malgady, R., Barcher, P., Towner, G., & Davis, J. (1979). Language factors in vocational evaluation of mentally retarded workers. *American Journal of Mental Deficiency, 83,* 432–438.

Manolson, A. (1983). *It takes two to talk.* Toronto: Hanen Early Language Resource Centre.

Marcell, M., & Armstrong, V. (1982). Auditory and visual sequential memory of Down syndrome and nonretarded children. *American Journal of Mental Deficiency, 87,* 86–95.

Marshall, N., Hegrenes, J., & Goldstein, S. (1973). Verbal interactions: Mothers and their retarded children vs. mothers and their nonretarded children. *American Journal of Mental Deficiency, 77,* 415–419.

McCarver, R. & Craig, E. (1974). Placement of the retarded in the community: Prognosis and outcome. In N. Ellis (Ed.), *International review of research in mental retardation* (Vol. 7). New York: Academic Press.

McDonald, E. (1980). Early identification and treatment of children at risk for speech development. In R. Schiefelbusch (Ed.), *Nonspeech language and communication: Analysis and intervention.* Baltimore: University Park Press.

McLean, J., & Snyder-McLean, L. (1978). *A transactional approach to early language training.* Columbus, OH: Charles E. Merrill.

McLeavey, B., Toomey, J., & Dempsey, P. (1982). Nonretarded and mentally retarded children's control over syntactic structures. *American Journal of Mental Deficiency, 86,* 485–494.

McNutt, J., & Leri, S. (1979). Language differences between institutionalized and noninstitutionalized retarded children. *American Journal of Mental Deficiency, 83,* 339–345.

Meacham, M.J., & Jones, D. (1967). *Utah test of language development.* Utah: Communication Research.

Mehrabian, A., & Williams, M. (1971). Piagetian measures of cognitive development for children up to age two. *Journal of Psycholinguistic Research, 1,* 113–126.

Menyuk, P. (1974). Early development of receptive language: From babbling to words. In R. Schiefelbusch & L. Lloyd (Eds.), *Language perspectives—Acquisition, retardation and intervention.* Baltimore: University Park Press.

Mercer, C., & Snell, M. (1977). *Learning theory research in mental retardation.* Columbus, OH: Charles E. Merrill.

Miller, A., & Miller, F. (1973). Cognitive developmental training with elevated boards and sign language. *Journal of Autism and Childhood Schizophrenia, 3,* 65–68.

Miller, J. (1980). *Assessing language production in children.* Baltimore: University Park Press.

Miller, J., & Yoder, D. (1974). An ontogentic language teaching strategy for retarded children. In R. Schiefelbusch & L. Lloyd (Eds.), *Language perspectives—Acquisition, retardation, and intervention.* Baltimore: University Park Press.

Miller, S., & Sloan, H. (1976). The generalization effects of parent training across stimulus settings. *Journal of Applied Behavior Analysis, 9,* 355–370.

Millett, A., & Newhoff, M. (1978). Language disordered children: Language disordered mothers? Paper presented at the American Speech and Hearing Association Annual Conference. San Francisco.

Mindell, C., & Budd, K. (1977). Issues in the generalization of parent training across settings. Paper presented at the annual meeting of the American Psychological Association.

Mittler, P. (1974). Language and communication. In A. Clarke & A. Clarke (Eds.), *Mental deficiency: The changing outlook.* London: Methuen.

Mittler, P. (1976). Assessment for language learning. In P. Berry (Ed.), *Language and communication in the mentally handicapped.* Baltimore: University Park Press.

Montague, J., Hutchinson, E., & Matson, E. (1975). Comparative computer content analysis of the verbal behavior of institutionalized and noninstitutionalized retarded children. *Journal of Speech and Hearing Research, 18,* 43–57.

Morehead, D. (1972). Early grammatical and semantic relations: Some implications for a general representational deficit in linguistically deviant children. *Papers and Reports of Child Language Development, 4,* 1–12.

Muma, J. (1978). *Language handbook: Concepts, assessment, intervention.* Englewood Cliffs, NJ: Prentice-Hall.

Musselwhite, C., & St. Louis, K. (1982). *Communication programming for the severely handicapped: Vocal and non-vocal strategies.* Houston: College-Hill Press.

Naremore, R., & Dever, R. (1975). Language performance of educable mentally retarded and normal children at five age levels. *Journal of Speech and Hearing Research, 18,* 82–95.

Nelson, K. (1973). Structure and strategy in learning to talk. *Monograph of the Society for Research in Child Development, 38.*

Newfield, M. (1966). A study of the acquisition of English morphology by normal and EMR children. Master's thesis, Ohio State University, Columbus.

Newfield, M., & Schlanger, B. (1968). The acquisition of English morphology in normal and educable mentally retarded children. *Journal of Speech and Hearing Research, 11,* 693–706.

O'Connor, N., & Hermelin, B. (1978). *Seeing and hearing and space and time.* New York: Academic Press.

O'Regan-Kleinert, J. (1980). Pre-speech/language therapeutic techniques for the handicapped infant. Paper presented at the American Speech-Language-Hearing Association Convention, Detroit.

O'Regan-Kleinert, J., Rosenwinkel, P., & Robbins, R. (1979). Remediation of severe language disorders: A pre-speech sensorimotor developmental model. Paper presented at the American Speech-Language-Hearing Association Convention, Atlanta.

Osofsky, J., & O'Connell, E. (1972). Daughter's effects upon mother's and father's behavior. *Developmental Psychology, 7,* 157–168.

Owens, R. (1982). *Program for the acquisition of language with the severely impaired (PALS).* Columbus, OH: Charles E. Merrill.

Owens, R. (1984). *Language development: An introduction.* Columbus, OH: Charles E. Merrill.

Owens, R., & House, L. (1984). Decision-making processes in augmentative communication. *Journal of Speech and Hearing Disorders, 49,* 18–25.

Owens, R., & MacDonald, J. (1982). Communicative uses of the early speech of nondelayed and Down syndrome children. *American Journal of Mental Deficiency, 86,* 503–510.

Owings, N., & Guyette, T. (1982). Communication behavior assessment and treatment with the adult retarded: An approach. In N. Lass (Ed.), *Speech and language: Advances in basic research and practice* (Vol. 7). New York: Academic Press.

Papania, N. (1954). A qualitative analysis of vocabulary responses of institutionalized mentally retarded children. *Journal of Clinical Psychology, 10,* 361–365.

Petersen, G., & Sherrod, K. (1982). Relationship of maternal language to language development and language delay of children. *American Journal of Mental Deficiency, 86,* 391–398.

Phillips, I., & Williams, N. (1975). Psychopathology and mental retardation: I. Psychopathology. *American Journal of Psychiatry, 132,* 1265–1271.

Phillips, J., & Balthazar, E. (1979). Some correlates of language deterioration in severely and profoundly retarded long-term institutionalized residents. *American Journal of Mental Deficiency, 83,* 402–408.

Piaget, J. (1954). *The construction of reality in the child.* New York: Basic Books.

Pickett, J., & Flynn, P. (1983). Language assessment tools for mentally retarded adults: Survey and recommendations. *American Journal of Mental Deficiency, 21,* 244–247.

Polk, X., Schilmoeller, G., Embry, L., Holman, J., & Baer, D. (1976). Prompted generalization through experimenters' instructions: A parent training study. Paper presented at the annual meeting of the Midwestern Association of Behavior Analysis.

Prater, R. (1982). Functions of consonant assimilation and reduplication in early word productions of mentally retarded children. *American Journal of Mental Deficiency, 86,* 399–404.

Prior, M., Minnes, P., Coyne, T., Golding, B., Hendy, J., & McGillivray, J. (1979). Verbal interactions between staff and residents in an institution for the young mentally retarded. *Mental Retardation, 17,* 65–70.

Prutting, C. (1979). Process: The action of moving forward progressively from one point to another on the way to completion. *Journal of Speech and Hearing Disorders, 44,* 3–30.

Realon, R., Lewallen, J., & Wheeler, A. (1983). Verbal vs. verbal feedback plus praise: The effects on direct care staff's training behaviors. *Mental Retardation, 21,* 209–213.

Rees, N. (1978). Pragmatics of language: Applications to normal and disordered language development. In R. Schiefelbusch (Ed.), *Bases of language intervention.* Baltimore: University Park Press.

Rees, N. & Wellner, S. (1981). Toward a taxonomy of pragmatic abilities in children. Paper presented at the ASHA Northeast Regional Conference, Philadelphia.

Reich, R. (1978). Gestural facilitation of expressive language in moderately/severe retarded preschoolers. *Mental Retardation, 16,* 113–117.

Reid, B., & Kiernan, C. (1979). Spoken words and manual signs as encoding categories in short-term memory for mentally retarded children. *American Journal of Mental Deficiency, 84,* 200–203.

Reid, G. (1980). Overt and covert rehearsal in short-term motor memory of mentally retarded and non-retarded persons. *American Journal of Mental Deficiency, 85,* 69–77.

Reiss, S., Levitan, G., & Szyszko, J. (1982). Emotional disturbance and mental retardation: Diagnostic overshadowing. *American Journal of Mental Deficiency, 86,* 567–574.

Reiter, S., & Levi, A. (1980). Factors affecting social integration of noninstitutionalized mentally retarded adults. *American Journal of Mental Deficiency, 85,* 25–30.

Rheingold, H., & Eckerman, C. (1975). Some properties for unifying the study of social development. In M. Lewis & M. Rosenblum (Eds.), *Friendship and peer relations.* New York: Wiley.

Rice, M. (1983). Contemporary accounts of the cognition/language relationship: Implications for speech-language clinicians. *Journal of Speech and Hearing Disorders, 48,* 347–359.

Richmond, G., & Lewallen, J. (1983). Facilitating transfer of stimulus control when teaching verbal labels. *Education and Training of Mentally Retarded, 18,* 111–115.

Robinson, N., & Robinson, H. (1976). *The mentally retarded child: A psychological approach* (2nd ed.). New York: McGraw-Hill.

Rondal, J. (1976). *Maternal speech to normal and Down's syndrome children matched for mean length of utterance* (Research Report 98). BEH Contract No. 300–76–0036. Washington, DC.

Ross, D., & Ross, S. (1979). Cognitive training for the EMR child: Language skills prerequisite to relevant-irrelevant discrimination tasks. *Mental Retardation, 17,* 3–7.

Rushakoff, G., & Johnson, P. (1979). The use of published language tests with the mentally retarded: A national survey. Paper presented at the American Speech-Language-Hearing Association Convention, Atlanta, GA.

Russell, A., & Tanguay, P. (1981). Mental illness and mental retardation: Cause or coincidence? *American Journal of Mental Deficiency, 85,* 570–574.

Russo, J., & Owens, R. (1982). The development of an objective observational tool for parent-child interaction. *Journal of Speech and Hearing Disorders, 47,* 165–173.

Ryan, J. (1975). Mental subnormality and language development. In F. Lenneberg & E. Lenneberg (Eds.), *Foundations of language development* (Vol. 2). New York: Academic Press.

Salzberg, C., & Villani, T. (1983). Speech training by parents of Down syndrome toddlers: Generalization across settings and instructional contexts. *American Journal of Mental Deficiency, 87,* 403–413.

Schiefelbusch, R. (Ed.) (1963). Language studies in mentally retarded children. *Journal of Speech and Hearing Disorders, Monograph Supplement No. 10.*

Schlesinger, I. (1971a). Learning grammar: From pivot to realization rules. In R. Huxley & E. Ingram (Eds.), *Language acquisition: Models and methods.* New York: Academic Press.

Schlesinger, I. (1971b). Production of utterances and language acquisition. In D. Slobin (Ed.), *The otogenisis of grammar.* New York: Academic Press.

Seitz, S., & Riedel, G. (1974). Parent-child interactions as the therapy target. *Journal of Communication Disorders, 7,* 295–304.

Semmel, M. (1967). Language behavior of mentally retarded and culturally disadvantaged children. In J. Magary & R. McIntyre (Eds.), *Distinguished lectures in special education.* Berkeley: University of California Press.

Semmel, M., Barritt, L., & Bennett, S. (1970). Performance of EMR and non-retarded children on a modified cloze task. *American Journal of Mental Deficiency, 74,* 681–688.

Semmel, M., & Herzog, B. (1966). The effects of grammatical form class on the recall of Negro and Caucasian educable retarded children. *Studies of Language and Language Behavior, 3,* 1–9.

Shane, H., & Bashir, A. (1980). Election criteria for the adoption of an augmentative communication system: Preliminary considerations. *Journal of Speech and Hearing Disorders, 45,* 408–414.

Shane, H., Lipshultz, R., & Shane, C. (1982). Facilitating the communicative interaction of nonspeaking persons in large residential settings. *Topics in Language Disorders, 2,* 73–84.

Shane, H., & Wilbur, R. (1980). Potential for expressive signing based on motor control. *Sign Language Studies, 29,* 331–347.

Share, J. (1975). Developmental progress in Down's syndrome. In R. Koch & F. de laCruz (Eds.), *Down's syndrome.* New York: Bruner Mazel.

Shepard, G., & Marshall, J. (1976). Perceptions of interpersonal communication of EMR adolescents and their mothers. *Education and Training of Mentally Retarded, 11,* 106–111.

Siegel, G. (1975). The use of language tests. *Language, Speech & Hearing Services in the Schools, 6,* 211–217.

Silverman, F. (1980). *Communication for the speechless.* Englewood Cliffs, NJ: Prentice-Hall.

Simic, J., & Bucher, B. (1980). Development of spontaneous mending in language deficient children. *Journal of Applied Behavior Analysis, 13,* 523–528.

Sinclair, H. (1970). Transition from sensorimotor behavior to symbolic activity. *Interchange, 1,* 119–126.

Sinclair, H. (1971). Sensorimotor action patterns as a condition for the acquisition of syntax. In R. Huxley & E. Ingram (Eds.), *Language acquisition: Models and methods.* New York: Academic Press.

Skinner, B.F. (1957). *Verbal behavior.* New York: Appleton-Century-Crofts.

Slobin, D. (1970). Suggested universals in the ontogenis of grammar. *Language Behavior Research Laboratory: Working Paper, 32.*

Snart, F., O'Grady, M., & Das, J. (1982). Cognitive processing of subgroups of moderately mentally retarded children. *American Journal of Mental Deficiency, 86,* 465–472.

Snell, M. (1979). Higher functioning residents as language trainers of the mentally retarded. *Education and Training of Mentally Retarded, 14,* 77–84.

Snow, C., & Ferguson, C. (1977). *Talking to children.* New York: Cambridge University Press.

Snyder, L. (1978). Communicative and cognitive abilities and disabilities in the sensorimotor period. *Merrill-Palmer Quarterly, 24,* 161–180.

Sommers, R., & Starkey, K. (1977). Dichotic verbal processing in Down's syndrome children having qualitatively different speech and language skills. *American Journal of Mental Deficiency, 82,* 44–53.

Spiegel, B. (1983). The effect of context on language learning by severely retarded young adults. *Language, Speech & Hearing Services in Schools, 14.*

Spitz, H. (1966). The role of input organization in the learning and memory of mental retardates. In N. Ellis (Ed.), *International review of research in mental retardation* (Vol. 2). New York: Academic Press.

Spitz, H. (1979). Beyond field theory in the study of mental deficiency. In N. Ellis (Ed.), *Handbook of mental deficiency: Psychological theory and research.* Hillsdale, NJ: Lawrence Erlbaum.

Spradlin, J. (1963). Language and communication of mental defectives. In N. Ellis (Ed.), *Handbook of mental deficiency.* New York: McGraw-Hill.

Spradlin, J., & Siegel, G. (1982). Language training in natural and clinical environments. *Journal of Speech and Hearing Disorders, 47,* 2–6.

Stephens, B., & McLaughlin, J. (1974). Two-year gains in reasoning by retarded and nonretarded persons. *American Journal of Mental Deficiency, 79,* 116–126.

Stephens, W. (1972). Equivalence formation by retarded and nonretarded children at different mental ages. *American Journal of Mental Deficiency, 77,* 311–313.

Sternberg, L., Pegnatore, L., & Hill, C. (1983). Establishing interactive communication behaviors with profoundly mentally handicapped students. *TASH Journal, 8,* 39–46.

Stevenson, M., and Lamb, M. (1979). Effects of infant sociability and the caretaking environment on infant cognitive performance. *Child Development, 50,* 340–349.

Stoneman, Z., Brody, G., & Abbott, D. (1983). In-home observations of young Down syndrome children with their mothers and fathers. *American Journal of Mental Deficiency, 87,* 591–600.

Switsky, H., Rotatori, A., Miller, T., & Freagon, S. (1979). The developmental model and its implications for assessment and instruction for the severely/profoundly handicapped. *Mental Retardation, 17,* 167–170.

Szymanski, L., & Tanguay, P. (Eds.). (1980). *Emotional disorders of mentally retarded persons.* Baltimore: University Park Press.

Taenzer, S., Bass, M., & Kise, L. (1974). The young child, a language explorer: A Piagetian-based approach to language therapy. Paper presented to the American Speech & Hearing Association, Las Vegas.

Taylor, A., & Turnure, J. (1979). Imagery and verbal elaboration with retarded children: Effects on learning and memory. In N. Ellis (Ed.), *Handbook of mental deficiency: Psychological theory and research.* Hillsdale, NJ: Lawrence Erlbaum.

Tizard, B., Cooperman, O., Joseph, A., & Tizard, J. (1973). Environmental effects on language development: A study of young children in long stay residential nurseries. *Annual Progress in Child Psychiatry & Child Development,* 705–728.

Trotter, R. (1983, August). Baby face. *Psychology Today, 17,* 14–20.

Ullman, D. (1974). Breadth of attention and retention in mentally retarded and intellectually average children. *American Journal of Mental Deficiency, 78,* 640–648.

Van Biervliet, A. (1977). Establishing words and objects as functionally equivalent through manual sign training. *American Journal of Mental Deficiency, 82,* 178–186.

Vanderheiden, G. (1982). *Computers can play a dual role for disabled individuals.* Madison: University of Wisconsin, Trace Center.

Vihman, M. (1978). Consonant harmony: Its scope and function in child language. In J. Greenberg (Ed.), *Universals of human language, Vol. 2: Phonology.* Stanford: Stanford University Press.

Volpe, R. (1976). Orthopedic disability, restriction, and role-taking activity. *The Journal of Special Education, 10,* 371–381.

Watkins, O., & Watkins, M. (1980). The modality effect and echoic persistence. *Journal of Experimental Psychology: General, 109,* 251–278.

Welch, S., & Pear, J. (1979). Generalization by autistic-type children of verbal responses across settings. *Journal of Applied Behavior Analysis, 12,* 273–282.

Westby, C. (1980). Assessment of cognitive and language abilities through play. *Language, Speech, & Hearing Services in Schools, 11,* 154–168.

Whatmough, J. (1956). *Language: A modern synthesis.* New York: American Library.

White, B., Watts, J., Barnett, I., Kaban, B., Marmor, J., & Shapiro, B. (1973). *Experience and environment: Major influences on the development of the young child* (Vol. 1), Englewood Cliffs, NJ: Prentice-Hall.

Wilcox, M., & Campbell, P. (1983). Assessing communication in low-functioning multihandicapped children. Paper presented at the American Speech-Language-Hearing Association Annual Convention, Cincinnati, OH.

Windle, C. (1962). Prognosis of mental subnormals. *American Journal of Mental Deficiency,* (Monograph Supplement).

Winitz, H. (1983). Use and abuse of the developmental approach. In H. Winitz (Ed.), *Treating language disorders.* Batimore: University Park Press.

Wolfensberger, W. (1967). Counseling the parents of the retarded. In A. Baumeister (Ed.), *Mental retardation: Appraisal, education, and rehabilitation.* Chicago: Aldine.

Wolfensberger, W., Mein, R., & O'Connor, N. (1963). A study of the oral vocabularies of severely subnormal patients: III, Core vocabulary, verbosity and repetitiousness. *Journal of Mental Deficiency Research, 7,* 38–45.

Woodward, M., & Stern, D. (1963). Developmental patterns of severely subnormal children. *British Journal of Educational Psychology, 33,* 10–21.

Wulbert, M., Inglis, S., Kreigsmann, E., & Mills, B. (1975). Language delay and associated mother-child interactions. *Developmental Psychology, 11,* 61–70.

Wulz, S., Hall, M., & Klein, M. (1983). A home-centered instructional communication strategy for severely handicapped children. *Journal of Speech and Hearing Disorders, 48,* 2–10.

Yoder, D., & Miller, J. (1972). What we may know and what we can do: Input toward a system. In J. McLean, D. Yoder & R. Schiefelbusch (Eds.), *Language intervention with the retarded.* Baltimore: University Park Press.

Zeaman, D., & House, B. (1963). The role of attention in retardate discrimination learning. In N. Ellis (Ed.), *Handbook of mental deficiency.* New York: McGraw-Hill.

Zeaman, D., & House, B. (1979). A review of attention theory. In N. Ellis (Ed.), *Handbook of mental deficiency: Psychological theory and research.* Hillsdale, NJ: Lawrence Erlbaum.

Zetlin, A. & Gallimore, R. (1983). The development of comprehension strategies through the regulatory function of teacher questions. *Education and Training of Mentally Retarded, 18,* 176–183.

Zigler, E. (1967). Mental retardation technical comment. *Science, 157,* 578.

Zigler, E. (1971). The retarded person as a whole person. In H. Adams & W. Boardman (Eds.), *Advances in experimental clinical psychology.* New York: Pergamon Press.

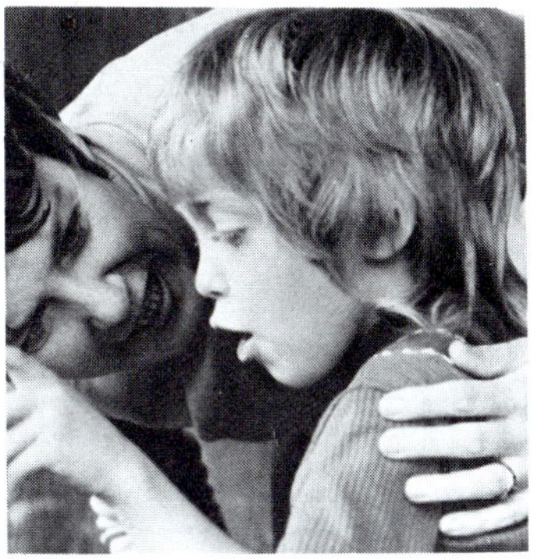

9

Autism: Learning to Communicate

Each autistic child has unique learning needs. Just as there are differences in normal language learners, so are there individual differences in disordered language learners. It is unrealistic, therefore, to view a population of language-disordered children as a single entity. The autistic population includes such a broad range of children who evidence language, cognitive, communicative, behavioral, and social learning problems that many researchers have suggested that perhaps it is not one group. Some researchers question whether there is a single cause or etiology for the disorder. The issue relates to how children are classified. Within the medical model, the underlying cause for a disorder is considered of primary importance. Historically, this point of view has carried over to the public school domain. As a result, disordered children are classified into handicapping areas and assigned to classes based upon etiological labels (i.e., mental retardation, autism, neurological impairment, etc.). Certainly, there are advantages and disadvantages to both the etiological and the nonetiological models. One advantage to a nonetiological approach to disorders in the schools might be the classification of children by characteristics such as communication and language behaviors. In this chapter, autistic children are described in terms of their communication and language behaviors. These behaviors represent an important insight into the unique needs of this population within the educational system.

More than any other population, autistic children highlight the many theoretical and therapeutic changes that have occurred recently in the area of child language acquisition. The following changes represent an organizational structure for the chapter:

This chapter was written by Dr. Ellenmorris Tiegerman, Adelphi University.

1. The theoretical and etiological perceptions of the underlying cause(s) of autism
2. The therapeutic programming provided for autistic children
3. The setting(s) within which the autistic child is trained
4. The role of the speech-language pathologist vis-à-vis the autistic child
5. The role of the parent of the autistic child
6. Our expectations of how the autistic person can function within society
7. The relationship between autism and language acquisition theory

THEORY AND TERMINOLOGICAL ISSUES

Psychiatrists who diagnose infantile autism are troubled by problems of agreement on terms and diagnostic reliability. The same difficulties confront neurologists and language pathologists who diagnose developmental aphasia or central language disorders. Diagnostic problems and terminological differences create formidable complications in placement and remediation. Specific theories relating to the cause of autism have been proposed but not proven. The range of etiological views of autism extends from a psychoanalytic perspective of the parent-child relationship to organic, genetic, and biochemical causes. Criteria for classification of children as autistic are not completely similar across authors and researchers. The following theories highlight how the underlying "cause" of the disorder has changed in recent years. In reading the theories, consider the therapeutic orientation that would result.

Etiology: A Psychological-Psychoanalytic Perspective

Kanner (1943) was the first to describe autistic children as being in a distinct category. Since that time, autism has been the subject of much clinical investigation and research; yet the nature of its causes, manifestations, and treatment remains in dispute. Kanner (1943) defined the cause as an innate inability to form biologically affective contact with people. He attributed this inability to an emotional deprivation resulting from rigidity of the parents. The parents of the children studied were characterized by obsessive-meticulousness and intellectualization. This theory was supported by Eisenberg (1956) who categorized the mothers of autistic children as cold and distant.

Bettelheim, in *The Empty Fortress* (1967), proposed a similar perspective. He suggested that the mother does not produce autism, rather it is the child's reaction to her attitudes. The autistic child fears maternal destruction and rejects the mother. When the child withdraws, the mother becomes indifferent or angry. The child retreats within himself even further, and reality becomes so fearful that inactivity is the only available response—autism develops. Thus, the symptoms of autistic children have been attributed to problems with early interpersonal relationships, motivation, and emotionality resulting in a diagnosis of emotional disturbance.

Controlled studies have failed to demonstrate significant differences in parental psychopathology and early mother-child interaction between groups of psychotic and nonpsychotic brain-damaged children (Alpern & Yang, 1969; DeMyer, Pontius, Norton, Barton, Allen, & Steele, 1972). For a long time, the psychoanalytic view that the mother-child relationship was the cause of autism was widely accepted; however, recently, several researchers have proposed an organic, etiological basis.

Etiology: A Neurological Perspective

The unusual behavioral characteristics typical of autistic children have led many researchers to look for a neurological explanation for the disorder. Ornitz and Ritvo (1968) posited a neurological basis for the disorder. Their theory emphasized the importance of a defective perceptual apparatus, manifested by a heightened awareness of sensory stimuli. The defective perceptual apparatus results in the children's distorted perception of reality which, in turn, affects their ability to establish appropriate object relations and reality contact.

Dalgleish (1975) posited that research on information processing in autistic children has revealed difficulties in integration of sensory functioning and in sequencing processes. These functions are basic to the acquisition of communication and linguistic systems. Several experimental studies have highlighted the difficulties of the autistic child in sensory integration. Conditioning experiments provide information on integration functioning in situations where simultaneous input from different sources is precisely controlled. Lovaas, Schreibman, Koegel, and Rehm(1971) attempted to condition three groups of children (autistic, retarded, and normal) to respond to a complex stimulus involving the simultaneous presentation of auditory, visual, and tactile elements. Once this discrimination was trained, the components of the complex stimulus supposedly had acquired control over the child's behavior. The autistic subjects responded primarily to only one of the cues; the normal children responded to all three cues; and the retarded children functioned between the two extremes. The data did not indicate that any one sense modality was impaired in autistic children. Rather, when presented with a complex stimulus, they revealed a marked preference for one of the components. The researchers referred to this pattern of responding as *stimulus overselectivity* or *overselective attention.* It indicates that autistic children have difficulties in learning situations requiring shifts in stimulus control.

Etiology: Central Language Disorder

Churchill (1978) presented a different theoretical model from which to analyze the autistic child. He posited that psychotic children with a psychiatric diagnosis of autism have a central language deficit which is more severe than that found in children with central language disorders. In addition, the three most prominent and clinically significant features of childhood psychosis are impairment of communicative interaction, social interactions, and appropriate object manipulations. Churchill presented some general similarities in responding for the autistic children involved in his experimental language investigation. Some of the autistic children evidenced channel-specific deficits (i.e., they indicated a conditioning preference for one stimulus modality). Some children displayed a difficulty in responding to two familiar elements simultaneously. Children also displayed difficulties in generalization, classification, cross-referencing, and syntactic/linguistic manipulations. The most important information may be that each child was *unique* (i.e., autistic children are a heterogeneous group of disordered children). Churchill concluded that each child generated a different profile of linguistic abilities and disabilities.

Baltaxe and Simmons (1975) proposed that the autistic child utilizes bizarre communicative and interactional strategies in the language learning process. Often there is no demonstration of speech production ability, which often indicates deafness of dysphasia. The strikingly aberrant aspect of language behavior is the *pattern* of language learning and language usage. Language is often learned without any appreciation of the nonlinguistic environment. The major sources of learning are frequently impersonal, such as television (Chase, 1972). A central language disorder may well be the necessary and sufficient cause of autistic behavior.

Resulting Clinical Problems

The lack of communicative speech and severe problems in the area of interpersonal relationships tend to limit the use of standard evaluative measures (i.e., language as well as psychological tests) as diagnostic and research tools with this clinical population. Alternative techniques must be devised in evaluating these children, assessing changes in behavior, and obtaining measures of behavioral differences which may exist between them and other populations (Clune, Paolella, & Foley, 1979). The literature described in this section illustrates that diagnosis and description of autistic children have been complicated. In the absence of a generally accepted theory, diagnostic classifications often vary among theoreticians or researchers. As a result, many autistic children are misdiagnosed during their early years.

Related Factors

Four factors have contributed to the changing ways in which the autistic child has been viewed in the past several years. First, the National Society for Autistic Children has heightened society's awareness of the needs of autistic children. This awareness has affected the direction of legislation in state and federal funding of educational programs. Second, Public Law 94-142 has had profound implications in the development of curricula for the handicapped in the "least restrictive" educational environment. As a result, there have been expanding funds available for the development of educational programs for autistic children, particularly in public school settings. Third, new developments in research have suggested neurological differences in processing (visual, auditory, linguistic, and cognitive) between autistic children and other populations of children. Neurological differences suggest an etiological explanation other than emotional disturbance; specifically, that the underlying cause for the disorder has a neurological basis. The fourth and final factor involves the recent research in child language development. The changing perspectives in language theory and therapy have affected the view that the communication and language deficits in children are of critical importance. The view that communicative and social aspects underlie language development, more clearly highlighted the pragmatic deficits in autistic children. The interplay among these factors has resulted in the progressive attempt to develop language and educational programs for the autistic within various learning contexts: home, school, intermediate care facility (ICF), etc.

Because the goal of this chapter is to describe autistic children in terms of characteristic behaviors, many aspects of developmental learning are presented: behavioral characteristics, language, cognition, play, social interaction, and so forth. These characteristics provide a comprehensive picture of the autistic child as a child who has communication and language learning problems. The chapter compares the developmental differences between autistic and normal language learners.

Chapter 9

BEHAVIORAL CHARACTERISTICS

The behavioral characteristics of the autistic child were originally presented by Kanner (1943, 1944). Many of the same characteristics are used today to describe the autistic child. The classic autistic child, as described by Kanner (1943) and Bettelheim (1967), exhibits most or all of the characteristics. The autistic population, however, is very heterogeneous. Children vary in the number and severity of characteristics exhibited, and the classic autistic child is probably a rarity. For the sake of description, all of the characteristics presented will be discussed in terms of Adam, who has been diagnosed as a classic autistic child. As children exhibit fewer of the characteristics, they become more autistic-like rather than autistic. Some of these characteristics will be discussed more fully in later sections dealing with communication and language.

Gaze Aversion

Perhaps the most salient characteristic of autism is the lack of eye contact with other people during the communication exchange process. This characteristic more than any other has caused autistic children to be described as aloof, distant, withdrawn, and nonrelating. What many people are describing is the fact that autistic children do not look at or facially orient their gaze at another person. Autistic children avert their eyes when someone talks to them. In fact, attempts to get the child to look at you are met with physical resistance, particularly when the autistic child is physically near another person. Hutt and Ounsted (1956) noted that as autistic children get farther away from another person, they exhibit a greater number of gazes oriented to that person. Another difference concerns the physical orientation of the child. Unless one is sneaking a look, the bodies of both speaker and listener are normally lined up shoulder to shoulder. With autistic children, the entire body (and head) is turned away from the speaker, and the children emit infrequent, fleeting gazes from the corners of their eyes. Consider Adam's gaze pattern during an interactional exchange.

> Adam: Even after Adam had been trained to look at the speaker, he would change the orientation of his body. The more he focused on the speaker facially, the more of his body was turned away. When holding his head so that *en face* interaction could take place, his eyes shifted from corner to corner (side to side).

Ritualistic Behavior

Rituals are a normal part of the daily routines and patterns of life. Normal children and adults exhibit ritual patterns. There are, however, differences between the rituals exhibited by normal and autistic children. The autistic child's ritual is a sequence or pattern of behavior which *must* be exhibited in the same way, in the same order, over and over again. There is very little room for any kind of change. The chair must be placed just so in the living room. The child can only drink from the Snoopy cup. When there is a change in the environment, autistic children attempt to reorder and recreate the sameness that they seek to maintain.

Rituals also involve the ways in which children manipulate objects within the environment. Autistic children spin records, twirl wires, bang objects, and turn lights on and off incessantly. They do not manipulate objects appropriately in a functional way. The performances with an object are repeated over and over again for hours. There are also rituals in which the child rocks back and forth in a corner. These repetitive behaviors are frequently referred to as *self-stimulatory* behaviors. They are presumably the child's attempt to maintain sameness or perhaps to repeat something salient. Let us consider several rituals.

> Poppy's ritual: Come home. Kiss the boys. Go into the office, turn on the answering machine to note recorded messages. Change into jeans. Read the newspaper. Have dinner. (Ritual pattern exhibited every night.)
>
> Jeremy's ritual: Take bottles and binkys (pacifiers) upstairs. Put bottles and binkys in bed. Put Superdog in bed. Cover Superdog. Give Superdog his bottle. Give Superdog his binky. Jeremy drinks bottle. Jeremy takes binky. (Ritual pattern exhibited every night.)
>
> Ellenmorris' ritual: Hi, Adam, Come on, let's go play. Offers hand to Adam. Walk hand-in-hand to therapy room. (Ritual pattern exhibited before every therapy session.)

What are the differences between the ritual patterns exhibited by the normal and autistic children? The first difference concerns the fact that for the normal child, the ritual pattern represents only a small part of the child's performance or interaction repertoire. Because autistic children have very limited and restricted performance repertoires, the ritual pattern represents a much larger proportion of the repertoire. Much of what autistic children do involves performing or developing a ritualized pattern of some kind. "Everything becomes a ritual," noted Adam's mother.

The second difference concerns the fact that it is very difficult to change autistic children's ritualized patterns. Any minute change in a ritual can result in a catastrophic reaction from the child. Many parents note that the resulting violent temper tantrums are so aversive that they hesitate to, and often do not, change the child's ritualized patterns. Poppy and Jeremy might balk a bit if something were performed differently within the sequence, or if some behavior (or object) were left out of the sequence (i.e., we did not give Superdog his binky); but, the result would not be a catastrophic reaction.

The third difference is that in normal children these ritualized patterns, referred to as *adultomorphisms* by Piaget (1962), indicate the child's relational knowledge of experiences and events within the environment. These sequences in the normal child show progressive and developmental changes. They incorporate the child's changing perceptions and conceptions of the world. Therefore, the ritual in the normal child indicates an attempt to integrate and synthesize observed environmental sequences. Not so for the ritualized pattern in autistic children. The ritual represents their attempt to maintain a systematic order within the environment.

Temper Tantrums

There are aspects of the natural environment which tend to develop and maintain ritualized patterns, albeit unwittingly. Let us reconsider Ellenmorris' ritual described previously with regard to the next section.

> Ellenmorris' ritual: One afternoon therapy was running late. As the clinician was getting ready for Adam, a graduate student volunteered to get him from the waiting room in

> the Speech and Hearing Center. A few minutes later, Adam was wildly screaming in the hallway. The clinician walked into the hallway to see Adam screaming and pounding the side of his head with his fists. The therapy session was, to say the least, difficult. Before Adam's mother left, she was asked if anything had happened on the way to the Center, and if Adam were feeling all right. She said that he was perfectly all right until the graduate student had picked him up in the waiting room.

For the 2 years that Adam had been enrolled at the Speech and Hearing Center, the clinician had gone to the waiting room to bring him to the therapy room. In essence, a ritualized pattern had developed. As a result of this experience, the clinical staff attempted to identify if other ritual patterns existed. The focus of the investigation was to identify and modify the clinician's patterns of behavior and interaction. Adam's response (a temper tantrum) was typical of how an autistic child reacts to attempts to introduce change of any kind into his world. The temper tantrum is the autistic child's catastrophic reaction to change.

Temper tantrums can be either self-abusive or aggressive in form. Self-abusive and aggressive behaviors exhibited by the autistic child can include any of the following: pulling hair, biting, scratching, head banging, pinching, head-butting, etc. The difference between self-abusive and aggressive behaviors is the direction or orientation of the behavior—towards self or towards another person. One of the difficulties related to temper tantrums involves the intensity of the child's reaction to even a slight environmental change. A minute change in the environment or in a ritual can result in a violent outpouring of behavior. The children are uncontrollable physically; and, obviously, the older and bigger they get, the harder it is for the parents to manage them.

The onset of these tantrums can be remarkably sudden. Many times the parent or teacher asks in frustration, "What happened?" Sometimes the answer to that question is not easily determined. Sometimes the answer is a tiny, or what seems to be a tiny, change (i.e., putting the cup in a different place). Part of the frustration with the temper tantrum is the inability of those involved to figure out or identify what happened. Another difficulty is that the child is not easily comforted. These violent tantrums can occur for an extended duration. Adam's mother often noted that it was almost impossible to make him stop once he got started, "He's like a steamroller coming down a hill." For all of these reasons, parents are rather hesitant to introduce change, especially in public places such as restaurants, supermarkets, parks, etc.

Self-stimulatory Behavior

Self-stimulation includes high-frequency behaviors that have been traditionally described as noncommunicative and noninteractional. They are often emitted when the child seeks to withdraw from the environment.

This withdrawal pattern occurs when the autistic child cannot cope with direct input from teaching or instruction. Self-stimulatory behaviors are nonprogressive. They interfere in the child's learning, especially in the classroom. What should the clinician or teacher do about these behaviors? Behavioral approaches to training the autistic child have proposed eliminating or decreasing the frequency of these interfering behaviors by means of aversive consequences. However, so much of the autistic child's repertoire includes these self-stimulatory behaviors, that if they were eliminated, there would not be much emitted behavior left. The problem involves the autistic child's limited and restricted behavioral repertoire; there is no definitive solution to the problem.

Hypo- versus Hyper-sensitivity to Stimuli

Hyposensitivity to stimuli in the environment describes the fact that autistic children do not indicate the same threshold level of responding as normal children. Parents often say that they could "clap a pair of cymbals next to the child's ear and he would not blink." What parents are referring to is that autistic children do not react, respond, or seem to recognize certain sounds consistently. It is not surprising that many autistic children at some point in their history have been identified as hearing impaired or deaf. The general pattern of unawareness in terms of environmental stimuli is inconsistent. Many parents describe the autistic child as being "here" and "there." When Adam was responsive during a therapy session, Adam's mother would say, "He's come in for a landing." The inconsistency in the child's responding is made more complicated by the inconsistency in the extreme reaction (hypersensitivity) to the slightest change in input. Adam would place his hands over his ears and eyes to block out input. The inconsistency in responding with the possibility of the catastrophic temper tantrum always present, makes the attempts at child "assessment" (i.e., determining how he is going to react) a guessing game for parents, clinicians, and teachers.

Mutism

Mutism seems to include a range of behavior going from total periods of silence to the production of sounds which are meaningless (i.e., not used for communicative exchange but rather for self-stimulatory purposes). Most, if not all, autistic children progress through a period of mutism. Some autistic children remain mute all of their lives. Eisenberg (1956) has posited that there is a critical speech period. If speech has not developed by 6 years of age, there is little probability that functional speech will develop after that critical period. If the autistic child becomes verbal, the initial words or phrases are quite intelligible. There seems to be a quantum leap or change in the child's performance that cannot as of yet be explained. The autistic child does not evidence the gradual developmental changes in pragmatics, phonology, semantics, and syntax during the first 36 months that are seen in the normal child. Fay and Schuler (1980) noted that most of the information accumulated about this period of time comes from parental reports, which are affected by "an emotional climate that can best be defined as a developmental hope countered by fear" (p. 22). We are not clear about why some children progress to the next stage, echolalic behavior, and some do not. We are not clear about what changes occur within the child that result in the transition to the next stage. Adam's developmental history represents a dramatic and unexplainable change from one stage to another.

> Adam: Adam was mute for the first 3 years. The only sounds he produced were meaningless grunts. When he started to "speak" his productions were long imitated utterances: open door please, time go home now. His productions were as his mother described, "as clear as a bell."

There are some autistic children who never develop speech and/or language. The incidence of muteness ranges from 28% (Lotter, 1967) to 61% (Fish, Shapiro, & Campbell, 1966). The variability is a function of the difficulties with terminology and issues discussed at the beginning of this chapter. Bartak and Rutter (1976) found that approximately 80% of all autistic children were identified or misdiagnosed as deaf at one time in their developmental history. DeMyer, Barton, DeMyer, Norton, Allen, and Steele (1973) noted that about 65% of the children who were mute at age 5 were still mute several years later. A large proportion of the autistic population never develops conventional communicative and/or linguistic interactions within the environment. Why do so many autistic children remain nonverbal? Why is the development of speech so delayed?

Echolalia

Echolalia has been defined traditionally as the meaningless repetition of someone else's words. As a result, some researchers have advocated the elimination or decrease in the frequency of occurrence of this behavior. Is the autistic child's imitation meaningless? If it is not meaningless and random, what function does it serve? Prizant and Duchan (1981) noted that to determine what echolalic utterances mean, one must analyze the utterance within the natural communicative environment. Echolalia also has been described traditionally as a transition period between muteness and the evidence of linguistic knowledge. Knowledge of how autistic children progress through various stages is limited. It is important to understand how the child functions within the communicative context; specifically, how autistic children use *whatever* behavior they have developed for the purpose of communication.

Prizant and Duchan (1981) described seven functional categories of echolalia, indicating various communicative and cognitive functions that echolalia may serve for the autistic child: nonfocused echolalia, turn-taking echolalia, declarative echoic utterances, rehearsal utterances, self-regulatory echoes, yes-answer category, and request echoes. These categories indicate that to determine the communicative intent of the autistic child's message, the researcher and clinician must analyze the communicative context within which the utterance occurs. In such cases, the elimination of echolalia would actually be a decrease in the occurrence of communicative behavior. It thus becomes important to determine if the echolalic form represents the child's communicative intention.

The following interactions illustrate that Adam's dramatic and, perhaps, quantum jump to an echolalic period, revealed the need to assess the child's meaning within context. The examples indicate how *this* autistic child manipulated various linguistic and nonlinguistic behaviors to convey communicative intentions.

Adam's mother was, to say the least, thrilled when her son started to "talk." However, her exuberance quickly wore away. She described Adam as her "talking shadow." A typical exchange between mother and child is presented to highlight the difficulty, confusion, and frustration in an exchange with a child who is echolalic.

Mother: Adam, are you ready?

Adam: Adam, are you ready?

Mother: Go open the door.
Adam: Go open the door.
Mother: Where is your coat?
Adam: Your coat

To determine if Adam's imitations were meaningful, several aspects of his behavior could be analyzed within the context. For example, let us analyze the following exchange:

Mother: Go open the door
Adam: Go open the door
Nonverbal Behavior: Adam looks at the door, then gets up and opens the door.

Adam indicated by means of his behavior that, although he echoed mother's production, he understood the meaning of the message and the related action. The child's nonverbal behavior (i.e., gaze behavior, gestures, actions) provides an indication of the child's understanding of the speech message and whether the echoic utterance was meaningful.

Mother: Where is your coat?
Adam: Your coat
Nonverbal behavior: Adam looks at the coat, then goes to pull on the coat, which is lying across a chair.

In the second interchange, there was not a difference between the form of the child's echoed utterance and mother's production. Adam's nonverbal behavior indicated his interpretation of the context. In *this* situation, Adam's echoed utterance was different from his mother's production in several ways. First, the linguistic form of Adam's production was slightly different. His intonation pattern, which was different from his mother's (upward inflection), indicated his ability to make changes in suprasegmental features. He also exhibited nonverbal behaviors which signalled that he understood his mother's message. This interchange indicates several other ways in which the child can manipulate some of the components of the language process.

These interchanges indicate how the form and function of the autistic child's communicative behavior can be analyzed within the ongoing natural context. There are many questions about the echolalic period that still remain unanswered. Does the echolalic period incorporate several progressive stages? Does echolalic behavior change structurally and/or functionally? Does the echolalic period contribute to language and communication development in the autistic child?

Impaired Relational Behavior

In the early chapter on normal language acquisition, it was emphasized that the child's experiences within the environment with agents, actions, and objects were important to the language learning process. Baltaxe and Simmons (1975) noted that autistic children exhibit deficits in their relationships with people and objects. These object deficits manifest themselves in terms of a limited toy-play repertoire, self-stimulatory behavior, bizarre manipulation behaviors, and nonprogressive play skills. The interpersonal deficits manifest themselves in terms of lack of gaze interaction, decreased physical interaction, severe limitations in cooperative play, and social interactional skill behaviors. The autistic child has difficulty relating to and interacting with the environment. Many autistic children withdraw from the approach and touch of others and become rigid or stiff when held or cuddled. Because communication and social learning involve interactional exchanges with peers and adults in the environment, one can only wonder about the effect the autistic child has on the parent. Interaction implies reciprocity; there must be some reaction or response from the child. If the autistic child does not respond or withdraws from the adult's initiations, what is the adult's reaction? Is it a feeling of rejection? Is it a feeling of frustration? Consider how Adam's mother and Jeremy described their interaction with Adam. Notice that Adam's lack of responsiveness negatively affected the communicative initiations of these two individuals. Autistic children, who need to learn about the social context, manage to isolate themselves further.

> Adam's mother: It is difficult to get close to a child who always pushes you away. Interaction is totally nonreinforcing.
>
> Jeremy: Him no like me.

Onset Before 30 Months

Identification of autistic children usually occurs before age 3. Some parents describe their early awareness of a problem during the infant's first months of life. They note that the infant could not "be comforted." The younger the infant, the more tenuous the determination of disorder unless there are neurological signs of impairment. Generally, parents proceed through the frustrations of a diagnostic battery or evaluation as the children approach their second birthdays. One of the most important diagnostic variables—language—is often difficult to evaluate by standardized means before this time. It is only within the past few years that early identification, which has focused on the child between 3 and 5 years, resulted in training and intervention within a clinic, center, or school placement. Educational options are still rather limited for the preschool autistic child.

Behavioral Characteristics: A Means of Discriminating Between Children?

The nine characteristics of autism described previously can differentiate between and among children. Table 9–1 highlights some of the performance differences between Adam's and Bryan's interaction within the environment.

There are *some* obvious developmental differences between the two children which might reflect neurological and processing differences. These differences are typical of children within the autistic population and highlight the fact that autistic children have very individual interactional patterns and styles. These learning differences ultimately affect therapeutic programming and the child's interactions in the environment.

In addition to behavioral characteristics, communication, play, and linguistic behaviors provide insight into the most critical variable in the autistic child—language functioning. Autistic children indicate severe deficits in language development. This inability to interact and to communicate imposes a restriction on learning about language as a social process. Communication, play, and linguistic behaviors provide a

TABLE 9–1
A Comparison of Behavioral Performances

Behavior	*Adam (40 mos.)*	*Bryan (40 mos.)*
Gaze aversion	Gaze aversion	Gaze aversion, but does track a moving object
Imitation	Lack of motor and vocal imitation	Lack of vocal imitation, limited motor imitation
Ritualistic behavior	Feeding, dressing, and washing rituals	Constantly rearranging furniture in the room (and house)
Self-stimulatory behaviors	Walks on toes, flaps hands, rocks back and forth, makes grunting/gutteral noises	Spins, opens and closes eyes rapidly, sticks finger down throat
Object performances	Nonfunctional and undifferentiated performances; spins, shakes, mouths, and bangs toys	Basically nonfunctional and undifferentiated; spins, shakes, mouths, and bangs toys. Some appropriate object related performances: picks up telephone receiver and makes noises into receiver, puts baby in bed, stacks rings on stick, can replace pieces in Simplex puzzle
Temper tantrums	Self-abusive behavior: headbanging, handbiting. Aggressive behavior; pulls hair and scratches	No self-abusive behavior. Aggressive behavior: bites, scratches, pinches, kicks, bunts his head, pulls hair, punches
Speech	Mute	Echolalic
Relational behavior	Turns and moves away when approached, stiffens when touched	Approaches people (adults and children), requests hugs, kisses, and tickles
Onset	Mother noted that something was wrong at 3 months of age. Psychiatric evaluation and diagnostic at 24 months	Mother states that child progressed "normally" until 12 months of age and then withdrew. Child's behavior deteriorated. Psychiatric evaluation and diagnosis at 30 months

more holistic picture of the autistic child's unique interactional style within a complex social environment.

COMMUNICATION BEHAVIORS

In the communication exchange between the adult and the child, the two are participants in an ongoing interactive event. The autistic child at 30 months does not evidence many of the communication behaviors evidenced by the normal infant at 6 months. The autistic child does not exhibit the normal developmental progression in gaze, vocal, and gestural communication behaviors, or the ability to coordinate these behaviors into complex patterns and sequences.

Often we are not aware that the child is autistic until after infancy (between 18 and 36 months). By this time, it has become clear that the child has not developed early communication and linguistic behaviors. The information concerning behavioral and communication development before the time of diagnosis is subjective and a function of the parents' interpretation and memory of the early experiences with the child.

The fact that communication behaviors *are* not present at 30 months, does not mean that the behaviors *were* not present earlier. It is possible that early communication behaviors did develop during the first 9 to 12 months, but due to neurological deficits, these behaviors and structures deteriorated. We do not have the diagnostic skills currently to identify the deficits that occur during infancy and early childhood that result in the disorder of autism. Infancy can provide some important insights into the early appearance and progression of this disorder. Gaze, vocal, and gestural communication behaviors may be critical in the early identification of the autistic child.

Play

It is generally acknowledged that play is important to the development of adaptability, learning, cognition, and social behavior (Weisler & McCall, 1976). Bruner (1967) has suggested that the function of play is to exercise and develop manipulative and interactional strategies which children will later integrate into more sophisticated task-oriented sequences. A more general theory suggests that in play, children learn to affect and control activities they are unable to execute or dominate in other contexts. In play, children develop control over animate and inanimate objects or contexts (Eckerman & Whatley, 1977). Recent analyses of early social interactions occurring during play suggest that play behavior also influences the actions of another child (Garvey, 1974). Play has a cognitive, social, and integrative function in development.

The theory underlying play indicates that play begins with action manipulations directed by the child. As manipulative and physical abilities expand, children develop an increasing capacity to deal with objects more actively. Autistic children, however, are limited in their interaction with the environment. Because of their restricted experience, they share with other disordered children many behavioral and learning problems, whether the specific diagnosis is mental retardation, cerebral palsy, brain damage, or autism. Autistic children withdraw from interactional experiences and learn to manipulate by means of temper tantrums and disruptive behaviors. Withdrawal from the environment makes it difficult to determine if they do not know how to play, if they lack the opportunity to do so, or both. Many researchers suggest that there is a cyclical relationship between the bizarre manipulative performance and autistic children's inability to integrate experiences within the environment, causing even further withdrawal. The child's creation of an "inner" world is an attempt to establish and maintain an internal order which cannot be established in the outside world. Self-stimulatory and ritualistic behaviors might be a result of such perceptions of the environment.

Michelman (1974) posited that when autistic children sit for hours rocking back and forth, their sensory, perceptual, and intellectual pathways are pathologically involved and development is delayed. Unlike normal children, autistic children cannot discover their relationships to objects and people within the environment. Basic skills such as banging, shaking, rolling, or throwing do not progress or develop in complexity. Self-stimulation does not lead to learning about the environment. The process of play that spontaneously results in learning about environmental control and manipulation relationships in the normal child does not occur in the autistic child.

The characteristic toy-play of autistic and psychotic children has been described by a number of authors. Black, Freeman, and Montgomery (1975) reported that these children become fixated with one kind of object performance, such as spinning objects, and retain these primitive manipulative patterns as a mode of play. Bakwin (1954) cited a disinterest in toys or play with one toy which continues for hours. Polan and Spencer (1959) characterized the toy-play behavior of autistic children as compulsive and perseverative.

LANGUAGE COMPONENTS

In describing autism as a communication and language-based disorder, I will discuss several components of language—pragmatics, semantics, syntax, phonology, and cognitive processes. Cromer (1981) has noted that it is important to understand these language components "as a means of focusing on the problems that may be faced by specific language-disordered groups" (p. 71). The interrelationship among these components in the autistic child can provide insight into the unique learning needs of this type of language-impaired child.

Learning and Integration of Language Components

Blank, Gessner, and Esposito (1979) described a language-disordered boy whose syntactic and semantic development were structurally and functionally on-target and whose language seemed to be conceptually appropriate and relevant to the environmental context. A syntactic or semantic analysis failed to indicate the language learning problems of this child. In investigating further, the researchers noted that within a social situation, the child's communication problems became evident. This child was unaware of the communicative responsibilities of speaker/listener roles. He did not respond appropriately to initiations from a speaker, so he could not function adequately or appropriately as a listener. As a speaker, the child could not monitor his listener to determine if his message had been received, noticed, or understood.

The researchers noted that this child's pragmatic communication skills could not be determined or detected outside the framework of the social context. From an interpersonal perspective, this child's language was aloof, detached, and socially inappropriate. Many autistic children are described in these terms. Thus, the language of autistic children may be analyzed in terms of a deficit in the pragmatic component of their language system. The preceding research highlights the fact that development within the language system can be uneven or different. In this case, the child evidenced normal developmental progressions in syntax and semantics which contrasted with a deficiency in pragmatics.

Curtiss (1981) suggested that semantic and syntactic development can progress independently from one another. A child may evidence more advanced or complex semantic skills, while syntactic abilities remain severely retarded. Language-disordered children can also evidence more advanced syntactic skills with severe deficits in semantic development. Autistic children evidence an uneven developmental pattern across the language components. Curtiss posited that different structures and functions of the nervous system control different language processes. Uneven development indicates that different areas within the central nervous system are more or less impaired, which determines the level of functioning and the language abilities developed within the child. Language represents an integrated system; all of the components contribute to the development of the whole.

To understand the learning needs of language-disordered children, particularly autistic children, it is important to compare and contrast development within and across components. The language and communication deficits evidenced in autistic children might be caused by:

- Uneven developments within/across the components of the learning system
- An inability to interface/exchange developmental information across the components of the learning system

Cognitive Processes

The relationships among perception, language, and cognition remain rather controversial. Current trends have been influenced by cognitive theories which stress the importance of early social and interactional experiences within the environment. Piaget described language development as based within the sensorimotor period. Such cognitive theories have described the development of the child's conceptual knowledge and the changing affect on the development of language. In discussing cognitive development in autistic children, it is important to consider perceptual and cognitive processes and environmental and social experiences.

Kanner (1952) indicated that autistic children evidence an absence of physical stigmata, good motor dexterity, an absence of motor developmental delays, and excellent rote memory. These characteristics in combination with near normal IQ scores led Kanner to propose that intellectual deficits were a function of an affective disorder. Although Kanner's criteria are still used for diagnostic purposes, serious questions have been raised about the cognitive potential of these children. Most clinical research indicates that a majority of autistic children function within the mentally retarded range of intellectual skills (DeMyer, Barton, Alpern, Kimberlin, Allen, Yang, & Steele, 1974). However, unlike mentally retarded children, autistic children evidence a wide variability of skills. Autistic children display significantly higher abilities on tasks that require the discrimination of concrete visual-spatial relations and significantly lower abilities on tasks that require abstraction or the ability to organize concrete information on the basis of subtle relationships between stimuli (Hermelin, 1978). Autistic children evidence uneven performances on intelligence tests; they achieve higher performances on the nonverbal subscale than on the verbal subscale (Lockyer & Rutter, 1970). Autistic children evidence integration deficits when stimuli increase in complexity and/or require cross-modal processing (Bryson, 1970). They have difficulties in identifying what is meaningful and relevant in a situation (Dalgleish, 1975). Autistic children utilize a rigidly imposed set of rules in interacting with the environment. In addition, they attend to, or fixate on, one aspect of a picture or story; often some irrelevant minutiae (Maltz, 1981). Processing deficiencies were identified in a series of experiments by Lovaas and Schreibman (1971) which indicated that autistic children tended to be overselective in their responding. All of these examples highlight an idiosyncratic pattern of interaction within the environment.

Autistic children also indicate difficulty in generalizing learned behaviors from one context to another (Koegel & Rincover, 1977). Because autistic children cannot identify the relevant information within the complexities of a situation, they cannot identify what is important and what is not, creating a further problem in establishing conceptual or perceptual relationships. The ability to establish categories of any kind depends upon the ability to discriminate differences as well as to determine how stimuli are associated and related to one another. Autistic children tend to fixate on irrelevant aspects of a situation. As a result, their perceptions of the environment are rather distorted and limited. These deficits contribute to the failure to generalize learning. Fay and Schuler (1980) suggested that the deficits in generalization indicate a cognitive impairment in autistic children. The problem imposes a serious limitation on the ability to learn spontaneously and to benefit from more structured and formalized learning within therapy.

The inability to identify the relationships among stimuli and to benefit from past learning experiences condemns autistic children to repeated learning experiences. These children are not able to extract and utilize the similarities across situations. Normal children are in search of rules. To establish rules, children must be able to identify relevant and related stimuli within conceptual categories. Generalization involves the ability to identify the relationship between situation A and B, and then to apply the rule to A^1 and B^1. Again, rule-governed behavior enables children to process, categorize, and interpret more effectively the complexities of stimuli within the environment. Otherwise, it is very difficult to make sense of all the impinging stimuli.

The uneven developmental pattern in autistic children is difficult to explain given our limited understanding of normal developmental processes. The autistic child's abilities are often contrasted with extreme delays in other areas of skill acquisition. Adam, for example, had an excellent memory and rote recall. His ability, however, should be viewed in terms of his use of the skill within the social context. The remarkable recall is often used for noncommunicative and self-stimulatory purposes. Information was frequently extracted as a whole and not used for interactional purposes. Adam would sit in a corner of his room and recite verbatim the news report presented by Walter Cronkite from the night before. Identifying strengths, skills, or assets is only an initial step. It is important, especially with autistic children, to determine how skills are *used* or *applied* within the learning context.

Little is known about how autistic children perceive their environments. Assumptions are made on the basis of their patterns of interaction in the environment; that is, the way in which they relate to agents, actions, and objects. The behavioral characteristics described previously provide some indication of the child's internal operations and the resulting reactions to the impinging world. What is it that the autistic child sees and hears? One can only infer about the child's difficulties and confusions on the basis of observed responses and reactions.

Very little of what autistic children see and hear makes any sense. Words, voices, faces, and gestures are just rapidly changing stimuli, like changes in color; it is all so transient and difficult to grasp. People handle the child, manipulate the child, do things to the child; what does it mean? All those faces, a sea of changing expressions; what do they mean? There is little that looks the same; everything is always changing. It is not surprising that the world is confusing. It is not surprising that the child maintains a ritualized ordered environment and indeed, struggles to continue that order and sameness; everything else is so elusive. Finally, when the environment impinges beyond the management point, the child fights back and throws tantrums. The tantrum is the result of frustrations and confusions. The inner world that the autistic child creates is more understandable and consistent. Self-stimulation can be seen as the child's attempt to reestablish sameness. Many parents describe the exhibition of self-stimulatory behavior when the child is exposed to a new situation or experience. In order to understand autistic children's behavior, it is essential to consider the way they perceive the world.

The perceptual deficits in the autistic child create further disturbance because they severely limit the child's interactional experiences within the environment. Children who see the world in a distorted manner, interact with the world in a distorted manner. This vicious cycle does not enable the child to experience the multiplicity of interactions that are the building blocks of conceptual development (Michelman, 1974). Because the roots of representational behavior are based upon the child's interactional experiences within the environment, it is important to examine the interrelationship between cognitive and communicative functioning. Future research might indicate that autistic children's unique acquisition and use of language results from a cognitive processing style different from normal children's.

Pragmatics

The area of linguistic pragmatics has received a great deal of attention in the past several years. The pragmatic component of language involves the way language is used for communication purposes. Because they possess a noncommunicative style of interaction, autistic children are described as "nonrelational." The autistic child's use of language for communication purposes remains severely impaired in spite of developments in other language areas. Part of the problem relates to the interrelationship between social interaction and communication. The autistic child's interactional behaviors are rather limited. In addition, the few behaviors that are interactive are often part of specific and unusual routines. As noted previously, the established routine allows the autistic child to maintain some control within the rapidly changing environment. The routine establishes predictability by maintaining a contextual sameness.

Although autistic children indicate a preference for building such routines, these ritualized patterns further restrict social interaction. This added social limitation maintains the communication deficit. By responding to a limited range of behaviors, autistic children selectively reinforce certain aspects of the adult's input. The dilemma for the adult is the limited interactional responsiveness. Frequently, for the sake of interaction, the adult continues to provide a highly restricted form of communication. As a result, social interaction tends to be inflexible, ritualistic, and rigidly routinized. In turn, these social and interactional patterns affect the communication behavior problems typically described in autistic children:

1. Initiating and terminating interaction
2. Maintaining conversational topics
3. Functioning within speaker and listener roles
4. Using behavior for the purpose of communication

Shapiro and Fish (1969) suggested that autistic children evidence severe deficits in communicative functions which contribute to their rigid and socially inappropriate language. Blank, et al. (1979) proposed that autistic children fail to produce or to understand gestural and communicative behaviors. The child, therefore, does not develop the earliest communicative interactions: gaze, vocal and gaze signalling, play, and social behaviors, all of which provide the underpinnings for interactional patterns of behavior.

Curcio (1978) noted from an analysis of sensorimotor and communicative behaviors of autistic children, that they did not use protodeclarative acts. Pointing as a behavior did not occur in the behavioral repertoire of autistic children. If there were some kind of extended reaching, it usually signalled a request for an object and never indicated the location or existence of an object. Part of the problem with pointing was the children's inability to determine their own limitations in space (i.e., where they begin and end) and then to signal something beyond the self. Pointing represents an awareness that something is beyond reach. It is an attempt to extend self.

Autistic children do not readily develop the range of communicative intentions produced by normal children because of an inability to develop and coordinate the interactional behaviors described previously. If and when linguistic skills do develop, communicative deficits remain. The linguistic pattern reflects problems with pronouns, definite articles, relative clauses, deictic forms, and social variables (Baltaxe, 1977). The language pattern in autistic children indicates severe deficits in the pragmatic component of language.

Communicative Acts

Does the autistic child communicate? If the autistic child does communicate, what is the nature of the interaction? The only way to determine intentional behaviors is to observe and analyze the autistic child's behavior within the social situation. What should the clinician look for in the autistic child's behavior? Even the most severely impaired child has behaviors which can be identified as communicative if they are analyzed within the context. Several incidents with Adam highlight this point.

Situation 1: Clinician places a tightly sealed container of Jahn's vanilla ice cream on the table.

Adam: Adam walks over to the container, turns it over, tries to pull open the top, bites on the container, and drops it on the table. He walks away for several moments. He walks back to the table and picks up the container. He brings the container to the clinician and puts it in her lap. He walks away from the clinician and looks at her from across the room. (The clinician of course does nothing.) Adam approaches the clinician from the side, takes her hand, and places it on the ice cream.

Interpretation: Adam is requesting that the clinician perform an action (i.e., open the ice cream) which he could not do himself.

Situation 2: Clinician approaches Adam and sits down next to him.

Adam: Adam gets up and moves away from the clinician.

Interpretation: Adam is rejecting interaction.

Situation 3: Clinician talks to Adam.

Adam: Adam puts his hands over his ears, turns away from the clinician, but does not move away. Periodically, he takes his hands off his ears. When the clinician stops talking, Adam turns back to the clinician.

Interpretation: Adam does not want to engage in verbal interaction. The clinician learned that during these periods, Adam would participate in activities that could be maintained without discourse (e.g., puzzles, blocks, coloring, etc.).

The preceding incidents can be identified in the repertoires of even the most impaired autistic children. Adam could communicate several different intentions, and evidenced different combinations of behavior to indicate his response to input and stimuli from the environment.

The clinician must learn to read children's behaviors within the contextual framework before attempting to interpret their reactions to the environment. In fact, the maternal variable of "rich" interpretation facilitates the communication exchange process. The mother assumes that her infant reacts to the environment and treats the infant as an active listener and communicator. Assumptions have been very different with regard to the abilities of autistic children. The assumption that they do not have the ability to communicate results in a self-fulfilling prophesy. Autistic children's behavior is not analyzed to identify communicative behaviors because they cannot communicate. Because they cannot communicate, they are not treated as communicators.

Autistic children may be at a prelinguistic and even precommunicative stage, but they do react to environmental occurrences. Their behaviors should be analyzed within context to determine the individual and/or idiosyncratic expression of intent.

Semantics

The linguistic term *semantics* refers to meaning as it is encoded in language. Semantic knowledge therefore, refers to the meaning within a language that is linguistically coded. Conceptual knowledge affects the acquisition of the semantic component of language. Cromer (1981) suggested that conceptual knowledge in normal children is transformed into semantic knowledge. The difficult task for children is to determine which aspects of concepts are encoded within their particular linguistic system. The interactional experiences with agents, actions, and objects develop the semantic relationships that code the content of language.

Tager-Flusberg (1981) commented that there are "no systematic studies of semantic development in autistic children" (p. 49). This lack is rather unfortunate because an understanding of the semantic component in autistic children could describe how they develop and organize their conceptual experiences into progressively more sophisticated linguistic structures.

Baltaxe and Simmons (1975) collected speech samples and noted that the most frequent errors were violations of semantic constraints. The researchers posited that autism involves a semantic deficit in language learning. Ricks and Wing (1975) suggested that autism involves a deficit in representational behavior and high-level abstractions. Autistic children have difficulty developing complex relationships and thus, establishing the underpinnings for symbolic forms of behavior, which provide the foundations for language. Menyuk (1978) suggested that the underlying deficit relates to an inability to establish meaningful and relevant perceptual-conceptual categories. These abilities and their interaction enable normal children to establish general categories; that is, to relate agents, actions, and objects to one another. The establishment of categories enables children to make some cohesive and consistent sense of an environment, stimuli in the environment, and experiences within the environment which would otherwise be continually novel and changing. The abilities identified by Menyuk provide normal children with the means of organizing what they see and experience into manageable and related categories. According to Schmidt (1976), autistic subjects could not understand how objects were functionally related or associated (e.g., needle-thread). Although the autistic children could identify the objects, they did not know how these objects related to one another in terms of functional usage. Tager-Flusberg (1981) suggested that autistic children are not able to translate their real world experiences into linguistic structures; they cannot make use of a semantically based processing strategy.

Table 9–2 describes Adam's development of lexical items to express his semantic knowledge and ideas about the world. Adam's semantic development at this time (4 years, 9 months) indicates the limited or restricted developmental use of functions. Adam developed lexical items within four semantic categories. Most of the lexical items were food related—specifically, desserts. There were fewer action performances than objects coded, and two of the action performances related to food (e.g., eat and drink). Analyzing the child's corpus in this way provides the clinician with insight into what is important to the child within the environment. Clinically, Adam's preferences were incorporated into therapeutic activities.

Phonology

Phonological development in autistic children seems to follow the same course as in normal children. The suprasegmental features of rate, prosody, rhythm, and quality however, represent deviant aspects of autistic children's speech.

Bartolucci, Pierce, Streiner, and Eppel (1976) suggested that the frequency of distribution of phonemes in autistic children was similar to that found in retarded children. In both groups of children, the highest percentage of errors involved phonemes that were generally acquired later in normal children. The order of phonemic acquisition seems to follow the normal developmental pattern, in spite of the delay in the onset of

TABLE 9–2
Adam's Early Lexicon

Semantic Functions	*Lexical Entries*
Object	car, cookie, pretzel, juice, ice cream, milk, chip, M & M, hot dog, lolly, soda, popcorn, puzzle, slinky, block, shoe, raisin, grape.
Action	open, push, eat, drink, throw, give
Negation: rejection	no
cessation	no
Recurrence	repeat of item label
Agent	—
Action + Object	—

speech. Fay and Schuler (1980) noted that autistic children's phonological ability contrasted markedly with the developmental delays in the other linguistic and communicative areas.

The use of suprasegmental features, such as stress and intonation, are often described as deviant in autistic children. Many clinicians have noted that autistic children have peculiar voice quality and sometimes speak in a monotone. The stress and pitch patterns used by autistic children are often inappropriate to the meaning of the linguistic utterance and the context of the situation. In addition, autistic children's lack of affect may be explainable by the inability to process and utilize intonational features (environmental cues). This explanation of autistic children's speech behavior is more parsimonious than the suggestion of emotional impairment. The flat affect and monotonic pattern which is so typical of autistic children may be the result of an inability to process, register, and generate suprasegmental features within the linguistic message (Fay & Schuler, 1980).

The following description illustrates how these variables appeared in Adam's developmental pattern. Adam's progression from a period of muteness and virtual silence to a period of intelligible imitative productions was remarkable. There are many questions concerning this transition. Did the transition from muteness to echolalia result from the therapeutic and environmental experiences, neurological development, or both? The change from muteness to speech is, to say the least, remarkable if not explainable.

> Adam: Adam remained mute until the age of 4 years, 3 months. The only sounds that he produced were self-stimulatory sounds used to block out input from the environment. During these occurrences, Adam would raise the intensity or loudness of his own voice to block out various types of input: speaker's voice, music, and environmental noises such as a telephone ringing, a fire engine, or an airplane. The only other sounds he uttered were whining and crying sounds of distress.
>
> When Adam started to speak, he evidenced echolalic behavior. Although the suprasegmental features were deviant resulting in robot-like, wooden productions, his articulatory productions were extraordinarily intelligible. At 4 years, 6 months Adam's phonological development:
>
> 1. Had progressed *further* than any other language component
> 2. Followed the normal pattern or progression more closely than any other component

Syntax

Curtiss (1981) proposed that language components emerge from developments in cognitive knowledge. The development of a normal linguistic system in which structure is related to meaning, requires an interfacing of linguistic and nonlinguistic cognitive development. Curtiss suggested that lexical and relational semantic abilities are linked to broader conceptual development but that morphological and syntactic abilities are not.

There are very few studies which provide detailed information about the syntactic developments in autistic children. Cunningham (1968) described a longitudinal analysis of an autistic child from 6 to 11 years of age. The child's language indicated a gradual increase in mean length of utterance from 1.9 words to 3.0 words over a 6-month period. Grammatical morphemes and function words (articles, copulas, auxiliaries, pronouns, and prepositions) were often omitted. Bartolucci, Pierce, Streiner, and Eppel (1976) described the particular difficulty autistic children have with the developmental use of verb endings, such as past tense and present progressive. The researchers did not interpret these findings as a difficulty with grammatical structure, but rather as a difficulty with semantic development. The more basic problem for autistic children is that they do not understand the underlying conceptual ideas (i.e., past occurrence) that contribute to the formulation of language. Autistic children have difficulties using or manipulating certain linguistic forms of language because they do not understand the semantic counterparts of these forms.

Bartak, Rutter, and Cox (1975) compared autistic and dysphasic children. The researchers found both groups comparable in mean length of utterance (one of the major measures of productive language development) and grammatical complexity. On a test of comprehension, however, the autistic children performed more poorly than the dysphasic children. The researchers suggested that autistic children indicate a difficulty in their understanding of language.

It seems that the syntactic delays in autistic children are related to the general developmental delays. These children present syntactic processing skills similar to those evidenced by other types of disordered children. Linguistic analyses indicate the use of rule-governed behavior in the autistic child's limited production and comprehension of language. "Autistic subjects display mastery of a variety of grammatical rules, similar to matched groups of retarded, schizophrenic, or developmental aphasic subjects" (Tager-Flusberg, 1981, p. 49).

Adam's productions are analyzed within the framework of various contextual and interactional situations to highlight his limited linguistic processing abilities. Consider Adam's use of the following morphemes: present progressive, past tense, personal pronouns, relative pronouns, copula, articles, and plurals.

Clinician: What is mommy doing?
Adam: Mommy is opening juice.

Within the framework of an interaction with the adult, Adam was able to use the copula and present progressive morphemes within his own speech. He also responded to the adult's question by altering the inflectional form of the adult's utterance (i.e., he did not imitate the question's inflectional pattern).

Clinician: What did you do?
Adam: Adam eat three cookie.

Within the framework of an interaction with the adult, Adam responded to the question. He did not use any of the personal pronouns, but referred to himself as Adam. He was not able to code (or use) the past tense form. When Adam was not able to code the morphemic structures presented within the adult's production, he reduced his own utterance or reverted to a string of content words. Plural forms were coded by the use of number without the plural -s.

In the preceding examples, there was a structural relationship between the linguistic input provided by the adult and the structure of the child's linguistic response. Adam patterned his response on the structure of the adult's input. The following interaction shows what happened to Adam's linguistic structure when adult input was not provided.

Clinician: (Has just poured Adam some juice)
Adam: Drink juice (describing his own action)
Adam: More (requesting more juice)
Adam: Pour juice (directing clinician to perform an action)
Adam: Give (requesting cup from clinician)

In this interaction, the clinician responded nonverbally to all of Adam's requests and directions. He did not, therefore, have the adult's linguistic input to rely on to structure his own utterances. The result was a reduction to the minimum use of forms that convey the communicative message, or "get the message across" effectively. This reduction process was quite typical of Adam's spontaneous, or self-initiated speech. In order to understand autistic children's structural/syntactic abilities, it is important to analyze if and how the language structure changes within various interactional situations. For Adam, the adult's input provided a syntactic framework for productions or responses. Finally, Adam's productions required a close analysis of the context in order to determine or disambiguate the meaning of his utterances. He *rarely* provided gestural support for his verbal productions.

THERAPEUTIC ISSUES AND STRATEGIES

Our view of the autistic child has changed in the past several years. The theoretical changes occurring in the area of child language development have affected dramatically the content and context of therapeutic programs. An analysis of *what* autistic children have been trained to *do* has changed from speech training to communication training. With the focus on communication learning, several related issues have been investigated by speech-language pathologists: parent language training, home training, alternative language systems, and language socialization in the classroom. These components present a more holistic approach to the language learning experience for autistic children.

Therapeutic programming varies from child to child, family to family, and clinician to clinician. It is this variety in training approaches and styles that provides our profession with its clinical strength.

The Operant Orientation

Because of the extensive behavioral difficulties characteristic of autistic children, many clinicians have used behavioral procedures to train targeted behaviors such as self-care and daily living skills, as well as speech behaviors. The behavioral approach has also been used as part of educational programs to deal with inappropriate and injurious behaviors exhibited within the classroom. The classroom teacher has relied on the modification model because of the need to operationalize classroom procedures and training goals. Underlying the behavioral approach is the identification of an observable and measurable targeted performance (i.e., sitting, looking, and vocalizing). The clinician or teacher would not target, for example, *attention* as a training performance.

Rather, the clinician would identify all of the descriptive behaviors of attention: sitting, physical orientation, eye contact, etc. These identified behaviors were then trained by means of a successive approximation procedure. The example of vocal training that follows shows such an orientation to develop speech. The emphasis in training was on a specific *form* of behavior.

> Adam at this time was mute; the only sounds he produced were self-stimulatory, guttural productions. The decision was made to train Adam to say /mama/. The primary reinforcer used was Jahn's vanilla ice cream. Adam was seated directly opposite the clinician. The clinician was seated in a child's chair so that she was at eye level with Adam. The sound targeted for initial training was the /a/. Adam had *already* been trained to sit in his chair and look at the clinician when instructed to do so. The procedure used to train these behaviors was a successive approximation procedure in which performances that gradually progressed in the direction of the targeted or final behavior were reinforced. Approximately 1,500 training trials were required to develop the production of /mama/.

The problems with this type of training procedure concern generalization and functional usage for autistic children. Autistic children have great difficulty in generalizing learned behavior to a new context or situation. In normal children, it could have been assumed that successive training would have decreased the training necessary to achieve the criterion for the next production. With Adam however, each training experience was a new one. This extensive and arduous training was difficult to justify (i.e., six "word" productions in one semester). Training resulted in an imitative response, not a behavior which the child could use communicatively, at least not at this point.

Function and Context

Functional usage for the child is a critical issue. Once having trained /mama/, what does the production mean to the child? Because the production resulted in ice cream in the training experience previously described, that is what it meant to Adam. There was not a relationship between what he said and a meaningful consequence in the environment. It would have been different if Adam had been trained to say ice cream and the result were ice cream.

The problem with the approach is *what* the children are being trained to do, not *how* they are being trained. The difference concerns content versus procedure. Vocal/speech training goals have been identified for autistic children by many researchers (Hartung, 1970; Hewett, 1965; Lovaas, 1977). Yoder and Calculator (1981) noted that when a primary reinforcer such as ice cream is the consequence of a child's behavior, there is an arbitrary relationship between the child's behavior and the environment. The procedure described was concerned with the form of the child's utterance rather than its function or intent. This procedure has frequently been used to train speech productions or productions which have little functional use for the child (i.e., shapes, colors, and numbers). Yoder and Calculator stressed the importance of the child's behavior within the framework of the communication context; they urged teaching the child how to interact within a social milieu.

Clinical Changes

Several researchers have noted that there might be a critical period for language learning. If this is the case, then it becomes more important as the child gets older to identify a training program, technique, or context that is directly suited to the needs of the child. In terms of autistic children, clinical research has indicated serious deficits in the areas of semantics and pragmatics. Developmental research has described that normal children acquire communication behaviors before semantic behaviors, and semantic behaviors before syntactic behaviors. Autistic children must be provided with the prerequisite social underpinnings if linguistic structure is going to develop meaningfully in relation to the other language components.

Learning Contexts

Adam's training was changed to reflect the theoretical issues raised in the literature during the 1970s and 1980s. In the following program, there was an attempt to incorporate each environment (school, after school therapy, and home) within the educational process. A set of operating principles was developed to coordinate intervention goals and therapeutic programming. The identified learning contexts represented a means of generalizing communication experiences for the child across the different educational environments. The communication behaviors learned in the classroom could be generalized to the home or the therapy room. The following operating principles were utilized to develop Adam's learning contexts:

1. A learning context was defined as any activity which provided an interactional framework, that is an opportunity for interchange between the adult and the child. The activity was then described in terms of the type of (*a*) interactions to be developed, (*b*) communicative behaviors to be learned, and (*c*) semantic functions to be coded (See Table 9–3).
2. Each learning context presented a format or routine.
3. Each learning context established a task structure to develop an anticipation and sequence of events in the routine.
4. The learning context facilitated action and interaction; it allowed for the development of reversible role relationships between adult and child.

TABLE 9–3
An Example of a Learning Context

Place	*Activity/Context*	*Materials*	*Routine*	*Communicative Behavior*
Therapy Room	Making bubbles	Bubbles Large bubble wand Fan	Get bubbles Open bubbles Get wand Pour bubbles Fan on Make bubbles	Point to object Gaze at object/adult Sign for object (or action) Consistent vocalization for object (or action) Word Some combination of these behaviors

5. A core lexicon within each learning context was developed to consistently and systematically focus communication and language training across all of the adults working with the child.
6. The core lexicon was based upon the development of those communicative behaviors that appear earliest in child language. These communicative behaviors were used across a variety of learning contexts to generalize language and communication relations.
7. Communicative interaction was stressed above production of stereotypic/routinized utterances.
8. Learning contexts developed were relevant and functional to the *child.* The adult focused on activities that the child preferred in order to facilitate interaction and communication.
9. Input to the child was limited in complexity and mean length of utterance. Adult input was functional and relevant to the immediate context and semantically related to the child's vocal, verbal, and nonlinguistic behavior.
10. The child was presented with a choice of learning contexts; at any time, he could maintain or terminate an activity. Verbal, vocal, and nonverbal behaviors were analyzed within the learning contexts, to determine communicative intentions.
11. The child was first trained to participate and interact within the context. Then the child was trained to produce behaviors that coded the next occurrence in the routine.
12. Every adult working with the child was given a copy of the communication/language description of each learning context. Thus, each adult provided consistent input within and across activities (See Table 9–4).
13. Echolalic behavior was used to develop language behaviors. With the knowledge that the child would imitate, the adult would code, for instance, a nonlinguistic event:
    Event: Adam opening the bubbles
    Adult: Adam open bubbles
    Adam: Adam open bubbles

Therapeutic Goals and Clinical Strategies

The clinical goals identified for training included:

1. Development of imitative interaction skills
2. Expansion of object manipulation skills (semantic knowledge)
3. Development of sign/gesture forms
4. Use of interactional behaviors that signal communicative intentions
5. Generalization of communication behaviors

The goals and procedures described in this section should be considered with regard for the need to individualize language and communication programming. However, the following procedures and issues are related to interactional deficits that are characteristic of autistic children.

TABLE 9–4
An Example of a Communication/Language Description of a Learning Context

Context—Bubbles

Materials

Bottle of bubbles

Bubble maker
Fan

Semantic Functions	*Forms Trained/Adult Input*
1. Object	Bubbles, fan
2. Action	Open, blow, give, turn-on
3. Agent	Ellen, Adam, Mommy, Daddy
4. Agent + Agent	Adam open, Ellen open Adam blow, Ellen blow
5. Action + Object	Make bubbles, pour bubbles, open bubbles
6. Recurrence	Bubbles . . bubbles . . bubbles, more, more bubbles
7. Negation rejection cessation (action)	No, no bubbles Stop, no more, no more bubbles No pour, no blow
8. Agent + Action + Object	Adam open bubbles Ellen open bubbles Mommy open bubbles Adam pour bubbles Ellen pour bubbles Adam blow bubbles Ellen blow bubbles Mommy blow bubbles

Imitation and Interaction

Given Adam's inability to imitate vocal, body-oriented (clap hands), and object-oriented (shake bell) behaviors, an imitation play procedure was utilized to stimulate primitive and primary adult-child interactions (Tiegerman, 1979). In this procedure, Adam was seated opposite the clinician at a table with various objects on it. Duplicate objects were placed before the clinician. As Adam manipulated his object, the clinician *imitated* Adam's movements with the object. The basis for interaction was controlled by Adam. What Adam did affected what the clinician did. The similarity in performance between Adam and the clinician was the manipulation of the same object, the same action on the object, and the same interaction time with the object. The contingency relationship established that adult imitation was a function of the child's object manipulation performances. Fifteen minutes of every clinical session involved the use of this procedure.

The imitation procedure resulted in an increase in the frequency and duration of two performances—gaze and object manipulation. Imitation provided a basis for the development of interaction with Adam. Imitating Adam's object-oriented performances emphasized the effect he had on the object and the adult. The child's initiations were reinforced through control of the adult's performances (Tiegerman & Primavera, 1981, 1984).

By using Adam's limited manipulation repertoire, it was possible to expand his interactions within the environment. Knowledge of the environment is a necessary and important part of the sensorimotor experience. Children learn about agents, actions, and people through direct manipulation experiences of the environment. Thus, expanding autistic children's interactional skills increases their knowledge of the world. One problem often described is that autistic children are very resistant to the stricture and structure of training. The imitation procedure placed the child in control of the situation and did not create a pressure to perform. It ensured that the development of object manipulations was not confounded by the presentation of manipulative performances not within the child's behavioral repertoire. Thus, the child's performances were used to develop adult-child interaction. Imitation of the child provided a natural training experience in which the autistic child learned first about the imitation process and then the rules in playing the game.

An Alternate System of Communication

The theory underlying the use of an alternate system of communication in the nonverbal, nondeaf child, concerns the nature of the alternative experience and the possible cross-modal deficits in the autistic child. The alternative systems used most frequently with autistic children are sign language and communication boards using pictures, Blissymbols, or words.

Hermelin and O'Connor (1970) described the autistic child's difficulties in information and stimulus processing. Given problems in the simultaneous processing of auditory and visual information, the researchers suggested that sign language might provide a more concrete, motorically based system. Aside from the issue of processing difficulties with this population, there is also the question and possible reality of a critical period for language learning. It thus becomes more important as the child gets older to develop a communication system of one kind or another. A communicative system should be developed first, and the form of the system (oral versus sign language) addressed later. These issues have provided the impetus for the use of alternative communication systems in autistic children.

There are, however, problems with the use of the alternative systems. Is it realistic to suggest that another form of language will be trained easily later on to a child who has initial difficulties learning a language system? Is it appropriate to train a sign system in an oral environment? How many people within the oral environment will be able to respond to the child? How generalizable is a sign language system for the autistic child? Adam's mother noted her concern.

> "My son is not deaf. Given the severity of his learning problem, will he be able to make the transition between what he hears and the sign form of language? Teaching him a nonstandard form of communication makes him even more different than other children; he's different enough as it is."

The parents' concerns and feelings must be addressed. Parents must believe in what they are doing if they are going to play a role in their child's training. In spite of these questions, sign language training has been utilized with many nonverbal populations of children to establish an initial communication system.

Adam's training was typical of the sign training experience provided to many autistic children (Bonvillian & Nelson, 1976). He was observed in the environment to note his interests and preferences for objects and actions. On the basis of his preferences, a training corpus of signs was developed. Adam, for example, was "into" Jahn's vanilla ice cream. During training, the sign was always paired with the presentation of the word, providing him with both forms of input. Although Adam was only required to initiate interaction by using sign forms, the simultaneous input (sign and word) was presented to facilitate the child's transition from sign to oral communication. A short-term clinical goal was to train Adam to communicate by using sign forms. A long-term clinical goal was to generalize sign communication to oral communication.

Miller and Miller (1973) described the development of sign usage as a function of the autistic child's need to change the physical environment. They described how the use of raised floor boards forced autistic children to focus on their environment. The child learned to remove physical obstacles by communicating with an adult. As a mediator, the adult changed the environment in some way for the child. This organization of the clinical context was used with Adam to facilitate communicative interaction. A corpus of 14 signs was developed in 15 weeks. The first 2 signs required the greatest number of training trials. Unlike the vocal training experience, the number of training trials needed to achieve a performance criterion level decreased dramatically and steadily for each new sign introduced.

> Adam was given the ice cream in a container that he could not open. He had to sign *open,* and then the clinician would open the container. A successive approximation procedure was used to gradually shape the child's productions of the sign. Once the ice cream container was open, Adam had to sign for *spoon* and then *eat* before he finally got the ice cream. In this way, a series of related events was linked or chained together to produce a series of signs which eventually resulted in the desired object, action, or person.

Echolalia and Communicative Intentions

Prizant (1983) suggested that echolalia should be viewed as a dynamic and integral part of autistic children's developmental pattern. Their echolalic behavior can provide a means for training communication interactions. Their imitative ability can be used to assimilate and coordinate a linguistic event with a related nonlinguistic event. By emphasizing the relationship between linguistic behavior and nonlinguistic environmental consequences, echolalic behavior can be embedded meaningfully within appropriate contexts. The development of communicative intentions should be actively stimulated by the adult initially using the children's echolalic tendencies to establish the relationship between language and environmental referents (objects, actions, and people). The adult language input model should be regulated in terms of linguistic complexity to the child's level of comprehension (Tiegerman & Siperstein, 1984). In addition, the adult's language model, which sets the occasion for the child's echolalic behavior, should always result in an immediate and observable environmental consequence. It is important to teach autistic children that language has an effect—it creates change. Whenever possible and relevant, the adult should manipulate the environment to produce the effect the child linguistically codes. The clinician's use of exaggerated gesture and intonation, linguistic simplification and repetition, and action repetition, are helpful in focusing the child on language that is relevant to an activity.

In attempting to teach autistic children to express their needs, the clinician should manipulate contextual events to create the need and facilitate its expression.

Context: Ice cream container that cannot be opened by the child

Adult: Ellen open ice cream

Adam: Ellen open ice cream

Consequence: Ellen performs action

It is important for the clinician to identify a number of situational contexts that create communicative need. These situations provide autistic children with the opportunity to direct intentionally the course of events within the environment. The ultimate goal involves teaching autistic children that language is a tool, a vehicle, a means to affect the behavior of other interactants. To achieve this goal, autistic children must experience themselves as effective communicators within the social context.

Although difficult to explain, the following sequence describes Adam's transition from the use of sign language to oral language forms. The end result of this period was echolalic behavior.

> Adam's mother described this occurrence as the child's "eureka" experience. Adam came to language therapy one day producing a verbal label (very clearly, I might add) in place of a learned sign. In the next 4 weeks, he replaced his sign productions with verbal productions. In Adam's case, sign training seems to have facilitated the development of verbal production. Once a sign was replaced with a verbal production, the sign was never used again. His communication system, therefore, consisted of several forms: words, sign forms, and interchangeable sign/verbal forms. These interchangeable forms indicated a transition—replacement of sign by word. Each new word form increased in usage as the sign decreased.

This replacement process emphasizes that even as an impaired learner, Adam indicated a systematic learning pattern. Perhaps the pattern represents a unique or idiosyncratic pattern of learning, but it was a pattern nonetheless, and when identified, provided some insight into how Adam learned.

Generalization of Communication Behaviors—Home Training

In the attempt to generalize the language learning experience to various environments, a home training program was developed. The home provided a training experience for Adam within a more natural learning environment. Part of the program included training parents and siblings as communication facilitators. In addition, a dedicated group of volunteers was trained to work within the framework of the program and to provide extensive training 7 days a week—after school and on weekends.

The home training program can be contrasted with the more traditional therapy experience provided for Adam in school. Family members could not participate in sessions during the school day. At home, the parent training model incorporated everyone's participation. His mother was present and integrated into the framework of each session. She was carefully trained by the speech-language pathologist to work with Adam at home.

The home and school training experiences were different in terms of the amount of stimulation provided. The home-based program was developed to be a language training program for as long as Adam was awake. In school, the speech-language pathologist provided language training outside the classroom 3 times a week for 30 minutes. Coordinating training goals with the classroom teacher was possible but difficult.

Another difference concerned the nature of the training experience itself. The home training program focused on the development of language and communication behaviors within all of the training contexts (See Table 9–3). Activities were identified to facilitate interaction and communication. The activity provided a means to an end—adult-child interaction. Nothing had to be simulated. Activities were meaningful and relevant to the child's daily living needs and the immediate context. The adult's input to the child and the child's language corpus were

1. Regulated to the child's level of communication functioning
2. Related semantically to the ongoing nonlinguistic experience
3. Sensitive to the child's interests and preferences

Traditional classroom activities with colors, shapes, numbers, beads, and pegs were never utilized because of their limited potential for facilitating communication and interaction.

As a language learning experience, the home training program presented certain advantages for Adam as a severely language-disordered child. First, family members were trained to function as communication facilitators. Second, the various activities within the home provided the means to integrate language behavior with relevant nonlinguistic experiences. Third, the use of communicative behaviors was generalized across training contexts. Fourth, the orientation of the program emphasized the child's language and communication needs. These components were not available to Adam within the traditional special education classroom. The home training program proved to be an important addition to traditional learning.

SUMMARY

This chapter has emphasized the unique language learning problems in autistic children. Traditionally, autistic children have been described as a single population. The research cited in this chapter has stressed the heterogeneity exhibited within this group, suggesting that the etiological label is misleading. In addition, the use of this label detracts from the central problem related to the disorder—the inability to integrate communicative function with other aspects of language. The research of Tager-Flusberg (1981) described a schism between "form and function" in autistic children; the basic disturbances in language are with pragmatic and semantic skills—phonological and syntactic skills develop relatively intact. In fact, the literature describing language evidenced in higher functioning autistic individuals, indicates severe communicative deficits in contrast to the acquisition of structural linguistic skills (Baltaxe, 1977). Such communicative incompetence included ongoing problems with initiating and terminating interaction, deficits in topic maintenance, and speaker/listener roles.

Autism as a disorder, emphasizes the need for language-based educational orientation. The changes in child language theory have contributed greatly to the new therapeutic approaches used with autistic children, such as Adam. In a way, Adam is a product of the pragmatic era and communication revolution. At this point, one can only wonder about the impact of these theoretical and therapeutic changes on autistic children.

Finally, the speech-language pathologist has a central role to play in the educational programming developed for autistic children. There is not another professional who can better understand the language and communication deficits underlying this disorder.

STUDY QUESTIONS

1. Describe the autistic child's interactional behaviors. How do these interactional behaviors affect the autistic child's language? Describe the unique communication characteristics related to the autistic child.
2. What purpose does the ritual serve? How is the autistic child's language affected by ritualized patterns?
3. How could the clinician analyze the interactive behaviors exhibited by an individual child?
4. What are the issues related to the use of alternative systems of communication?
5. Why should the speech-language pathologist play a central role in the educational programming of autistic children?

BIBLIOGRAPHY

Alpern, G., & Yang, E. (1969). *Objective personality differences between parents of brain damaged autistic children.* (Research report 9). Paper presented at the Clinical Research Center for Early Childhood Schizophrenia, Indianapolis.

Bakwin, H. (1954). Early infantile autism. *Journal of Pediatrics, 45,* 492–497.

Baltaxe, C. (1977). Pragmatic deficits in the language of autistic adolescents. *Journal of Pediatric Psychology, 2,* 176–180.

Baltaxe, C., & Simmons, J. (1975). Language in childhood psychosis: A review. *Journal of Speech and Hearing Disorders, 40,* 439–458.

Bartak, L., & Rutter, M. (1976). Differences between mentally retared and normally intelligent autistic children. *Journal of Autism and Childhood Schizophrenia, 6,* 109–120.

Bartak, L., Rutter, M., & Cox, A. (1975). A comparative study of infantile autism and specific developmental receptive language disorder. I. The children. *British Journal of Psychiatry, 126,* 127–145.

Bartolucci, G., Pierce, S., Streiner, D., & Eppel, P.T. (1976). Phonological investigation of verbal autistic and mentally retarded subjects. *Journal of Autism and Childhood Schizophrenia, 6,* 303–316.

Bettelheim, B. (1967). *The empty fortress—Infantile autism and the birth of the self.* New York: Free Press.

Black, M., Freeman, B., & Montgomery, J. (1975). Systematic observation of play behavior in autistic children. *Journal of Autism and Childhood Schizophrenia, 5,* 363–371.

Blank, M., Gessner, M., & Esposito, A. (1979). Language without communication: A case study. *Journal of Child Language, 6,* 329–352.

Bonvillian, J., & Nelson, K. (1976). Sign language acquisition in a mute autistic boy. *Journal of Speech and Hearing Disorders, 41,* 339–347.

Bruner, J. (1967). *On knowing.* New York: Atheneum.

Bryson, C. (1970). Systematic identification of perceptual disabilities in autistic children. *Perceptual and Motor Skills, 31,* 239–246.

Chase, A. (1972). Neurological aspects of language disorders in children. In J.V. Irwin & M. Marge (Eds.), *Principles of childhood language disorders.* Englewood Cliffs, NJ: Prentice-Hall.

Churchill, D. (1978). *Language of autistic children.* New York: Wiley.

Clune, C., Paolella, J., & Foley, J. (1979). Free-play behavior of atypical children: An approach to assessment. *Journal of Autism and Developmental Disorders, 9,* 61–72.

Cromer, R. (1981). Developmental language disorders: Cognitive processes, semantics, pragmatics, phonology and syntax. *Journal of Autism and Developmental Disorders, 11,* 57–74.

Cunningham, M. (1968). A comparison of the language of psychotic and nonpsychotic children who are mentally retarded. *Journal of Psychiatry, 9,* 229–244.

Curcio, F. (1978). Sensorimotor functioning and communication in mute autistic children. *Journal of Autism and Childhood Schizophrenia, 3,* 281–292.

Curtiss, S. (1981). Dissociations between language and cognition: Cases and implications. *Journal of Autism and Developmental Disorders, 11,* 15–30.

Dalgleish, B. (1975). Cognitive processing and linguistic reference in autistic children. *Journal of Autism and Childhood Schizophrenia, 5,* 353–361.

DeMyer, M., Barton, S., DeMyer, E., Norton, J., Allen, J., & Steele, R. (1973). Prognosis in autism: A follow-up study. *Journal of Autism and Childhood Schizophrenia, 3,* 199–216.

DeMyer, M., Barton, S., Alpern, G., Kimberlin, C., Allen, J., Yang, E., & Steele, R. (1974). The measured intelligence of autistic children. *Journal of Autism and Childhood Schizophrenia, 4,* 42–60.

DeMyer, M., Pontius, W., Norton, J., Barton, S., Allen, J., & Steele, R. (1972). Parental practices and innate activity in normal, autistic and brain-damaged infants. *Journal of Autism and Childhood Schizophrenia, 2,* 49–66.

Eckerman, C., & Whatley, J. (1977). Toys and social interaction between infant peers. *Child Development, 48,* 1645–1656.

Eisenberg, L. (1956). The autistic child in adolescence. *American Journal of Psychiatry, 112,* 607–612.

Fay, W., & Schuler, A. (1980). *Emerging language in autistic children: Language intervention series.* Baltimore: University Park Press.

Fish, B., Shapiro, T., & Campbell, M. (1966). Long-term prognosis and the response of schizophrenic children to drug therapy: A controlled study of trifluoperazine. *American Journal of Psychiatry, 123,* 32–39.

Garvey, C. (1974). Some properties of social play. *Merrill-Palmer Quarterly, 20,* 163–180.

Hartung, J. (1970). A review of functional speech in autistic children. *Journal of Speech and Hearing Disorders, 35,* 203–217.

Hermelin, B. (1978). Images and language. In M. Rotter & E. Schopler (Eds.), *Autism: A reappraisal of concepts and treatment.* New York: Plenum Press.

Hermelin, B., & O'Connor, N. (1970). *Psychological experiments with autistic children.* London: Pergamon.

Hewett, F. (1965). Teaching speech to an autistic child through operant conditioning. *American Journal of Orthopsychiatry, 35,* 927–936.

Hutt, C., & Ounsted, C. (1966). The biological significance of gaze aversion with particular reference to the syndrome of infantile autism. *Behavioral Science, 11,* 346–356.

Kanner, L. (1943). Autistic disturbances in affective contact. *Nervous Child, 2,* 217–250.

Kanner, L. (1944). Early infantile autism. *Journal of Pediatrics, 25,* 211–217.

Kanner, L. (1952). Emotional interference with intellectual functioning. *American Journal of Mental Deficiency, 56,* 701–707.

Koegel, R., & Rincover, A. (1977). Research on the difference between generalization and maintenance in extra-therapy responding. *Journal of Applied Behavior Analysis, 10,* 1–12.

Lockyer, L., & Rutter, M. (1970). A five to fifteen year follow-up study of infantile psychosis. IV. Patterns of cognitive ability. *British Journal of Social and Clinical Psychology, 9,* 152–163.

Lotter, V. (1967). Epidemiology of autistic conditions in young children: Some characteristics of parents and children. *Social Psychiatry, 1,* 163–181.

Lovaas, O.I. (1977). *The autistic child: Language development through behavior modification.* New York: Irvington.

Lovaas, O.I., Schreibman, J., Koegel, R., & Rehm, R. (1971). Selective responding by autistic children to multiple sensory input. *Journal of Olinormal Psychology, 71,* 211–222.

Lovaas, O.I., & Schreibman, L. (1971). Stimulus overselectivity of autistic children in a two-stimulus situation. *Behavior Research and Therapy, 9,* 305–310.

Maltz, A. (1981). Comparison of cognitive deficits among autistic and retarded children on the Arthur Adaption of the Leiter International Performance Scales. *Journal of Autism and Developmental Disorders, 11,* 413–426.

Menyuk, P. (1978). Language: What's wrong and why. In M. Rutter & E. Schopler (Eds.), *Autism: A reappraisal of concepts and treatment.* New York: Plenum Press.

Michelman, S. (1974). Play and the deficit child. In M. Reilly (Ed.), *Play as exploratory learning.* Beverly Hills, CA: Sage.

Miller, A., & Miller, E. (1973). Cognitive-developmental training with elevated boards and sign language. *Journal of Autism and Childhood Schizophrenia, 3,* 65–85.

Ornitz, E., & Ritvo, E. (1968). Perceptual inconstancy in early infantile autism: The syndrome of early infant autism and its variants including certain cases of childhood schizophrenia. *Archives of General Psychiatry, 18,* 76–98.

Piaget, J. (1962). *Play, dreams, and imitation in childhood.* New York: Nordon.

Polan, C., & Spencer, B. (1959). A checklist of symptoms of autism in early life. *West Virginia Medical Journal, 55,* 198–204.

Prizant, B. (1983). Echolalia in autism: assessment and intervention. *Seminars in Speech and Language, 4,* 63–78.

Prizant, B., & Duchan, J. (1981). The functions of immediate echolalia in autistic children. *Journal of Speech and Hearing Disorders, 46,* 241–249.

Ricks, D., & Wing, L. (1975). Language, communication and the use of symbols in normal and autistic children. *Journal of Autism and Childhood Schizophrenia, 5,* 191–220.

Schmidt, J. (1976). *Relations between paired-associate learning and utterance patterns in children with echolalia.* Unpublished doctoral dissertation, Boston University School of Education.

Shapiro, T., and Fish, B. (1969). A method to study language deviation as an aspect of ego organization in young schizophrenic children. *Journal of American Academy of Child Psychiatry, 8,* 36–56.

Tager-Flusberg, H. (1981). On the nature of linguistic functioning in early infantile autism. *Journal of Autism and Developmental Disorders, 11,* 45–56.

Tiegerman, E. (1979). *A comparison of three play procedures in the manipulation of gaze behavior and object use with autistic children.* Doctoral dissertation, City University of New York.

Tiegerman, E., & Primavera, L. (1981). Object manipulation. An interactional strategy with autistic children. *Journal of Autism and Developmental Disorders, 11,* 427–439.

Tiegerman, E., & Primavera, L. (1984, March). Imitating the autistic child: Facilitating communicative gaze behavior. *Journal of Autism and Developmental Disorders.*

Tiegerman, E., & Siperstein, M. (1984). Individual patterns of interaction in the mother-child dyad: Implications for the language disordered child. *Topics in Language Disorders, 4,* 50–62.

Weisler, A., & McCall, R. (1976). Exploration and play: Resume and redirection. *American Psychologist, 31,* 492–504.

Yoder, D., & Calculator, S. (1981). Some perspectives on intervention strategies for persons with developmental disorders. *Journal of Autism and Developmental Disorders, 11,* 107–124.

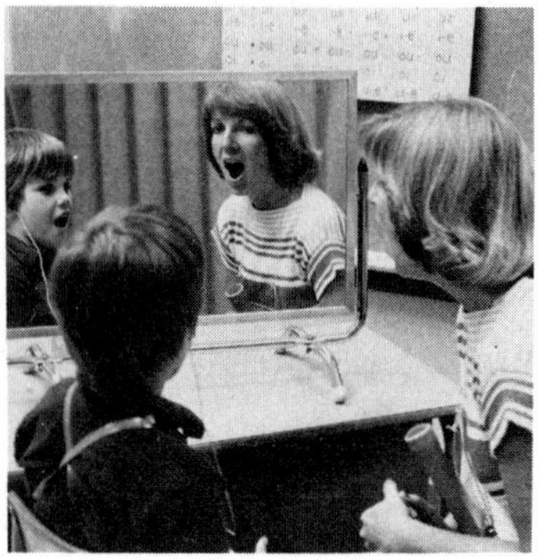

10

Hearing-Impaired Children: Language Acquisition and Remediation

Hearing-impaired children have been taught in a variety of educational settings including oral, acoupedic, and sign language programs. When evaluating the appropriate classroom placement, the most important issue relates to the hearing-impaired child's language proficiency. There are specific problems related to the speech-language profile of the hearing-impaired child. These problems must be identified appropriately by speech-language pathologists to enable the child to perform optimally in an educational setting. Significant to the child's progress will be the type of individual and group amplification used both at home and in the classroom.

Language input models have a profound effect on the child. Parents now have greater options concerning the type of educational setting best suited for their children. A parent can research and make an educated decision concerning placement into oral, manual, or total communication programs. Much of this freedom afforded to parents is a direct result of federal legislation passed in 1973 and 1974. Section 504 of the Rehabilitation Act and Public Law 94-142 mandated that all handicapped children are entitled to an appropriate education. This landmark decision changed countless school placements for hearing-impaired children.

Remediation for hearing-impaired children incorporates a variety of speech-language therapeutic techniques. To create optimum results, most approaches are combined and include speechreading, auditory training, and cued speech, as well as instruction in syntax, morphology, and pragmatics.

This chapter was written by Dr. Joan Braverman-Callahan, Adelphi University, and Christine K. Radziewicz, Adelphi University.

In addition to focusing on those problems specific to the hearing handicapped, this chapter will also examine the development of speech and language behaviors of the hearing impaired and will comment on the important research that has occurred during the last several years. This research has important implications for the teacher/speech-language pathologist working with hearing-handicapped children. The majority of this research refers to a severely hearing-impaired population, and for purposes of clarity we have used the terms *hearing-impaired* and *deaf* interchangeably. Both of these terms refer to a child who has a hearing threshold of 71 dB or above in the better ear.

Describing the speech and language behaviors of hearing-impaired children is a difficult task. The various factors or variables that influence the development of language in the presence of hearing loss (Quigley & Kretchmer, 1982) include:

- degree of hearing loss
- age of onset of loss
- slope of hearing loss
- age of identification of hearing loss
- age of habilitation
- amount of habilitation
- type of habilitation
- the nature of the language input—English or American Sign Language
- the nature of the communication mode—manual or oral

Degree of hearing loss refers to the severity of the hearing loss and is easily measured. According to Knauf (1972), the hearing threshold is frequently the first measurement available for estimating the impact of a child's hearing impairment. In the past, it had generally been assumed that the greater the hearing loss, the greater the impact on speech and language development. Although a severe hearing loss of 71 dB to 90 or 95 dB does have a devastating effect on speech and language development, we cannot assume that a mild hearing loss of 26 dB to 40 dB will always have a minimal effect or that a profound loss of 96 dB or above will have the most detrimental effect on speech and language development. To emphasize this point, Northern (1984) referred to a case report of a 13-year-old patient who had suffered from frequent bouts of otitis media. Over a period of 7 years, the air conduction thresholds fluctuated from normal to mild to moderate levels. Over the 7 years, five myringotomies were performed. However, a progressive sensorineural hearing loss had resulted from the repeated attacks of serous otitis media leaving this patient with an underlying mild to moderate sloping sensorineural hearing loss with bone conduction thresholds of 25 dB at 4000 Hz in one ear and of 30 and 45 dB at 2000 Hz and 4000 Hz in the other ear. In this case, not only the degree of hearing loss but the age of onset, the age of identification, and the type of habilitation were critical factors which resulted in the severity of the language deficit. Although this child's loss was not discovered until the age of 6, he probably had suffered from chronic otitis media earlier in his life. Age of onset could have occurred more than 5 years before age of identification, and therefore could have included the critical language-learning years. Furthermore, habilitation involved surgical myringotomies without habilitative speech and language therapy. Northern concluded his description of this case by stating that when the 13-year-old patient was given a hearing aid for habilitation, it was already 13 years too late. This child was evidencing a delay in speech and language that was irreversible.

The degree of hearing loss, although the most salient variable, is not necessarily the most critical. The combination and interplay of all the aforementioned variables determine the effect of hearing loss on speech and language development. Because of the interdependency of variables, one can never predict with certainty the detrimental effects of hearing loss on speech and language from degree of impairment alone. The only certainty is that hearing loss in any form (conductive, mixed, or sensorineural) and of any degree (mild to profound) can have a devastating effect on speech and language development.

HEARING LOSS—TYPES AND ETIOLOGY

Hearing loss may be viewed according to type. If the hearing loss is due to a condition existing in the external or middle ear, the loss is a conductive one. Conductive hearing impairments never exceed a hearing threshold level of 60 dB (ANSI) and are generally remediable through medical intervention. A common conductive impairment found in children 12 years and younger is otitis media, an inflammation of the middle ear space. Pashley (1984) stated that "otitis media is the most common problem (other than upper respiratory infection) for which a child is seen by a physician" (p. 103). There are two forms of otitis media: otitis media with effusion and purulent otitis media. When an inflammation of the middle ear space occurs without infection, liquid is still present within the middle ear cavity. This liquid may be thin (serous) or thick (mucoid). This form of otitis media is termed *otitis media with effusion.* It can occur when the eustachian tube becomes blocked and a closed middle ear space exists. Negative middle ear pressure will result, and fluid will ooze into the cavity.

When the inflammation of the middle ear space occurs as a result of infection, and pus is present, the eardrum may rupture and discharge otorrhea. This form of otitis media which involves pus behind the eardrum and/or rupture of the eardrum is called *purulent otitis media.* It is a progressive disease that changes the condition of the middle ear over a period of time. Pashley (1984) classified these changes according to stages: acute, which lasts up to 5 weeks; subacute, which begins at 6 weeks and lasts up to 11 weeks; and, chronic, which occurs from 12 weeks onward. Acute otitis media with accompanying ear pain occurs quite suddenly, and may subside suddenly when the tympanic membrane ruptures allowing the discharge of otorrhea.

Chronic otitis media often has its onset in early childhood, is a recurrent disease, and is a serious threat to speech and language development. Kaplan, Fleshman, Bender, Baum, and Clark (1973) studied the incidence of otitis media in Eskimo children and its effect on their speech and language development. This longitudinal study of approximately 500 children traced their development from birth to 7 through 10 years old. All the children were assessed using the Wechsler Intelligence Scale for Children (WISC), the Bender-Gestalt tests for perceptual problems, the Metropolitan Achievement Test, and the Draw-a-Person Test. Results of this study demonstrated that those children who had a history of otitis media before age 2 had suffered 5 to 7 attacks, had hearing levels of 26 dB or greater, evidenced a significant loss of verbal ability, and had deficits in reading, math, and language. From this study, it can be concluded that children who have recurrent episodes of otitis media beginning before the age of 2 are likely to be delayed in speech and language development. This delay can result later in poor academic performance.

Conductive hearing loss also can occur when there is obstruction in the ear canal. This condition can be caused from a congenital malformation such as atresia of the external canal, which is an abnormal constriction of the canal, or it can be caused from impacted cerumen, or wax.

Cholesteatoma is another cause of conductive hearing loss. A cholesteatoma is a cyst that is lined internally with squamous epithelium (scale-like skin). This cyst originates from the upper part of the tympanic membrane and forms a pouch. Eventually this cyst can cause perforation of the tympanic membrane and erode the ossicles (tiny bones) of the middle ear.

Any of these conditions which cause conductive impairment can also be present in a child who has a sensorineural loss. When both a sensorineural and a conductive loss exist, the child is said to have a mixed hearing loss.

A sensorineural hearing loss is a loss of hearing caused by damage to the nerve fibers and cochlear hair cells or damage to the auditory nerve. Sensorineural hearing loss can range from mild to profound. The following is an audiometric classification system suggested by Bess and McConnell (1981):

Hearing Threshold Level	*Classification*
26–40 dB	Mild
41–55 dB	Moderate
56–70 dB	Moderate Severe
71–90 or 95 dB	Severe
96 dB or above	Profound

These dB levels refer to the better ear pure tone average. The better ear pure tone average refers to the commonly used procedure of averaging hearing loss. The pure tone frequencies of 500 Hz, 1000 Hz, and 2000 Hz are known to be important for hearing speech and are frequently referred to as the speech frequencies. Therefore, audiologists have used the hearing level thresholds for the three frequencies to estimate the potential handicapping effects of the hearing loss. For example, if a child has a hearing loss of 40 dB at 500 Hz, 50 dB at 1000 Hz, and 60 dB at 2000 Hz in the left ear, the pure tone average is calculated by dividing the sum of the three dB level thresholds by three. This calculation results in a pure tone average of 50 dB. Likewise, if the right ear has thresholds of 40 dB at 500 Hz, 45 dB at 1000 Hz, and 50 dB at 2000 Hz, the pure tone average for that ear is 45 dB. In this case, the better ear pure tone average is 45 dB in the right ear, and this child would be classified as having a moderate hearing loss. Causes of sensorineural hearing loss can be genetic or hereditary, or nongenetic occurring to the child in utero, during birth, or after birth. Sensorineural hearing losses generally are not amenable to medical treatment.

An important aspect of hearing loss is the slope of the loss. This slope refers to the categories of audiogram configurations based on the shape of the recorded hearing thresholds. A flat loss means that the hearing loss is approximately equal at all frequencies. A gradually falling curve indicates a hearing loss that descends at 5 to 10 dB per octave. A sharply falling curve indicates a hearing loss that increases dramatically by 15

Figure 10–1. Sloping hearing loss

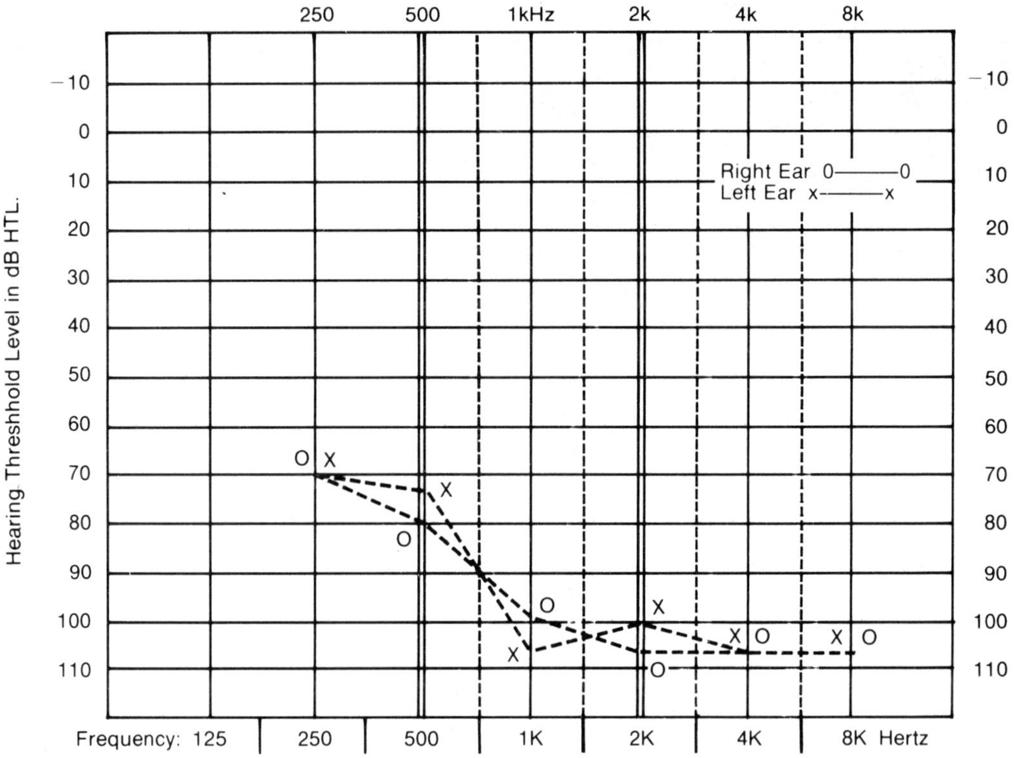

to 25 dB or more. Severely or profoundly hearing-impaired children generally have their greatest hearing loss at the high speech frequencies (1000 Hz, 2000 Hz, 4000 Hz), and the slope of their loss can sharply drop at these frequencies (See Figure 10–1).

Hearing loss is also classified according to age of onset. *Prelingual* means that the hearing loss occurred some time before language was acquired, and *postlingual* indicates that it occurred after language was acquired. *Congenital* refers to a hearing impairment present at birth, and *acquired* means that the hearing impairment occurred some time after birth. If a child is congenitally hearing impaired, prelingual hearing impairment is implied. However, if a child has an acquired hearing loss that occurred after the age of 3, this child is postlingually hearing impaired.

Etiology

There are numerous etiologies of prelingual hearing loss. Bergstrom (1974) devised a dichotic classification consisting of genetic and nongenetic categories. Included in the genetic category are all hereditary forms of hearing loss. There are over 60 types of hereditary hearing loss, and approximately 50% of childhood hearing loss is attributed to heredity (Bess & McConnell, 1981). Genetic hearing loss implies that the hearing impairment was genetically passed on through either a dominant, an x-linked, or a recessive or polygenic gene. Hearing loss alone or in a combination of traits could be inherited genetically. When a group of disorders are genetically inherited with hearing loss being one of the traits, the term *syndrome* is used to describe this grouping of disorders. There are many hereditary syndromes which are characterized by hearing loss. Usher's syndrome (retinitis pigmentosa with sensorineural hearing loss), Pierre Robin syndrome (craniofacial skeletal disorder, cleft palate, occasional mental retardation, conductive and/or sensorineural hearing loss), and Waardenburg's syndrome (white forelock, lateral displacement of medial canthi, mild to severe sensorineural hearing loss) are just a few. Each of these syndromes can include hearing loss as well as other impairments such as neurological impairment, cognitive deficits, or visual impairments. Children who evidence these syndromes are considered multihandicapped, and their hearing losses could range from mild to profound.

Nongenetic hearing loss implies that the hearing loss is not hereditary. Two prenatal factors causing nonhereditary hearing loss are maternal ototoxicity and rubella. Maternal ototoxicity refers to the ingestion of ototoxic drugs by the mother during pregnancy. Ototoxic drugs are medications which are poisonous or damaging to the ear and can injure the developing auditory system of the embryo. During the late 1950s and mid-1960s, rubella epidemics accounted for an increase in hearing losses in children born at that time. Later research has shown that other conditions associated with rubella include cataracts, salt and pepper retinopathy, and heart defects (Boughman & Shaver, 1982). Meningitis was another prevalent cause of hearing loss before the mid 1970s. Both of these conditions can cause severe sensorineural hearing losses.

Included in the nongenetic category is hearing loss of unknown etiology. In this instance, the cause of the deafness is not known and cannot be traced to any specific factors. Children whose hearing impairment is due to unknown causes comprise the largest percentage in the nongenetic category.

The presence of additional handicapping conditions in children with both genetic and nongenetic hearing losses is common. The multihandicapped hearing-impaired child is one whose hearing impairment is accompanied by other seriously handicapping conditions such as visual defects, emotional or behavioral problems, cognitive defects, heart defects, and perceptual-motor deficits. In the past, education of these children was neglected. With the enactment of the Education for all Handicapped Children Act of 1975 (PL 94–142), educational opportunities became available for them (Arkell, 1981). A demographic study of the deaf in the United States completed in 1972 (Gentile & McCarthy, 1973) concluded that almost one-third of the deaf population has at least one additional handicap. Monsees (1976) stated that a rule of thumb applied by professionals working with handicapped children is that when one abnormality is identified, look for a second. It is likely that the more severe the hearing impairment, the greater the chance for another handicapping condition.

EARLY IDENTIFICATION OF HEARING LOSS AND INTERVENTION PROGRAMS

Early identification of hearing loss and the delivery of appropriate services are critical factors in the habilitation of hearing-impaired children. Because language development begins from the time a child is born, there is an urgent need for an organized infant screening procedure to identify those infants who may have hearing losses. Identification of hearing-impaired infants can be facilitated through neonatal screenings of infants with a high risk of hearing loss. A high risk criteria compiled by the National Joint Committee on Newborn Screening in 1973 (Bess & McConnell, 1981) consisted of:

1. History of hereditary childhood hearing impairment
2. Rubella or other nonbacterial intrauterine fetal infection (e.g. herpes virus infection)
3. Defects of ear, nose, or throat
4. Birth weight less than 1500 grams
5. Bilirubin level greater than 20 mg/100 ml serum

An infant demonstrating any of these criteria should be referred for a complete audiological evaluation within the first 2 months of life.

In 1977, to further delineate the follow-up procedures for a high risk register, the National Maternal Child Health Conference generated guidelines for early screening (Northern & Downs, 1978, p. 207) recommending that:

1. Audiological follow-up of the high risk infants should be made as soon as possible, certainly by 7 months
2. The mother-child relationship in the first 4 months should be safeguarded by education and careful information
3. Informed consent should be obtained
4. Information on what to look for in later infancy should be given to the parents
5. Development and implementation of adequate identification and diagnostic procedures related to hearing impairments should be undertaken by public health agencies

Recently, investigations have focused on language development in the normal hearing infant within the first 2 years of life. These investigations have shown that normal hearing children have a basic capacity for perceiving speech behaviors in the environment, and also are sensitive to the social and affective aspects of the context of language (Eimas, 1974; Miller & Morse, 1976; Miller, Morse, & Dorman, 1977; Morse, 1972). Bloom and Lahey (1978) have stated that one of the precursors of language use occurs when infants begin to exchange gaze and vocalizations with their mothers. Bateson (1975) also described this mutual gaze or eye contact between mother and infant and called it *proto-conversation.* Jaffe, Stern, and Peery (1973) studied the infant-mother dyad and found mother-infant gazing to be analogous to the rhythms of adult dialogue. Behaviors such as these are all continuous with the eventual development of speech and language that begins in the 2nd year of life. Although hearing-impaired infants do not have the perceptual capabilities to receive and discriminate speech sounds as well as normal hearing children, they do have a residual amount of hearing that allows for some discrimination when amplification is utilized. In addition, they are able to extract the social and affective aspects of the context of language (Bloom & Lahey, 1978).

Brown (1975) stated that the most important form of concept learning for the infant is probably socially mediated. The first social contact of the infant is the parents. They are the most responsible for the development of the behaviors that lead to language growth in the normal child, and they are the major forces in the habilitation of the hearing-impaired child. Because studies have demonstrated that mothers of normal hearing children play a vital role in the development of speech and language, it becomes obvious that mothers of hearing-impaired infants play an even more crucial role.

Greenstein, Bush, McConville, and Stellini (1977) examined the mother-infant communication dyad and its effect on language acquisition in hearing-impaired infants. They found that affective aspects of mother-infant interaction were central to the language acquisition of the hearing-impaired child. All other aspects of the mother's language input to the child were far less significant than the existence of a good mother-infant bond. This bond frequently was broken by the mother's discovery of the child's hearing handicap. Vorce (1974) believed that the social relationships that exist between the mother and child stimulate the infant's early vocalizations, and therefore this relationship should be emphasized.

Because speech and language development begins with the earliest social exchanges between mother and infant, and because the affective aspects of mother-infant interaction are crucial to future language acquisition, programs which enhance mother-infant communication are invaluable in effective intervention for hearing-impaired children. Parent-infant programs, developed during the 1970s, educate parents about their critical role in the development of their hearing-impaired child. Parents are taught to make everyday experiences language-enhancing experiences. They learn to understand the implications of hearing impairment on speech and language development and how to deal with their feelings about the hearing loss in their child. Furthermore, they are taught how to incorporate auditory training into the child's daily life and how to employ language-learning strategies when they are interacting with their child. Parent and infant come to the parent-infant center at least once a week for training, and the teacher/speech-language pathologist makes weekly visits to the home. Parents frequently meet with other professionals such as psychologists and audiologists for additional training and support. A variety of training techniques is employed by the teacher/speech-language pathologist. A study is in progress now to assess the effectiveness of using a series of videotape presentations for parent training (Radziewicz, 1984). If these videotapes are proven to be effective training vehicles for parents of hearing-impaired infants, they would be one more tool that can be used to facilitate effective early intervention.

When hearing-impaired children and their parents are enrolled in a parent-infant program, that child's education begins during the critical speech and language learning years. Intervention before the age of 3 increases the child's chances of developing more normal speech and language. The parent-infant program also bridges the gap between early identification of hearing impairment and enrollment of the child into a preschool educational program (Elwood, Johnson, & Mandell, 1977).

SPEECH AND LANGUAGE BEHAVIORS OF THE HEARING IMPAIRED

There are few studies concerning the development and acquisition of language in hearing-impaired children. In order to fully understand the implications of the literature pertaining to speech and language development in the hearing impaired, one must be familiar with the normal processes of language development. These data can be found in Chapters 2 and 5. The remainder of this section reviews some recent research pertaining to speech and language behaviors of the hearing impaired.

Cognition

The cognitive development of deaf children has been examined and measured since 1900. Pinter (1920) and other researchers in the early part of the twentieth century conducted studies to evaluate intellectual abilities of deaf children. It was concluded from these studies that deaf children were retarded by 3 to 4 years when compared to normal hearing children. These early cognitive studies relied on measuring intellectual abilities with paper and pencil group tests (Moores, 1978).

In 1960, Myklebust proposed that deaf children were not intellectually inferior to hearing children. They were, instead, qualitatively different from normal hearing children in nearly every phase of development due to an organismic shift. According to Myklebust, language behaviors are acquired through experience with the environment, and can be viewed in terms of levels or hierarchies. These hierarchies follow the order of sensation, perception, imagery, symbolization, and conceptualization. When the lowest level, sensation, is impaired, as with hearing-impaired children, all higher levels are altered. An organismic shift occurs which consequently impedes the development of certain abstract behaviors. Therefore, because the deaf are highly dependent on vision as their primary sense of sensation, they are intellectually more concrete than the hearing population.

Myklebust's theory was refuted later in the 1960s and 1970s when several researchers (Furth & Youniss, 1965; Furth, 1966; Vernon, 1967) proposed that there is very little difference between the cognitive abilities of the deaf and hearing populations. Furth and Youniss (1965) examined the performance of deaf children on Piagetian tasks. They concluded that the deaf pass through the Piagetian cognitive levels of development in the same order as hearing children. However, in the later stages of development, such as the concrete operational stage and the formal operations stage, the deaf evidence a delay. In 1966, Furth further examined concept development in deaf children based on the Piagetian framework. He concluded that intelligence does not rely on a linguistic system, a system that deaf children are usually deficient in, and that performance deficits on intelligence tests result from communicative difficulties rather than lower intelligence.

Schlesinger and Meadow (1972) concluded that linguistic competence is an intervening variable that mediates between IQ and other indexes of cognitive functioning. This line of thinking suggests that there is an inextricable interplay between cognition and language that becomes evident once the child passes through the Piagetian sensorimotor stage and enters the preoperational stage. Thus, the child attains basic levels of cognitive and perceptual development before language develops, but once language develops, language and cognition become so intertwined it is impossible to extricate one from the other (Quigley & Paul, 1984).

Meadow (1980) stated that deaf children usually score within the normal range on intelligence tests, but that their mean scores are somewhat lower than those of hearing children when the tests are administered with nonverbal instructions and when the deaf do not have to respond verbally. She also ascertained that the research indicates that deaf children learn concepts in the same manner and in the same sequence but at a somewhat delayed rate when compared with hearing children. Furthermore, the influence of innate intellectual ability on the attainment of concepts is still questionable when the issue is confounded by the possible secondary effects of auditory and experiential deprivation. Deprivation may depress the ability to perform adequately on tests of intelligence.

Phonology

The methodology for studying speech and language development in the deaf has changed several times (Skarakis & Prutting, 1977), paralleling the methodologies used in studying normal language development. We will describe these methodologies and chronologically trace important research beginning with studies that examined the speech intelligibility of the deaf.

In 1942, Hudgins and Numbers studied the speech production of approximately 200 deaf children between the ages of 8 and 20 years. This descriptive study concluded that 21% of all consonants and 12% of all vowels were misarticulated by the deaf subjects. Specifically, errors included omission of initial and final consonants, errors in clustered consonants, voicing and nasality errors, numerous substitutions, and vowel distortions. In addition, the deaf subjects also evidenced severe disturbances in the prosodic features of speech production which included errors of intonation, duration, and rhythm.

Later, other researchers (Jensema, Karchmer, & Trybus, 1978; Markides, 1970; Nober, 1967) also investigated speech articulation among the deaf and found that a major portion of their speech production is unintelligible to the inexperienced and experienced listener alike. Smith (1975) examined the relationship of residual hearing and speech production in 40 congenitally deaf children. She found that speech intelligibility was related to hearing level for pure tones, but the measure most closely related to intelligibility was the test of phoneme recognition. The auditory recognition of speech features by the deaf children was directly reflected in their ability to produce intelligible speech. She further stated that there was an interaction between prosodic errors and speech intelligibility, and concluded that speech training of deaf children should emphasize improvement in the stress and intonation patterns of speech rather than on correct articulation. With improved stress and intonation in the speech of the deaf child, "listeners were able to compensate for omitted and substituted elements which resulted in better intelligibility" (p. 810).

During the 1970s, two other researchers examined the vocalizations of the deaf, but they focused on the development of very early vocalization (Mavilya, 1977; Menyuk, 1974). They compared and described the vocalizations of deaf infants, birth through 6 months, to those of normal hearing infants. It was found that at the babbling stage (approximately 4 months), the vocalizations of the deaf infants differed significantly from those of hearing infants. This difference was one of quantity and not of quality. At the babbling stage, normal hearing children engaged in increasing vocalizations, while the vocalizations of deaf infants lessened.

In the 1970s, a phonological approach was also employed to investigate the speech production of the deaf. Several researchers (Oller, Jensen, & Lafayette, 1978; Oller & Kelly, 1974; West & Weber, 1973) studied the speech of young hard-of-hearing children with mild to moderate hearing losses to determine if their phonology were rule-governed. All of these researchers concluded that the hard-of-hearing children demonstrate basically the same kind of phonological processes as those of younger, normal hearing children. Dodd (1976) sampled the spontaneous speech of ten profoundly congenitally deaf children, 9 to 12 years old, in order to derive phonological rules. It was theorized that if evidence of a phonological system exists in children with a moderate hearing loss, there may be some consistent phonological behavior in profoundly congenitally deaf children. Results of this study demonstrated that a partially rule-governed phonological system did exist in the congenitally deaf children, and that these children did use some phonological rules consistently. However, these phonological rules are somewhat dependent on the input modalities of the deaf children—lipreading and audition. This study suggested that deaf children gain information about phonological systems through lipreading as well as residual hearing, and that they use this phonological system in a manner similar to that of normal hearing children.

Syntax

Researchers also study the structure or syntax of language. Brannon and Murray (1966) compared the syntax of 30 hearing-impaired children to that of 30 normal hearing children. The hearing-impaired children were divided into two groups—15 children with hearing losses of 27 to 66 dB in the better ear (ASA, 1951) who were considered to be hard of hearing and 15 children with average losses greater than 75 dB in the better ear who were considered to be deaf. The children ranged in age from 12 to 13.5 years. The purpose of the study was to determine if relationships exist between hearing loss and certain measures of spoken language—total output of words, words per sentence, total errors, words per corrected sentences, and syntax. Results demonstrated that, in total output of speech, the normal hearing and the hard-of-hearing children were similar; however, the deaf children were significantly lower in this measure. The hard-of-hearing children were significantly worse than the normal children in structural accuracy, and the deaf children were worse than the hard of hearing. Most of the sentences spoken by the hard of hearing and deaf children were simple declarative sentences in the form subject-verb-object. This study represents an early attempt to describe the spoken syntax of hard of hearing and deaf children. Later in the 1970s, extensive studies of comprehension and production of syntactic structures of deaf children and youth were done (Power & Quigley, 1973; Quigley, Smith, & Wilbur, 1974). These later researchers were interested in answering the following questions (Quigley, Power, & Steinkamp, 1977):

1. What is the order of difficulty of various syntactic structures for deaf children?
2. Is this order of difficulty similar to that of hearing children?
3. How well established are the syntactic rules of English in the language of deaf children 10 to 18 years old?
4. Do these syntactical rules progress through developmental stages?
5. Are these developmental stages similar to those of hearing children?
6. Do deaf children acquire the same syntactic rules as hearing children but at a slower rate?
7. Do deaf children acquire syntactic rules that are idiosyncratic to only their population?

Their data revealed that the order of difficulty of syntactic structures was similar for both deaf and hearing children. Negation (easiest), conjunction, and question formation were the least difficult structures for the deaf. The same structures were least difficult for the hearing, but in the progression of question formation (easiest), conjunction, and negation. The most difficult structures for the deaf were relativization (most difficult), complementation, the verb system, and pronominalization. The most difficult for the normal hearing children were verbs (most difficult), relativization, complementation, and pronominalization.

The only syntactic rules that were relatively well established for the deaf subjects were negation, question formation, and conjunction; however, even these structures were not mastered to any significant degree. Hearing students at a comparable age had mastered most of the difficult structures.

Syntactic structures do progress through developmental stages. Deaf children reach these stages at a much delayed rate when compared to hearing children. Deaf children acquire the same syntactic rules as hearing children; however, certain syntactic structures appeared in the language system of the deaf that did not exist in the hearing children and are, in fact, not a part of English grammar. Obviously, the deaf children generated syntactic rules that were peculiar to themselves. These syntactic structures were a combination of English grammar and attempted approximations of English grammar. They were consistent in the written language of the deaf, and some of the structures were confined to particular language environments, thus supporting the fact that they were generated by rules. Several implications from these studies could be applied to remediation techniques. First, once knowledge of the deaf-specific syntactic structures is ascertained, teachers should remediate these rules to facilitate correct syntactic development rather than treating each syntactic deviation in isolation. Second, knowledge concerning the level of mastery of specific syntactic structures enables speech-language pathologists and teachers to construct language and reading materials appropriate to the child's knowledge of syntax and level of comprehension.

Wilbur, Goodhart, and Montandon (1983) investigated nine syntactic structures that had not been examined previously in the literature: why-questions, conditionals, nonlocative prepositions, indefinite pronouns, quantifiers, modal verbs, elliptical constructions, reciprocal pronouns, and comparative constructions. One hundred eighty-seven subjects, aged 7 to 23 years, were required to read comic book format material and to answer multiple choice questions. The results of the study provided guidelines to the relative difficulty of the structures, with why-questions being the easiest and comparatives being the hardest for the hearing-impaired subjects. The study results also indicated that performance improves as reading level increases. The authors suggested that many of the syntactic structures appeared to be learned in a piecemeal fashion, and that the syntactic structures that contained substructures (nonlocative prepositions, indefinite pronouns, quantifiers, modals, and comparatives) "seemed to be learned as separate lexical items rather than as unified syntactic structures" (p. 342).

Pragmatics and Semantics

Dore (1974) demonstrated that, at the level of the most basic and early communicative acts, there is no distinction between semantics and pragmatics. However, once the child passes through that very early communicative behavior stage, a difference does exist between the content of the act, semantics, and the intent of the act, pragmatics. Pragmatic categories include requesting, labeling, answering, and repeating (Dore, 1974). Semantic categories include the dative, locative, negation, action, etc. (Greenfield & Smith, 1976).

For organizational purposes we shall separate the recent literature on pragmatic and semantic development of the hearing-impaired into two categories—development in oral deaf children, and development in deaf children who use manually coded English. (See Language Input Models.)

Development in Oral Deaf Children. Skarakis and Prutting (1977) used a sociolinguistic approach to describe the semantic-pragmatic components in the communication of four 2- to 4-year-old hearing-impaired preschoolers. The children were enrolled in the John Tracy Clinic which uses an oral approach in educating deaf children. The children were observed for a period of 4 weeks. Results revealed that (*a*) the children did exhibit semantic functions and communicative intentions in spontaneous communication; (*b*) the semantic functions and communicative intentions expressed were the same as those in younger, normal hearing children 9 to 18 months old, (*c*) the hearing-impaired children communicated primarily by using prelinguistic behaviors such as gestures; and (*d*) the hearing-impaired children demonstrated that they had acquired the basic foundation for future language use.

Similar findings were reported by Curtiss, Prutting, and Lowell (1979) who also investigated early pragmatic-semantic communicative development of hearing-impaired children. The children, 22 to 60 months old were enrolled in the John Tracy Clinic. They also found that the hearing-impaired children had the ability to express a wide range of pragmatic intentions and several semantic categories through nonverbal means. However, the communicative ability, or pragmatics, and the development of semantic ability were clearly at different levels. The pragmatic abilities of the hearing-impaired children appeared to be developed by age 2 and were equal to the pragmatic abilities of hearing children of the same age. Specific semantic functions appeared to develop at a slower rate than did pragmatic functions. This finding is not surprising because the children used nonverbal behavior more frequently than verbal behavior, and it is extremely difficult to code meaning through nonlinguistic means.

Both of these studies demonstrate that hearing-impaired children develop the same semantic categories and communicative intentions as do young normal hearing children, although development of their semantic abilities occurs at a slower rate.

Development in Deaf Children Who Use Manually Coded English. Champie (1981) reported on the language development of a congenitally deaf child who participated in a preschool program which stressed total communication. This child entered the program at the age of 3 years. She had been fitted with a hearing aid at 28 months, and her parents began to learn sign language when she was 30 months. The child's language development was monitored for 2.25 years. The responses and utterances collected and analyzed were all spontaneous and were given in sign language. By the time the child was 5.5 years old, she was found to be using semantic relations that were restricted when compared to normal hearing children's. This finding could be attributed to the fact that intervention did not begin until she was 3 years old. Had she been exposed to signs earlier, her semantic development might not have been delayed.

Earlier, Newport and Ashbrook (1977) compared the development of semantic relations in deaf children learning ASL to that of hearing children. They concluded that the order of acquisition of semantic relations by the deaf children was similar to that of hearing children.

All of these studies seem to suggest that deaf children, whether they are exposed to manually coded English or oral English, demonstrate a delay in the development of semantic abilities. However, hearing-impaired children do evidence a similar pattern and rate of development of pragmatic abilities as do hearing children.

Implications

The recent literature on pragmatic, semantic, phonological, and syntactic development has important implications for the remediation procedures that should be used with the deaf. In the area of semantics and pragmatics, teachers and speech-language pathologists should be cognizant of the specific pragmatic intentions and semantic functions that are displayed in the communicative system of the young normal hearing child. They should then use this normal developmental model as the organizational framework from which habilitative procedures are adapted. For example, if one is working with a 3-year-old hearing-impaired child who expresses a wide range of pragmatic intentions through nonlinguistic means but who has limited linguistic abilities, it would be appropriate to teach that child a word that could be used to code several pragmatic categories (*want*—requesting and answering). Another strategy would be to teach that child to use his or her own name to code a number of semantic functions such as indicative object or agent.

The literature on phonological development indicates that deaf children can develop an extensive phonetic repertoire, and that they do develop a partially rule-governed phonological system (Dodd, 1976). This phonological system is only partially rule-governed because the children receive incomplete information due to their hearing loss. This phonological system is similar to one used by hearing children but at much younger ages. The teacher/speech-language pathologist can use this knowledge to determine the hearing-impaired child's phonological development and to devise an intervention program based on the normal phonological development model. Included in this program also would be very specific auditory training and speechreading training procedures.

Syntactic development in the deaf child also has been shown to be similar to that of the hearing child, although much delayed. The teacher/speech-language pathologist can apply this knowledge by ascertaining the child's stage of development and by then developing graduated remedial materials to enable the child to acquire increasing mastery of syntactic structures. Furthermore, the teacher/speech-language pathologist should rewrite existing materials to accommodate the syntactic level of the child (Quigley, Power, & Steinkamp, 1977).

The deaf population demonstrates the same innate abilities to acquire speech and language as the hearing population. However, because of the nature of their physical handicap, they cannot acquire language primarily through audition and must depend on vision as their language learning modality. This dependency results in an overall delay of speech and language development. It is up to researchers and educators alike to devise new methods and teaching techniques to enable the deaf population to develop and use their innate abilities to the fullest degree.

LANGUAGE INPUT MODELS

Hearing-impaired children are exposed to a variety of language input models from infancy to childhood. The relationship between the language input system and children's language development has been studied in an attempt to trace the development of language in hearing-impaired children (Quigley & Paul, 1984). Some of the most widely used models are included in this section.

The oral, or oral-aural, method is a multisensory approach used to teach speech and language to hearing-impaired children. In this method, hearing-handicapped children receive information through speechreading and the amplification of residual hearing. The oral method prohibits sign language and gesture because its proponents feel that the auditory avenue is the most influential in the development of speech and language. The goal of the oral approach is to facilitate integration of the hearing impaired into the world of the hearing.

Closely allied to the oral method is the acoupedic approach. This language input model is unisensory and is used primarily with young children. This method received a great deal of attention in the 1960s (Pollack, 1964). The acoupedic approach emphasizes the hearing-impaired child's maximum use of residual hearing for audition without the added visual and tactile component found in the oral method. The mother's involvement in the child's education is a paramount component for successful treatment. As the child grows older, the emphasis on audition, however, is more difficult to control. Young children growing up can't help but rely on tactile and visual stimuli to help them better understand their environment. The popularity of this approach is constrained by the need for excessive parental involvement and extensive speech and audition therapy. Advocates of the acoupedic approach firmly believe that the hearing-impaired child will utilize speech and language best in a method emphasizing audition.

The auditory global approach is similar to the acoupedic method (Calvert & Silverman, 1975; Simmons-Martin, 1972). The emphasis of this approach is on the maximum use of residual hearing combined with intervention and fluent connected speech.

Another critical input model is manual communication. Manual communication models include a variety of systems and approaches. A manual method is nonverbal by definition and consists of fingerspelling and sign language. This method utilizes a physical representation of letters, words, and concepts made with the hands or fingers. Many educators of the deaf feel that it is an extremely efficient way of teaching communicative language skills to the hearing impaired.

One method involving fingerspelling of individual letters of the alphabet is called the Rochester method. It is used as a method unto itself and as an adjunct to an oral approach. Quigley (1969) compared the Rochester and the oral method in two preschool deaf education programs. He found that the Rochester method produced superior students in fingerspelling, reading, and written language. In a second study, Quigley (1969) examined the Rochester method in elementary and secondary school children with hearing impairments and compared these children to those in a school using a simultaneous approach (signs, fingerspelling, and oralism). In this study, the

Rochester method produced students who received superior scores on the subtests of the Stanford Achievement Test. The students using the Rochester method also did better in fingerspelling, but there were no appreciable differences in their speech and speechreading skills. Quigley concluded that fingerspelling, as demonstrated in the Rochester method, has important positive implications for instructing hearing-impaired children.

A popular language system currently used with the hearing impaired is sign language. There are various signing systems, including American Sign Language (ASL), Seeing Essential English (SEE 1), Signing Exact English (SEE 2), Manual English, Signed English (SE), and Total Communication (TC), a system incorporating sign language, speech, and speechreading.

American Sign Language (ASL) is considered the language of the deaf and is the third most widely used non-English language in the United States (Wilbur, 1979). Most researchers in the field of linguistics and deaf education agree that ASL is a language unto itself with specific grammatical rules. (Liddell, 1980; Siple, 1982; Wilbur, 1979). Stokoe (1958), a pioneer in the study of ASL, examined the formation of signs called *cherology* and found it to be similar to the phonological system used in spoken language. The term *cheremic* refers to hand positions and movements. Hearing-impaired children use signs at an earlier age than hearing children utter their first words. (Hoffmeister & Wilbur, 1980). It has been suggested that the motor control needed for hand movements is more easily attainable than the motor control needed for speech. There is little research on the children who have learned ASL in their early years and its effect on their subsequent learning of English. Most research has involved deaf children of deaf parents who used ASL initially with their children. The children of this group scored higher than deaf children of hearing parents in both psychological and educational tests (Meadows, 1968).

Another form of sign language used in educational settings is Seeing Essential English (SEE 1), a system developed by David Anthony. SEE 1 is used primarily by hearing parents and teachers of deaf children. It conforms to the English language with additional signs added to represent English concepts. One sign represents many meanings of a single word in English. The system classifies English words into three groups: basic, compound, and complex (Quigley & Paul, 1984). Researchers have examined grammatical relationships in SEE 1 as compared to English in normal hearing children. Schlesinger and Meadow (1972) studied three subjects who had been exposed to SEE 1 and found, for example, that young deaf children code agent-object relationships. Although deaf children acquire language at a slower rate than their hearing peers, they seem to develop grammatical competence in the same sequential manner as hearing children (Menyuk, 1963).

Signing Exact English (SEE 2) was developed by Gustason, Pfetzinger, and Zawolkow (1972). The SEE 2 method is widely used in educational settings. Both SEE 1 and SEE 2 are comparable to spoken English, and both methods are generally easier to learn than ASL, especially for hearing parents.

Manual English was developed at the Washington State School for the Deaf in 1972 (Wilbur, 1979). This method utilizes many ASL signs but incorporates more fingerspelling than the SEE approaches. Manual English is used to reinforce the structure of normal English. The morphology of English presents some difficulty when sign language plus fingerspelling are used in conjunction with spoken English. Many hearing people who are not familiar with ASL, but who have a large sign vocabulary are proponents of Manual English. Manual English conforms in many ways to spoken and written English, and it is often used as the initial system for teaching deaf children. The syntax of Manual English parallels that of hearing society. Therefore, many educators feel that deaf children will read and write with greater clarity if taught this method of communication.

Signed English (SE) was investigated by Bornstein, Saulnier, and Hamilton (1980). This method utilizes ASL signs with a variable amount of fingerspelling. It is similar to spoken English with 14 markers and fingerspelling used to represent sign language with English construction (Wilbur, 1979). In SE, contractions have their own signs and are treated as individual words. Bornstein, Saulnier, and Hamilton examined twenty 4-year-old prelingually deaf children in a 4-year longitudinal study. Using the Peabody Picture Vocabulary Test and the Northwestern Syntax Screening Test, Bornstein, Saulnier, and Hamilton found that morphological structures and vocabulary growth were similar in hearing children, although the rate of growth was slower.

The sign system of choice in many schools for the deaf and in many mainstreamed settings is the Total Communication (TC), or the Pidgin Sign English (PSE) system. This method combines some of the ASL signs and uses them in a standard English word order. The system, in its purest sense, incorporates sign language, fingerspelling, speech, and speechreading. It is usually demonstrated in school settings where the teacher and the hearing-impaired child are signing and speaking English simultaneously. Problems limiting the success of the method are not inherent to the system itself. In order for the deaf child to succeed with such a system, extensive training is needed in speech, speechreading, and auditory discrimination. A synthesis of these input avenues is necessary to make optimum use of TC (Wilbur, 1979).

PERSONAL AND GROUP AMPLIFICATION SYSTEMS

The child who is successful in a school setting must have the ability to use residual hearing to its greatest advantage. A variety of amplification systems have been devised to facilitate auditory comprehension in the hearing-impaired child. The most common amplification devices involve individual hearing aids which can be worn at school or at home with ease and comfort. Educational amplification units are widely used today. Both types of amplification will be reviewed in this section.

The Body Aid. Wearable hearing aids come in a number of styles and degrees of power. Hearing aids are chosen with both the audiometric configuration and the specific hearing-related problems in mind. The body aid is generally secured by a harness or clip to the chest of a hearing-impaired child. The aid is about the size of a small crayon box and contains a microphone, amplifier, and a battery compartment. A receiver button is worn in the ear and is attached to the aid by a flexible cord. Body aids are often recommended for multiply handicapped deaf children because of their durability and the ease in which the controls can be adjusted. This type of aid is also used with young profoundly deaf children, although the behind-the-ear aid is gaining greater acceptance and is generally the hearing aid of choice.

Postauricular Hearing Aids. The behind-the-ear, or postauricular hearing aid is often recommended by the educational audiologist. All the component parts of the hearing aid are contained within its plastic casing, including the amplifier, microphone, receiver, and the battery. A flexible tube connects the earmold to the postauricular casing. Many schools for the deaf and most mainstreamed programs fit their children with this type of hearing aid because it is rather inconspicuous and has a high level of performance. It also provides directionality because the fitting is at ear level.

In-the-ear. In-the-ear aids are gaining acceptability among educators, but they are still not commonly used with hearing-impaired children. The entire aid, including the battery, fits into the outer ear. Increased amplification has been made possible during the past few years; however, the controls remain small and individual adjustments to the aid remain difficult. These aids are gaining increased popularity with hearing-impaired adults, and undoubtedly they will be a more acceptable fitting for children as technology advances.

Eyeglass Aids. The eyeglass hearing aid is not routinely fitted to young children. The hearing aid is built into the temple of the eyeglass frame. It is recommended only for children who wear glasses all day and who can tolerate using a hearing aid and eye glasses simultaneously.

Auditory Training Units. Auditory training units are routinely used in schools for the deaf because they provide the best signal to noise ratio in a background of classroom noise. Auditory training units have become an integral part of an aural rehabilitation program and are routinely used to provide maximum benefits from a hearing-impaired child's residual hearing.

Portable Auditory Trainers. The portable auditory trainer is widely used by speech-language pathologists in the public school setting. The system should provide binaural hearing, although monaural and pseudobinaural units are available. This desk-top auditory training unit amplifies all sounds, including background noises, equally. Therefore, the quieter the listening situation, the more effective the auditory capacity of this trainer. Individual speech-language pathologists also find this unit effective in working with the hearing-impaired child.

FM Systems. Schools that can afford more expensive equipment for their hearing handicapped population generally choose the FM auditory group trainer, a wireless unit which uses a specific FM radio frequency band for transmission. The FM system resembles a radio, and amplification occurs when the teacher transmits sound to the student's receiver which is then amplified through the child's personal hearing aid or a set of small earpieces. Because installation is not needed in this system, it also has popular appeal in mainstreamed settings. Units are recharged nightly, making battery burnout less of a problem. At present, there are 32 frequencies available for transmission, allowing various teachers to use the units simultaneously. This feature is especially effective at the middle and high school levels, when a child may change classes and need amplification throughout the day in different classrooms. One major advantage of this system is that the child can pick up auditory clues from the teacher/speech-language pathologist and can also hear other students through the microphone intended for environmental pick-up of auditory signals. The teacher/speech-language pathologist can be heard clearly from a variety of distances when the teacher's microphone is properly used. Noise levels can be decreased by turning off the student's environmental microphone, allowing a clear signal from teacher to student. The quality of the message transmitted is excellent and the FM system has proven to be valuable instrumentation in schools for the hearing-impaired as well as in mainstreamed settings. The freestanding FM system is most desirable and widely used because (*a*) children can wear their personal hearing aid, (*b*) no installation is required, (*c*) it is inconspicuous in design, and (*d*) it improves the listening conditions in the classroom making learning an easier task for the hearing-impaired youngster.

Loop Systems. The modern loop system operates with a wire or loop placed around the physical parameters of the classroom. In this system, children wear their own hearing aids set to the telephone (T) position, and the teacher wears an individual microphone. Students can hear through the directional or nondirectional microphones placed strategically around the classroom. When students want to communicate with each other, they use the environmental microphones built into their individual hearing aids. The loop system is gaining renewed popularity for group settings, i.e. libraries, meeting rooms, theaters, and auditoriums. In the classroom setting, the loop system is complicated by interference from adjacent classrooms (spillover). The loop system must be carefully installed to avoid dead spots. Because this system is economical, many theaters and movie houses are providing the loop system for their hearing-impaired clientele (Callahan, 1984).

Infrared Light Systems. A system of auditory transmission currently under investigation involves the use of an infrared light. The advantage of this system is that the teacher/speech-language pathologist does not need to be concerned about the microphone cable. The teacher/speech-language pathologist uses a regular FM microphone equipped with an FM transmitter. The FM receiver is attached to the infrared transmitter. This system still has acoustic and environmental flaws usually attributed to excessive sunlight in classrooms resulting in noise interference. Most of these problems will be solved with advancing technical knowledge, and the wireless FM system remains the auditory trainer of choice in most classroom settings.

ASSESSMENT: INTELLIGENCE TESTS AND TESTS OF LANGUAGE AND ACADEMIC ACHIEVEMENT

Before remediation is begun, it is important to adequately assess the hearing-impaired child. Because many tests of intelligence and academic achievement are in fact tests of language, the speech-language pathologist should be familiar with procedures and techniques which are appropriate for assessing the hearing-impaired population. Tests which are normed on the hearing impaired are far more likely to give educators a better indication of a child's cognitive abilities. We will evaluate applicable tests, with consideration given to those normed on hearing-impaired youngsters in the sections which follow.

One of the most widely used tests of cognitive ability is the Hiskey-Nebraska Test of Learning Aptitude. This test was designed and standardized on the hearing impaired. It is comprised of 12 subtests which correlate with academic achievement tests such as the Stanford-Binet, the Gates-MacGinitie Reading Test, and the Metropolitan Achievement Test (Kretschmer & Quigley, 1981).

The Wechsler Intelligence Scale and the WISC-R are also popular intelligence tests. The WISC-R has been normed on hearing-impaired children, and a good deal of research has been completed on this test. The performance section of the Wechsler test is free from the language component which makes achievement so difficult on the verbal section. Scoring well on the verbal section of the WISC-R tends to be an indicator of academic success, but may have little validity with hearing-impaired children who are by nature of their handicap, language impaired.

Another test of intelligence is the Knox Cube Test which was designed for the hearing impaired. Although it is administered nonverbally, it lacks established norms which makes it a somewhat less effective tool.

The Harris-Goodenough Draw-a-Man Test is often used with the hearing-impaired population. Research indicates that hearing-impaired children perform within average limits through 13 years of age on this test (Myklebust, 1960).

The Metropolitan Achievement Test is a standardized test designed to measure a pupil's achievement in a variety of content areas including reading, arithmetic, word knowledge, and word analysis. The language area includes pronunciation, capitalization, punctuation, parts of speech, and locational skills. The reading tests do not assess linguistic competence, but they do suggest areas of weakness, such as vocabulary and grammatical skills. Scores can be inflated by the grammatically correct choices a student is given (Moores, 1978). It is the educator's responsibility to evaluate the scores as they relate to the hearing-impaired child's classroom performance. The Metropolitan Achievement Test consists of a battery of eight performance levels from kindergarten through 12th grade. It provides no specific guidelines for the hearing impaired, and no norms have been established for this group. However, it is a useful tool in helping to establish remedial academic guidelines.

Two other instruments developed to assess language in the hearing-impaired population include the Test of Syntactic Abilities (Quigley, Steinkamp, Power, & Jones, 1978) and the Grammatical Analysis of Elicited Language: Simple Sentence Level (Moog & Geers,1979). The Grammatical Analysis of Elicited Language (GAEL) can be administered to hearing-impaired children from ages 5 to 9. It evaluates 16 grammatical categories and was standardized on children educated in oral programs. The Test of Syntactic Abilities (TSA) includes an in-depth battery geared to hearing-impaired children from 10 to 19 years of age. This test evaluates the syntactic abilities of hearing-handicapped children.

The Stanford Achievement Test has a special edition for hearing-impaired children. This test consists of six different levels and four subject areas including vocabulary, reading comprehension, mathematical concepts, and mathematical computation. The results of the Stanford Achievement Test help the educator with grade placement and prescriptive educational planning. Norms are based on a random sample of 6,873 hearing-impaired students (Zieziula, 1983).

The Gates-MacGinitie Reading Test can be used to test hearing-impaired children in grades 1 through 10. Although there are no special instructions for this test, and it is not normed on hearing-impaired children, it is suggested that children being tested be given instructions through an appropriate communication channel.

Test results help the educator achieve a degree of accountability in judgments concerning hearing-impaired children. Although not comprehensive, they provide useful information on the child's cognitive abilities and potential academic achievement.

REMEDIATION APPROACHES

There are several useful approaches to speech/language remediation with hearing-impaired children. Successful results depend on a variety of variables including (*a*) degree of hearing loss, (*b*) age of onset of the hearing problem, (*c*) parental and school support and involvement, and (*d*) general IQ levels.

Speechreading is one of the oldest remediation processes used consistently with the hearing impaired. Yet, despite the accepted use of this methodology, little applied research is available on this topic. Early research was an outgrowth of the development of speechreading tests used to evaluate speechreading ability in hearing-impaired children. Such tests include the Costello Test of Speechreading (Costello, 1957), the Children's Speechreading Test (Butt & Chreist, 1968), the Craig Lipreading Inventory (Craig, 1969), and the Utley Speechreading Test (1946). Speechreading requires a level of language comprehension as measured by vocabulary level and educational achievement (Jeffers & Barley, 1980). Speechreading has always been a difficult skill to master because many of the sounds in the English language are invisible, and the English consonants are homophenous in nature. Homophenous sounds refer to those that look alike on the lips such as /p/, /b/ and /m/. Therefore, without the aid of contextual clues, the auditorily-impaired child would find it impossible to differentiate /pen/, /Ben/, and /men/. This element of confusion makes speechreading a difficult, if not impossible, task for the profoundly hearing-impaired population.

Synthetic approaches to speechreading were first advocated by Nitchie in the early 1900s and are still popular today. Many exercises and materials currently in use are a direct result of Nitchie's concern with synthesizing speechreading into real life situations including social situations and academic subject matter. Materials most beneficial to the hearing impaired should be geared to the interest and speechreading abilities of individual students. The speech-language pathologist in the schools must integrate a child's academic subject matter and social circumstances into applicable speechreading lessons. Some of the materials best suited to hearing-impaired children are those devised specifically to meet their interests. Although there is a need for drill work and recognition exercises, the synthesizing of speechreading material will probably be of greatest benefit to the hearing-impaired child.

Speechreading is one of the oldest remediation techniques used with the hearing impaired. Early research was primarily concerned with assessment techniques, and a number of speechreading tests were developed. With emphasis on linguistic performance, much of the newer information involves recognition and identification of sounds to better understand and synthesize language. Speechreading is to be used as an adjunct to other language remediation techniques.

Auditory Training

A second approach to speech and language remediation involves the appropriate use of auditory training. One of the earliest approaches to auditory training was proposed by Wedenberg (1951). Wedenberg became one of the original proponents of an unisensory methodology which emphasized audition over visual and kinesthetic modalities. The emphasis in the Wedenberg method was the advancement of language and speech skills. Other early investigators in the training of the auditory channel include Goldstein (1939) and Whitehurst (1955). These approaches, however, were multisensory in nature, although great importance was placed on the auditory modality.

The greatest influences on auditory training came with the advent of the electronic hearing aid. Originally, listening practice was separate from the child's daily experiences, limiting the integration of daily speech and language into the auditory training sessions. Once hearing aids became common, hearing-impaired children had the benefit of constant exposure to language and environmental sounds. Most children, however, continue to need specialized instruction in coding meaningful stimuli.

Originally, instructional procedures involved four major areas. These were outlined by Carhart (1960) and included (*a*) awareness to sound, (*b*) development of gross discrimination, (*c*) broad discrimination using simple speech patterns, and (*d*) finer discrimination for speech.

Many auditory training programs employed today are patterned after the earlier work of Carhart. Sanders' (1971) approach, although similar, adds an audiological component concerning the knowledge of the child's audiometric configuration, hearing aid usage, and maintenance information.

Since these early approaches, there have been advances in the area of aural rehabilitation. Kretschmer (1974) has applied the use of linguistic rules rather than gross discrimination of environmental sounds. Almost all input material used with the hearing-impaired child is based on linguistic principles. The sequential development of Kretschmer's program adheres to language growth in the normal hearing child.

This approach is similar to the methodology advocated by Ling (1976) which also combines auditory training with speech and language therapy. Linguistic growth is an integral aspect in assessing this methodology. Important to the development of an organized auditory training curriculum is the five-sound test which was developed by Ling. The test consists of the following vowels and consonants: /u/, /a/, /i/, /ʃ/, and /s/. The five phonemes are plotted on an audiogram and represent the span of the speech range. When the aided thresholds are plotted, the parents and teachers have a visual representation of the child's hearing loss. The importance of hearing aids and amplification systems in the child's social and educational settings is emphasized (Ling, 1984). It is expected that hearing-impaired children with some residual hearing should be able to hear these five sounds at a distance of 5 yards. With better hearing, they should be able to increase the distance, while those with less residual hearing would have to remain closer to the speaker. The five-sound test is easy to administer, helps to establish an effective listening distance for the child, and verifies the functioning of the hearing aid without which effective auditory training becomes an impossible task.

Organizing an effective aural rehabilitation program is often left to the creative speech-language pathologist. Most rehabilitation programs contain some, if not all, of the following elements: (*a*) a form of assessment procedure, typically Ling's five-sound test, (*b*) a general check of the hearing aid, mold, and batteries, especially if the child's performance on the five-sound test differs from previous performance, (*c*) auditory discrimination of phonetic and phonologic material, (*d*) experience stories to check for semantic, syntactic, and morphological rules, (*e*) pragmatic situations to check areas of comprehension, and (*f*) home practice assignments for reinforcement (Paterson, 1982 p. 265).

It must be reemphasized that the use of optimal residual hearing in the framework of speech and language development is the primary goal of auditory training. It is the speech-language pathologist's professional responsibility to be familiar with the latest technological advances so that each child might be given a prescriptive plan to develop maximum auditory potential. These children must also be taught to synthesize visual, tactile, and auditory skills. Early intervention should provide improved developmental skills in speech and language for the hearing-handicapped child.

Cued Speech

In 1965, Cornett developed a communication system called *cued speech* (Lykos, 1971). This method was designed to maximize speech and language skills in the context of natural language communication. Cued speech is a means of clarifying oral communication and is used as an adjunct to speechreading, which is an ambiguous system. The hand is used to supplement information on the lips. Eight hand signals are utilized to indicate groups of consonants that can be distinguished on the lips. In Cornett's cuing system, there are 36 cues for the 44 phonemes in English. Vowels are represented by the position of the hand, and consonants are represented by the hand configuration. The teacher is encouraged to cue all information to facilitate the learning of language patterns and concepts. An element of naturalness is added to the hearing-impaired child's language system. Words are not changed to meet limited language constraints; rather, the language is expanded as with normal hearing children.

Cued speech has been critically reviewed by Moores (1969) and Wilbur (1979) who found a lack of distinction in cued speech between speech and language. Wilbur (1979) remarked that Cornett's theory is based on a child's ability to imitate a role model. Bloom (1970) found, however, that for many children, imitation does not facilitate language acquisition. This could make cued speech particularly difficult for some hearing-impaired children. There are also certain intrinsic phonetic problems within the cued speech method. These include problems in a transference to reading and dialect problems (Wilbur, 1979).

Ling and Clarke (1975) studied 12 hearing-impaired children using cued and noncued phrases and sentences. Their results indicated that more cued than noncued material was identified correctly when used as a supplement to speechreading. The children, however, demonstrated a low level of speech reception. When analyzing sentences, the mode of communication did not seem to be an influencing factor. However, the addition of cues made it easier for children to identify words in phrases rather than in sentences. Cued speech has potential in teaching pronunciation, vocabulary, and morphology. Additional research is needed before making judgments concerning this approach.

A follow-up study completed by Clarke and Ling (1976) indicated that cuing facilitated speechreading for phrases, words, and sentences. Audition did not seem to play a significant role in the speech perception of the subjects under investigation, and they did no better when integrating visual and auditory stimuli with or without the presence of cues. Further research on the effect of acoustic information on cued speech is suggested by these investigators.

In 1983, an additional study was completed on cued speech. Mohay (1983) studied the language development of three prelingually deaf children by examining videotapes of their performances. Each child's communication profile was analyzed with respect to frequency of gestures, cues, and speech. Mohay also examined the lexical development of these children and compared the data with children enrolled in an oral deaf education program. She concluded that cued speech as applied to young children is not a significant factor to spoken language development.

The case history of Leah, the daughter of Mary Elsie Henegar is carefully reviewed in *Cued Speech Handbook for Parents* (Henegar & Cornett, 1971). This case study provides interesting information on aspects of expressive language as it relates to cued speech. Leah's receptive language comprehension exceeded her expressive language abilities. However, empirical research was not part of this study, and much of the information is subjective in nature.

Gallaudet College published a teachers' handbook related to cued speech in 1971. The handbook includes a number of interesting activities and formal cued speech lessons. Cued speech, however, has had limited use in the United States, compared to other modalities. Moores (1969) emphasized that the system is not geared toward initial language learning but rather toward speech therapy. Danish schools have been using a cuing system for some time, but this system's primary application has been articulation training (Borrild, 1972). There is a need, however, for more objective research studies concerning the benefits of cued speech.

CASE STUDY

Jenny exhibits a profound hearing impairment (See Figure 10–2). Although intervention began before the age of 3 years, she may never achieve adequate speech and language

Figure 10–2. Jenny's audiogram

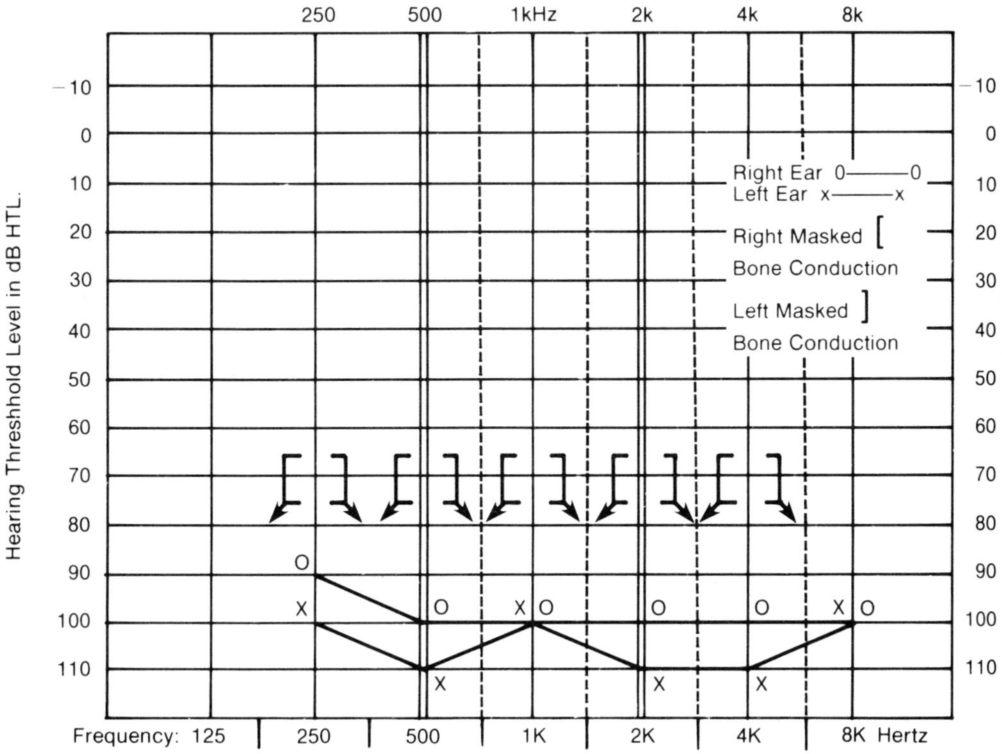

through the oral auditory modality and will have to rely on alternative communication systems (ASL, SEE 1, and SEE 2). Delay in language development could have an adverse effect on academic learning. Jenny might be placed in a special school for the hearing impaired which has specific academic curricula geared to meet the needs of individual students. She might be placed in a mainstreamed program with a strong network of support services such as audiological monitoring, speech and language therapy, counseling, tutoring, note-taking services, and interpreter services.

In Figure 10–2, Jenny's audiogram reveals a pure tone average of 100 dB in the right ear (AD) and 105 dB in the left ear (AS). Bone conduction testing could not be performed because it is beyond the limits of the audiometer. No bone conduction responses were available in either ear at a level of 70 dB.

SUMMARY

Language remediation strategies are perhaps the most important information needed by speech-language pathologists working with hearing-impaired children. In order to devise appropriate intervention programs, professionals must have an adequate understanding of normal speech-language development and the development of speech-language behaviors in the hearing-impaired population. They must know that children with conductive losses may perform quite differently than those with severe sensorineural losses. Likewise, the effects of prelingual deafness can be of such a magnitude that the hearing-impaired child can never develop an adequate level of language functioning. Furthermore, other variables such as linguistic environment, method of communication, and type of educational program are also critical factors which influence speech-language development.

The importance of early identification and intervention cannot be stressed enough. We must take full advantage of deaf children's innate capacity for language acquisition by providing them with adequate amplification and a home environment that provides optimum opportunity for language learning.

Personal and group amplification systems have greatly enhanced the auditory abilities of hearing-impaired children. These systems have been discussed in some detail in this chapter.

Language input models include oral, manual, and total communication systems. Each has a place in the habilitation of hearing-impaired children. Individual preferences will depend on the results of assessment obtained prior to the onset of therapy.

The component parts of the remediation process are within themselves complicated. Teacher and speech-language pathologists must have very refined skills to develop speechreading and auditory functioning in the hearing-impaired child. Furthermore, they must develop strategies that are effective techniques in developing the hearing-impaired child's phonological, syntactical, pragmatic, and semantic systems.

There are no easy answers when it comes to educating hearing-impaired children. The more that is known about the topics covered in this chapter, the better equipped the teacher/speech-language pathologist will be to deal with many problems unique to hearing-impaired children. The teacher/speech-language pathologist must be cognizant of all variables that relate to language growth. Certainly the task is not an easy one.

STUDY QUESTIONS

1. What is the etiology of hearing loss?
2. What are the differences and similarities among an oral communication approach, a total approach, and an acoupedic approach?
3. What are the most widely used approaches to speech and language remediation with the hearing impaired?
4. What are the advantages and disadvantages of the (*a*) portable auditory trainer, (*b*) the FM system, (*c*) the loop system, and (*d*) the infrared system?
5. What means are available for early infant identification and what kind of intervention is appropriate?
6. Of what importance is a basic understanding of normal speech and language development when working with hearing-impaired children?
7. How does American Sign Language differ from Total Communication?
8. Explain cued speech. How is this method used in remediation?
9. What general statement can be made regarding the speech and language behaviors of the hearing-impaired child?
10. How is speechreading used as a remediation technique?

BIBLIOGRAPHY

Arkell, C. (1981). Assessment of multiply handicapped deaf students for program developments. *American Annals of the Deaf, 126,* 526–532.

Bateson, M.C. (1975). Mother-infant exchanges: The epigeness of conversational interaction. In M. Aaronson & R. Reiber (Eds.), *Developmental psycholinguistics and communication disorders annals of the N.Y. Academy of Sciences.*

Bergstrom, L. (1974). *Handling the human communication sequelae.* Paper presented at the International Symposium on Human Communication, Mexico City.

Bess, F.H., & McConnell, F.E. (1981). *Audiology, education and the hearing impaired child.* St. Louis, MO: Mosby.

Bloom, L., & Lahey, M. (1978). *Language development and language disorders.* New York: Wiley.

Bornstein, H., Saulnier, K., & Hamilton, L. (1980). Signed English: A first evaluation. *American Annals of the Deaf, 125,* 467–481.

Borrild, K. (1972). Cued speech and the mouth-hand system. In G. Funt (Ed.), *International symposium on speech communication ability and profound deafness.* Washington, DC: Alexander Graham Bell Association for the Deaf.

Boughman, J.A., & Shaver, K.A. (1982). Genetic aspects of deafness: Understanding the counseling process. *American Annals of the Deaf, 127,* 393–404.

Brannon, J.B., & Murray, T. (1966). The spoken syntax of normal, hard of hearing, and deaf children. *Journal of Speech and Hearing Research, 9,* 604–610.

Brown, R. (1975). *Social psychology.* New York: Free Press.

Butt, D., & Chreist, F.M. (1968). A speechreading test for young children. *The Volta Review, 70,* 225–235.

Callahan, J. (1984). Cinema radio and FM systems for the hearing impaired. *Hearing Instruments, 35,* 7.

Calvert, D., & Silverman, S.R. (1975). *Speech and deafness: A text for learning and teaching.* Washington, DC: Alexander Graham Bell Association for the Deaf.

Carhart, R. (1960). Auditory training. In H. Davis & R. Silverman (Eds.), *Hearing and deafness,* (2nd ed., pp. 368–386). New York: Holt, Rinehart & Winston.

Champie, J. (1981). Language development in our preschool deaf child. *American Annals of the Deaf, 126,* 43–48.

Clarke, B., & Ling, D. (1976). The effects of using cued speech: A follow up study. *The Volta Review, 78,* 23–25.

Costello, M.R. (1957). A study of speechreading as a developing language process in deaf and in hard of hearing children. (Doctoral dissertation, Northwestern University, 1957.) *Dissertation Abstracts International, 17,* 3119. (University Microfilms No. 23493).

Craig, W.N. (1969). *Craig lipreading inventory.* Pittsburgh, PA: University of Pittsburgh, School of Education.

Curtiss, S., Prutting, C., & Lowell, E. (1979). Pragmatic, semantic development in young children with impaired hearing. *Journal of Speech and Hearing Research, 22,* 534–552.

Dodd, B. (1976). The phonological systems of deaf children. *Journal of Speech and Hearing Disorders, 41,* 185–198.

Dore, J. (1974). A pragmatic description of early language development. *Journal of Psycholinguistic Research, 3,* 343–350.

Education for All Handicapped Children Act of 1975 (PL 94–142). 20 USC Sec. 401 (Supp. 1975).

Eimas, P. (1974). Auditory and linguistic processing cues for place of articulation by infants. *Perceptual Psychology, 16,* 513–521.

Elwood, P.C., Johnson, W.L., & Mandell, J. (Eds.). (1977). Parent-infant program for the hearing impaired: A research guide. Washington, DC: Bureau of Education of the Handicapped, Department of Health, Education, and Welfare/Office of Education.

Furth, H. (1966). *Thinking without language: Psychological implications of deafness.* New York: Free Press.

Furth, H. (1973). *Deafness and learning: A psychosocial approach.* Belmont, CA: Wadsworth.

Furth, H., & Youniss, J. (1965). The influence of language and experience on discovery and use of logical symbols. *British Journal of Psychology, 56,* 381–390.

Gentile, A., & McCarthy, B. (1973). *Additional handicapping conditions among hearing impaired students.* United States: 1971–72 (Series D, No. 14). Washington, DC: Gallaudet College, Office of Demographic Studies.

Goldstein, M. (1939). *The acoustic method for the training of the deaf and hard of hearing.* St. Louis: Laryngoscope Press.

Greenfield, P.M., & Smith, H. (1976). *The structure of communication in early language development.* New York: Academic Press.

Greenstein, J.M., Bush, B., McConville, K., & Stellini, L. (c.1977). Mother-infant communication and language acquisition in deaf infants. New York: Lexington School for the Deaf.

Gustason, C., Pfetzing, D., & Zawolkow, E. (1972). *Signing exact English.* Silver Spring, MD: Modern Signs Press.

Henegar, M.E., & Cornett, R.O. (1971). *Cued speech: Handbook for parents.* Washington, DC: Gallaudet College Press.

Hoffmeister, R., & Wilber, R. (1980). The acquisition of sign language. In H. Lane & F. Grosjean (Eds.), *Recent perspectives on American Sign Language.* Hillsdale, NJ: Lawrence Erlbaum.

Hudgins, C.V., & Numbers, F.C. (1942). An investigation of the intelligibility of the speech of the deaf. *Genetic Psychology,* Monograph *5,* 289–392.

Jaffe, J., Stern, D., & Perry, J. (1973). "Conversational" coupling of gaze behaviors in prelinguistic human development. *Journal of Psycholinguistic Research, 2,* 321–329.

Jensema, C.J., Karchmer, M.A., & Trybus, R.J. (1978). *The rated speech intelligibility of hearing impaired children: Basic relationships.* Washington, DC: Gallaudet College, Office of Demographic Studies.

Kaplan, G.K., Fleishman, J.K., Bender, T.R., & Clark, P. (1973). Long-term effects of otitis media: A 10 year cohort study of Alaskan Eskimo children. *Pediatrics, 52,* 577–585.

Katz, J. (Ed.). (1972). *Handbook of clinical audiology.* Baltimore: Williams & Wilkins.

Knauf, V.H. (1972). Meeting speech and language needs for the hearing impaired. In J. Katz (Ed.), *Handbook of clinical audiology* (pp. 733–777). Baltimore: Williams & Wilkins.

Kretschmer, R. (1974). Auditory training procedures with hearing impaired preschool children. In E. Donnelly (Ed.), *Interpreting hearing aid technology.* Springfield, IL: Charles C. Thomas.

Kretschmer, R.E., & Quigley, S.P. (1981). The psycho-educational assessment of hearing-impaired children. In R.J. Rosser & M.P. Downs (Eds.), *Auditory disorders in school children.* New York: Thieme-Stratton.

Liddell, S. (1980). *American sign language syntax.* The Hague: Mouton.

Ling, D. (1976). *Speech and the hearing impaired child: Theory and practice.* Washington, DC: Alexander Graham Bell Association.

Ling, D. (1984). *Early intervention for hearing-impaired children: Oral options.* San Diego, CA: College Hill Press.

Ling, D., & Clarke, B. (1975). Cued speech: An evaluative study. *American Annals of the Deaf, 20,* 480–488.

Lykos, C. (1971). *Cued speech handbook for teachers.* Washington, DC: Gallaudet College.

Markides, A. (1970). The speech of deaf and partially hearing children with special reference to factors affecting intelligibility. *British Journal of Communication Disorders, 5,* 126–140.

Mavilya, M. (1969). *Spontaneous vocalization and babbling in hearing-impaired infants.* Doctoral dissertation, Teacher's College, Columbia University, New York.

Meadow, K. (1968). Early manual communication in relation to the deaf child's intellectual, social and communicative functioning. *American Annals of the Deaf, 113,* 29–41.

Meadow, K.P. (1980). *Deafness and child development.* Los Angeles, CA: University of California Press.

Mehr, A.S. (1983). *Auditory visual synchrony difference limen and speechreading ability in adolescence with severe to profound sensorineural hearing loss.* Unpublished doctoral dissertation, Adelphi University, Garden City, NY.

Menyuk, P. (1963). A preliminary evaluation of grammatical capacity in children. *Journal of Verbal Learning and Verbal Behavior, 2,* 429–439.

Menyuk, P. (1974). Early development of receptive language: From babbling to words. In R. Schiffelbusch & L. Lloyd (Eds.), *Language perspectives—Acquisition, retardation, and intervention* (pp. 213–235). Baltimore: University Park Press.

Miller, C., & Morse, P. (1976). The "heart" of categorial speech discrimination in young infants. *Journal of Speech and Hearing Research, 19,* 578–589.

Miller, C., Morse, P., & Dorman, N. (1977). Cardiac indices of infants' speech perception: Orienting and burst discrimination. *Quarterly Journal of Experimental Psychology, 29,* 533–545.

Mohay, H. (1983). The effects of cued speech on the language development of three deaf children. *Sign Language Studies, 38,* 25–47.

Monsees, E.K. (1976). The multiply involved child: A personal perspective. In P. Elwood, W. Johnson & J. Mandell (Eds.), *Parent-centered programs for young hearing impaired children.* Upper Marlboro, MD: State Department of Education.

Moog, J.S., & Geers, A.E. (1979). Grammatical analysis of elicited language: Simple sentence level (GAEL-S). St. Louis: Central Institute for the Deaf.

Moores, D. (1969). Cued speech: Some practical and theoretical considerations. *American Annals of the Deaf, 114,* 23–27.

Moores, D. (1978). *Educating the deaf: Psychology, principles, and practice.* Boston, MA: Houghton Mifflin.

Morse, P. (1972). The discrimination of speech and speech stimuli in early infancy. *Journal of Experimental Psychology, 14,* 477–492.

Myklebust, H.R. (1960). *The psychology of deafness.* New York: Grune & Stratton.

Newport, E., & Ashbrook, E. (1977). The emergence of semantic relations in American sign language. *Papers and Reports on Child Language Development, 13,* 16–21.

Nober, E. (1967). Articulation of the deaf. *Exceptional Child, 33,* 611–621.

Northern, J. (Ed.). (1984). *Hearing disorders* (2nd ed.). Boston: Little, Brown.

Northern, J. & Downs, M. (1978). *Hearing in children.* Baltimore: Williams & Wilkins.

Oller, D.K., Jensen, H., & LaFayette, R. (1978). The relatedness of phonological processes of a hearing impaired child. *Journal of Communication Disorders, 11,* 97–105.

Oller, D.K., & Kelly, C.A. (1974). Phonological substitution processes of a hard-of-hearing child. *Journal of Speech and Hearing Disorders, 39,* 65–74.

Pashley, N.R.T. (1984). Otitis media. In J. Northern (Ed.), *Hearing disorders* (pp. 103–110). Boston: Little, Brown.

Paterson, M. (1982). Integration of auditory training with speech and language for severely hearing impaired children. In D. Sims, G. Walter, & R. Whitehead (Eds.), *Deafness and communication.* Baltimore: MD: Waverly Press.

Pinter, R., Eisenson, J., & Stanton. (1946). *The psychology of the physically handicapped.* New York: Crofts.

Pinter, R., & Reamer, J. (1920). A mental and educational survey of schools for the deaf. *American Annals of the Deaf, 65,* 277–300.

Pollack, D. (1964). Acoupedics: A uni-sensory approach to auditory training. *The Volta Review, 66,* 400–409.

Power, D.J., & Quigley, S.P. (1969). Deaf children's acquisition of the passive voice. *Journal of Speech and Hearing Research, 16,* 5–11.

Quigley, S.P. (1969). *The influence of fingerspelling on the development of language, communication and education of achievement of deaf children.* Urbana: University of Illinois.

Quigley, S.P., & Kretschmer, R.E. (1982). *The education of deaf children.* Baltimore: University Park Press.

Quigley, S.P., & Paul, P.V. (1984). *Language and deafness.* San Diego, CA: College Hill Press.

Quigley, S.P., Power, D.J., & Steinkamp, M.W. (1977). The language structure of deaf children. *The Volta Review, 79,* 73–84.

Quigley, S.P., Smith, N.L., & Wilbur, R.B. (1974). Comprehension of relativized sentences by deaf students. *Journal of Speech and Hearing Research, 17,* 325–341.

Quigley, S.P., Steinkamp, M.W., Power, D.J., & Jones, B. (1978). *Test of syntactic abilities.* Beaverton, OR: Dormac.

Radziewicz, C. (1984). *The use of videotapes as a means of parent training for parents of hearing-impaired infants.* Doctoral dissertation in progress, Adelphi University, Garden City, NY.

Sanders, D. (1971). *Aural rehabilitation.* Englewood Cliffs, NJ: Prentice-Hall.

Schlesinger, H., & Meadow, K. (1972). *Sound and sign: Childhood deafness and mental health.* Berkeley: University of California Press.

Simmons-Martin, A. (1972). The oral/aural procedure: Theoretical basis and rationale. *The Volta Review, 74,* 541–551.

Siple, P. (1982). Signed language and linguistic theory. In L. Obler & L. Menn (Eds.), *Exceptional language and linguistics.* New York: Academic Press.

Skarakis, E., & Prutting, C. (1977). Early communication: Semantic functions and communicative intentions in the communication of the pre-school child with impaired hearing. *American Annals of the Deaf, 122,* 382–391.

Smith, C. (1975). Residual hearing and speech production in deaf children. *Journal of Speech and Hearing Research, 18,* 4, 795–811.

Stewart, J., Pollack, D., & Downs, M. (1964). A unisensory approach for the limited hearing child. *ASHA, 6,* 154–161.

Stokoe, W. (1958). *Sign language structure.* (Occasional Paper No. 8). University of Buffalo: Studies in linguistics.

Utley, J.A. (1946). A test of lipreading ability. *Journal of Speech and Hearing Disorders, 11,* 109–116.

Vorce, E. (1974). *Teaching speech to deaf children.* Washington, DC: Alexander Graham Bell Association for the Deaf.

Wedenberg, E. (1951). Auditory training of deaf and severely hard of hearing children. *Acta Oto-Laryngolgica.* (Supplementum), *110,* 1–82.

West, J., & Weber, J. (1973). A phonological analysis of the spontaneous language of a four-year-old, hard-of-hearing child. *Journal of Speech and Hearing Disorders, 38,* 25–35.

Whitehurst, M. (1955). Auditory training manual. *Hearing Rehabilitation,* North Merrick, NY.

Wilbur, R.B. (1979). *American sign language and sign systems.* Baltimore: University Park Press.

Wilbur, R.B., Goodhart, N., & Montandon, E. (1983). Comprehension of nine syntactic structures by hearing-impaired students. *The Volta Review, 85,* 328–345.

Zieziula, F.R. (1983). *Assessment of hearing-impaired people.* Washington, DC: Gallaudet College Press.

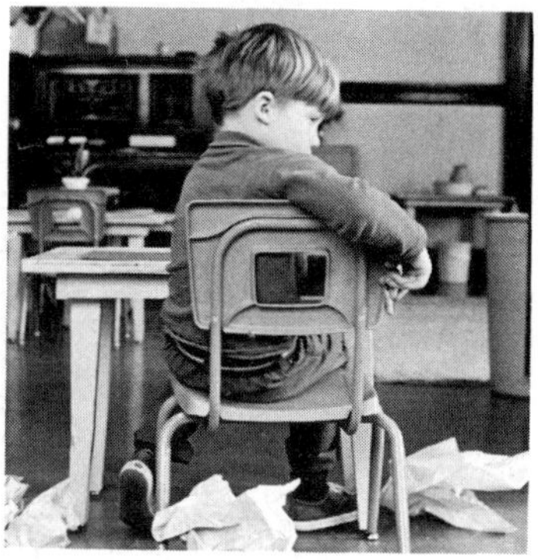

11

Understanding Learning Disabilities

THE CONCEPT OF LEARNING DISABILITIES

Historical Origins

Learning disabilities is the most recent classification to be included as a category of the handicapped. Since its introduction, the use of the term has become widespread in education, but many educators still remain unsure about the nature of this category of handicapping condition. Currently, the learning disability field still includes concepts such as perceptual-motor problems, hyperactivity, minimal brain damage, and psychoneurological disorders that have their roots in the origins of the field. The struggle to understand and define learning disabilities has characterized the field since its inception.

Lerner (1981) and Wiederholt (1974) divided the history of learning disabilities into four distinct phases:

1. *Foundation* phase (about 1800–1930), a period devoted to scientific investigation of brain function
2. *Transition* phase (about 1930–1960) during which it was assumed that children who were not learning possessed brain function deficits resulting in disordered behaviors. Professionals (Cruickshank, Bentzen, Razburg, & Tannhauser, 1961; Orton, 1937; Strauss & Lehtinen, 1947) began to develop assessment and treatment methods for these children

This chapter was written by Dr. Pearl L. Seidenberg, Long Island University.

3. *Integration* phase (about 1960–1980), a period characterized by increased interest in learning disabilities with a subsequent increase in school programs for the learning disabled, research, assessment practices, and teaching methods
4. *Contemporary* phase (1980 to the present) in which the direction is toward widening the definition of individuals served and the integration of services provided across school programs

One of the first to propose the term *learning disability* was Samuel Kirk (1963) who used the term to describe a group of children with specific learning deficits. He stated that a learning disability refers to a retardation, disorder, or delayed development in one or more of the processes of speech, language, reading, spelling, writing, or arithmetic. The learning disability results from a possible cerebral dysfunction and/or emotional or behavioral disturbance, not from mental retardation, sensory deprivation, or cultural or instructional factors. Kirk explained that these disabilities refer to a discrepancy between the child's achievement and apparent capacity to learn as indicated by aptitude tests, verbal understanding, and arithmetic computational skills.

Although the concept covered diverse learning handicaps, the term established a frame of reference for thinking about a child with specific learning disorders. The term avoided placing the blame for failure to learn solely on dysfunctions within the child who was assumed to have more intellectual ability than the child who is mentally retarded. Because the term did not specify a cause (i.e., minimal brain dysfunction or brain damage), it focused attention on the educational problems that the child faces and laid the framework for educational decision making and special education services.

In 1963 when the Association for Children with Learning Disabilities (ACLD) was formed, the term *learning disability* was adopted as a substitute term for such etiological labels as *brain-injured* and *perceptually handicapped.* In 1969 the following definition was presented to Congress by the National Advisory Committee on Handicapped Children:

> The term "children with specific learning disabilities" means those children who have a disorder in one or more of the basic psychological processes involved in understanding or in using language, spoken or written, which disorder may manifest itself in an imperfect ability to listen, think, speak, read, write, spell or do mathematical calculations. Such disorders include such conditions as perceptual handicaps, brain injury, minimal brain dysfunction, dyslexia and developmental aphasia. The term does not include children who have learning problems which are primarily the result of visual, hearing or motor handicaps, of mental retardation, of emotional disturbance, or of environmental, cultural or economic disadvantage. (Federal Register, 1977)

This definition served as the basis of the 1969 Learning Disabilities Act and later in 1975 was included in the Education for All Handicapped Children Act, Public Law 94–142.

In 1981, the National Joint Committee on Learning Disabilities revised the definition (Hammill, Leiger, McNutt, & Larsen, 1981), and agreed on the following:

> Learning disability is a generic term that refers to a heterogeneous group of disorders manifested by significant difficulties in the acquisition and use of listening, speaking, read-

> ing, writing, reasoning, or mathematical abilities. These disorders are intrinsic to the individual and are presumed to be due to central nervous system dysfunction. Even though a learning disability may occur concomitantly with other handicapping conditions or environmental influences, it is not the direct result of those conditions or influences. (p. 336)

This definition has been accepted by the Council for Learning Disabilities, the International Reading Association, the Division for Children with Communication Disorders, the Orton Society, and the American Speech-Language-Hearing Association.

The most basic and important difference from the definition included in Public Law 94–142 is the elimination of the phrase, "basic psychological processes." The joint committee agreed that the original purpose of the statement, which was to emphasize the *intrinsic* nature of learning disabilities, had been confounded by the controversy that resulted from the association of the term with the perceptual-motor and specific abilities training models that were in use at the time the original definition was adopted. Currently, explanations of the kinds of *cognitive, metacognitive,* and *ability* deficits that characterize the nature of the intrinsic disorders of the learning-disabled population are based on linguistic science and information-processing theory.

Defining Learning Disabilities

Because human behavior and learning is complex, learning disabilities may be difficult to define; but they are usually readily identifiable and distinguishable from other handicaps. Although professionals may be unable to agree on a single definition, in practice, most do not deny the validity of the condition.

The term is used to describe children and adolescents who are not learning at an expected rate despite the fact that they have experienced traditionally adequate instructional programs. The term *learning disability* does not identify a specific dysfunction or a syndrome of dysfunctions. The decision to describe a child as learning disabled is made by eliminating other causes of school failure such as emotional disturbance, mental retardation, or environmental or cultural disadvantage. The label encompasses a heterogeneous group of learners with diverse characteristics who have common problems with learning and who do not present a clearly identifiable reason for their learning deficits. Although the label is descriptive rather than diagnostic and does not denote a specific etiology or a specific cluster of characteristics, there are a number of behavioral characteristics that are often attributed to learning-disabled children.

Characteristics of Learning-Disabled Children

Although the characteristics associated with learning disability are not likely to be present in all or even many learning-disabled children, the behavioral characteristics are useful for helping us to understand the category. The following nine characteristics are mentioned most frequently:

1. *Hyperactivity*—inappropriate excessive motor activity such as tapping of finger or foot, jumping out of seat, or skipping from task to task
2. *Attention deficits*—distracted by irrelevant stimuli or perservation, or attention becomes fixed upon a single task or behavior which is repeated over and over
3. *Motor deficits*—general coordination problems resulting in awkward or clumsy movements

4. *Perceptual-motor deficits*—difficulty in integrating a visual or auditory stimulus with a motor response
5. *Language deficits*—delays in speech and difficulty in understanding and/or formulating spoken language
6. *Impulsivity*—lack of reflective behavior
7. *Cognitive deficits*—deficits in memory and concept formation
8. *Orientation deficits*—poorly developed spatial or temporal concepts
9. *Specific learning deficits*—problems in acquiring reading, writing, or arithmetic skills

These characteristics, for the most part, are *process* oriented as opposed to *effect* oriented. That is, they focus on the deficit behaviors exhibited by children with learning problems. The identification of the effect of the learning deficits (e.g., oral language, concept formation, etc.) directs attention to the child's deficiencies in level of performance or skill acquisition in academic areas. These effect-oriented characteristics are the only performance indicators that are useful in helping to develop appropriate educational interventions.

Because we would expect that an individual with known learning problems would also exhibit problems in other areas, the reported presence of many of these behaviors (i.e., short attention span, perceptual-motor difficulties) is not unexpected. These behavioral characteristics associated with a learning disability, however, are not the *cause* of the disability.

AN INFORMATION-PROCESSING PERSPECTIVE

Current characterizations of the intrinsic disorders manifested in learning-disabled children's ability deficits are based on information-processing theory. Attention has shifted from an interest in identifying and remediating discrete processing ability deficits to a focus on the inefficient, or maladaptive, information processing skills of learning-disabled children.

Psychological Processes

For some time, learning disabilities were considered to be the result of various types of specific ability deficits. Historically, the research in learning disabilities centered on various psychological processing tasks involving attention, perception, and memory. Comparisons were made between learning-disabled and nonlearning-disabled students. These tasks were considered to be measures of underlying cognitive abilities and were used to assess separate discrete functions (i.e., visual closure, visual and/or auditory figure-ground differentiation, auditory discrimination, visual and/or auditory memory, etc.). Because early theorists contended that these factors had to be adequately developed before learning could occur, training programs and materials were designed to remediate specific processing deficits (Frostig, 1968; Kephart, 1971; Kirk & Kirk, 1972).

An assumption underlying the processing abilities deficit model was that the areas were distinct from each other and that their component parts could be identified and assessed. Therefore, one could measure one of the systems without regard for any of the others. The interactive nature of the processes of perception, attention, and memory was not considered. Also, the role of the learner in cognitive processing was not viewed as an active one and, therefore, such confounding variables as meaningfulness of material or organizational abilities were not taken into consideration. The passive view of the child led to the belief that what was to be attended to, perceived, or memorized was "out there." Modification of the demands of tasks rather than attempts to influence the child's approach to a problem was emphasized.

From an information-processing perspective, perception, attention, and memory are considered interactive cognitive processes whose functioning reflects the influence and control of higher-order, integrated, goal-directed cognitive structures (Anderson, 1975). We develop control mechanisms, "a plan to execute a plan" (Miller, Galanter, & Prebam, 1960) which organize and direct the lower-order processes. Therefore, the learning difficulties experienced by some otherwise normal children have come to be recognized as related to the higher-order cognitive controls that regulate attention, perception, and memory. The most important and useful feature of information-processing theory is in enhancing our understanding of the learning-disabled child's problems. A much more complex picture of the learning process is emerging, which focuses attention on the strategies a child uses in approaching learning tasks and suggests very different educational interventions.

The Information-Processing Model

In 1969, Chalfont and Scheffelin described learning disabilities as a problem involving deviation in the ability to process information and as an inefficiency in the reception, analysis, synthesis, and symbolic use of information. Since then, information-processing concepts have provided a useful framework for understanding learning disabilities.

The conceptual model arising from information-processing theory enables us to describe systematically the way students who exhibit learning deficits process information. Cognitive psychology or information-processing psychology deals with the study of mental processes and begins with the idea that we have the innate capacity to make sense of our experiences. We pick up information, organize it, retain it, and retrieve it. We can call upon previously stored information to help us in managing new information. The fact that we make sense of our experience, even though nothing ever happens to us in exactly the same way twice, must mean that we are organized in some systematic way (Farnham-Diggory, 1980). Figure 11–1 is a sample of an information-processing model.

Auditory, visual, and tactile stimuli (sensory data) are transmitted to the central-processing mechanism (brain) where they are analyzed, integrated, and stored. The behavioral responses of the individual serve as an additional input source (feedback) for correcting or further modifying the responses. The input is always into a dynamic, organized, interactive system. Behavioral responses are determined not only by the actual stimulus but also by the ongoing programs, the result of past experiences that are already stored in the system.

Modern information-processing theory suggests that individuals may differ from one another cognitively in two broad areas. First, they may differ in the basic structure of their information-processing systems. These structural or architectural (Campione & Brown, 1978) features are the elements of the system that operate outside of the conscious control of the individual. Such things as capacity of short-term memory,

Figure 11–1. Information-Processing Model

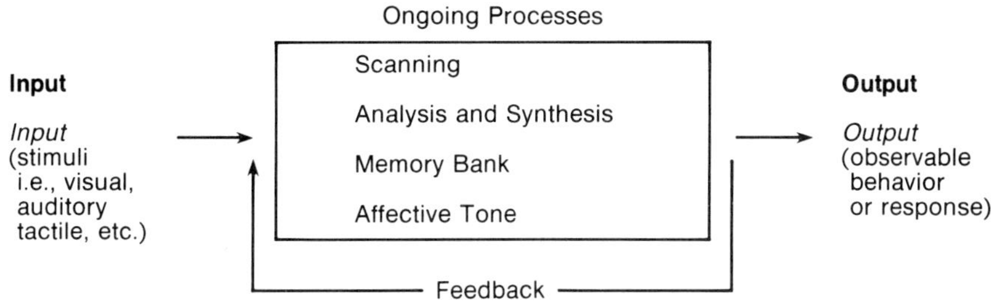

duration of memory traces, and speed of operations of various processes are all part of the structure of the system.

Individual differences are also the result of differences in information and skills that are *learned* as a result of experience. These are the content of long-term memory (i.e., programs already in the system), and are made up of general organized knowledge of the world (i.e., hierarchical semantic structures), habitual ways of thinking (i.e., concrete vs. abstract), and rules and strategies that guide performance and adaptation to tasks. The content of long-term memory and the functional features of the system are modifiable by instruction and are under our conscious control (Torgeson, 1982).

The distinction between structural and functional areas of cognitive performance made by information-processing theorists has led to new ways of thinking about the learning-disabled child's cognitive system. Traditionally, learning-disabled children's academic problems and poor performance on experimental tasks were explained in terms of specific ability deficits necessary for normal processing of information. A large number of disabilities such as perceptual-motor deficits, intermodel integration deficits, and psycholinguistic processing problems were considered to be relatively enduring cognitive deficits that restricted information processing. In information-processing terms, these earlier explanations claimed that all problems with learning were due to differences in the structural features of the system. Concepts derived from information-processing theory have greater explanatory power. They provide a framework for analyzing learning deficits which differentiates between the structural and functional elements of the system, that is, between the system and the programs that use the system. In the learning-disabled child, some information-processing components are not operating effectively for certain tasks. Therefore, the primary problem appears to be one of programming, and although there may also be some system defects, we can search for ways to develop programs that will compensate for them. A major assumption that underlies the information-processing view of disabled learners is that the rules and specific strategies used by learning-disabled children do not appear to be appropriate to their intellectual ability. They appear to have knowledge that they are unable to access under certain conditions, to have strategies that they fail to use, or to have not learned when to select particular strategies.

A number of information-processing models have been generated involving metacognitive and metalinguistic variables such as a verbal processing deficit (Vellutino,

1977), a phonological recoding deficit (Shankweiler, Lieberman, Mark, Fowler, & Fischer, 1979), a rehearsal deficiency (Bauer, 1977), a selective attention deficit (Hallahan & Reeves, 1980), and a deficit in active learning (Torgeson, 1977) in order to account for learning-disabled children's poor task performance. These metacognitive and metalinguistic variables have important implications for our understanding of the three major areas of learning disabilities: (*a*) deficiencies in oral language, (*b*) deficiencies in cognitive abilities, and (*c*) deficiencies in written language.

MAJOR AREAS OF LEARNING DISABILITIES

Deficits in Oral Language

Failure to develop adequate verbal language skills results in subsequent failure in many other areas of learning. It is important to understand the interdependencies of language disorders and learning disabilities. The history of the field of learning disabilities generally has not emphasized the role of language processes. Because of the origins of the field, an interest in perceptual motor functioning and other nonverbal tasks has dominated both the literature and educational programs until recently.

Currently, many researchers believe that language deficits are implicated in learning disabilities (Mattingly, 1972; Shankweiller et al., 1979; Vellutino, 1977; Vogel, 1975). They propose that these deficits also have an impact on reading ability and on academic success. I will present a brief overview of language problems representative of learning-disabled children. The reader is referred to Wiig and Semel (1976, 1980) for a more comprehensive review of this topic.

Preschool Language Deficits. Preschool children who exhibit language deficits or delays are generally "at-risk" for later school failure. Early language disorders are demonstrated in a number of areas. At-risk children frequently show no interest in verbal activities, are unable to follow a story line, and do not enjoy being read to. Although nouns, verbs, and most prepositions are understood, these children may have word retrieval difficulties or difficulty in following a series of oral directions. There is often a sustained delay in speech and language development, and syntax may be primitive with incidence of inadequate morphological pattern acquisition. Overall verbal concept development may be slow, and the children are often still unable to name colors, letters, or days of the week when they enter school.

In a comprehensive review of the research regarding young language-impaired children, Leonard (1979) presented a description of the at-risk children's linguistic problems. In general, the language skills of language-delayed preschoolers are similar to those of younger, normal children. Syntactically, the structures used by these children seem to be the same as those used by younger normal children, although at-risk children appear to use them less frequently and in more limited contexts. The size of their vocabulary and the length of their utterances (MLU) also resemble those of younger children. Similar findings relate to the areas of pragmatics and phonology. There is evidence of greater delays in the language-impaired child's use of the pragmatic and phonological features of language.

Because inadequate language development is often the precursor to learning problems during the school years, there is an urgent need for early identification of children who evidence developmental language delays. Early intervention can prevent later learning problems from developing and can offset the negative emotional consequences of school failure.

Language Deficits of the School-age Child. Many learning-disabled children exhibit a number of language deficits that affect both language comprehension and production. The linguistic demands of a classroom require a level of abstractness and complexity much greater than that needed for ordinary social communicative competence. The mismatch between the linguistic demands of instructional language and the poor linguistic abilities of many learning-disabled children may account in part for the hyperactive, impulsive behaviors and attentional deficits often attributed to these children.

Generally, language-impaired, learning-disabled children have difficulty in comprehending language involving Wh- questions, and in processing and using pronouns and possessives. Other aspects of syntax that cause difficulty for many learning-disabled children are the passive construction, negative constructions, relative clauses, negations, contractions, and adjective transformations (Vogel, 1975; Wiig & Semel, 1973, 1974, 1975). There is evidence of reduced mastery of the grammatical inflections for adjectives, verb tense markers, and possession (Vogel, 1975, Wiig, Semel, & Crouse, 1973). Specific difficulty with verb tense markers was found primarily in irregular past tense forms (Moran & Byrne, 1977) and with more complex grammatical structures (Edwards & Kallail, 1977).

Linguistic concepts expressing comparative, spatial, and temporal relationships are also problems for learning-disabled children. Wiig and Semel (1976) have demonstrated that the ability to process these structures follows a developmental course, with comparative relations being easiest, followed in difficulty by temporal and spatial relationships. It is important to note that not all learning-disabled children will have the same difficulties with the same linguistic concepts.

An extensive description of areas of possible difficulty with different form classes including nouns, verbs, adjectives, adverbs, and prepositions has been provided by Wiig and Semel (1980). The authors related many of the linguistic problems to more primary cognitive difficulties. They suggested that if relationships are not accurately perceived by children in their interactions with their environment, they will not be able to comprehend these relationships when they are coded linguistically. In addition, they believed that a child who has difficulty in generalizing and has a tendency toward concreteness will maintain narrower word meanings and have problems processing sentences containing multiple-meaning words and figurative language.

In development of their semantic system, learning-disabled children generally have been found to equal normal children in tasks of receptive vocabulary (Wiig & Semel, 1973; Vogel, 1975), but they do exhibit word-finding difficulties (Denckla & Rudel, 1976; Johnson & Myklebust, 1967). They demonstrate specific deficits in rapid naming tasks, naming pictures, naming opposites, and giving word definitions (Wiig & Semel, 1976).

The primary productive syntactic language problems evidenced by learning-disabled children appears to be a delay in the acquisition of basic transformational operations such as negative, interrogative, or passive transformations. In sentence repetition tasks, learning-disabled children appear to maintain the basic meaning or semantic relations of a sentence without difficulty, but they repeat the sentence in a reduced fashion

(Menyuk & Looney, 1972). In general, learning-disabled children appear to be performing similarly to younger normal children in this area.

Generally, the phonological problems of language-impaired children are more complex than the problems exhibited by the child with only an articulation disorder. The problems appear to be related more to morphosyntactic delays than to simple production difficulties. Often the language learning-disabled child evidences inconsistencies in sound production. Sounds may be produced accurately in simple sentences, but when the sentences become longer and more complex, production difficulties become evident. The language-delayed child appears more vulnerable to the syntactic demands of more complex structures, where the motor patterning and greater demands on idea formulation, appear to create organizational problems (Berry, 1980).

Finally, learning-disabled children may have deficits in pragmatics, the understanding of the rules governing the use of language in social contexts. In a review of a series of studies dealing with pragmatic competence, Bryan (1981) presented an overview of the deficits evidenced by learning-disabled children. In general, they did *not* differ from nondisabled children in conversational turn-taking or in referential communicative competence when a required response was unambiguous. However, when a situation was ambiguous or socially complex, the performance of the two groups differed. In these situations, learning-disabled children have difficulty with such pragmatic skills as asking questions, responding to inadequate messages, disagreeing, supporting an argument, and sustaining or monitoring a conversation. The studies also indicated that the relationships among syntactic-semantic knowledge, social knowledge, and development of communicative competence are interactive and complex and may be dependent upon the development of both linguistic skills and cognitive abilities.

Deficits in Cognitive Abilities

Any attempt to understand the performance of learning-disabled children in academic learning must consider the interaction of language and thought and the cognitive correlates of such an interaction. In processing written language, the learner is confronted with a combination of both abstract concepts and complex language. Without adequate development in both language and cognitive strategies for processing information, a serious mismatch between the child's ability and the academic task demands can result. The cognitive functions of perception, attention, and memory are related to each other, as well as to the acquisition of language. Understanding the nature of these interactions in the processing of verbally encoded information contributes to our understanding of the problems experienced by many children with learning disabilities.

According to current theory in cognitive psychology, perception, attention, and memory are interactive processes that reconstruct, organize, and internalize information. Cognitive development is continually emerging through stages of newly acquired strategies for actively processing environmental information. The child becomes increasingly able to attend selectively to critical attributes during perception and to hold more than one aspect of perceived information in memory simultaneously to perform cognitively on that information. There is evidence that as age increases, memory abilities are enhanced by the use of categorization and verbal rehearsal strategies (Ring, 1976). Similarly, with maturation, children develop increased ability to focus attention on the relevant aspects of learning tasks and to diminish attention to incidental stimuli (Tarver, Hallahan, Kaufman, & Ball, 1976).

Memory, attention, and perception interact and are interdependent. The individual actively analyzes and processes information by developing strategies that tap previously stored information acquired through past experience and organizational structures. Also, there appears to be a reciprocal relationship between language development and the development of cognitive abilities. This interactive nature of the relationship is viewed within the broader framework of the child's overall ability to organize, plan, monitor, and integrate information. The view that is generally held is that the development of cognitive strategies complements linguistic development in a way that facilitates the processing of verbally encoded information. Also, increased linguistic abilities contribute to the development of a number of cognitive functions such as memory and attention.

Many learning-disabled children exhibit deficits in the use of such elaborative encoding strategies as verbal grouping and verbal rehearsal (e.g., reauditorization or repetition of the information in order to support recall). This deficit appears to reduce the effectiveness of attention and memory in processing information. At the same time, they exhibit inadequate use of the organizational structure of syntax and of category clustering of verbal material. These deficits appear to be related to problems in processing verbal material (Bauer, 1977; Hallahan, Gajar, Cohen, & Tarver, 1978; Ring, 1976; Tarver, et al., 1976).

In a number of the previously reported studies, learning-disabled children's performance improved as a result of training in the use of selected processing strategies. These observed changes in behavior have led to the conclusion that learning-disabled children have more ability than can be presumed by their performance. Some of their learning deficits are not due to an inability to acquire effective cognitive strategies, but to other factors that interfere with their development. One factor that appears to result in poor performance is that learning-disabled children tend to be externally controlled; that is, they regard what happens to them as unrelated to what they themselves do. This view of themselves and the world may keep these children from actively using appropriate learning strategies (Hallahan, et al., 1978).

Many aspects of the relationships between cognition and language have still to be examined. Many of the behaviors reported in learning-disabled children, however, appear to support a hypothesis of a delay in cognitive development. Their cognitive development indicates deficits in the use of higher-order cognitive strategies such as (*a*) simultaneous processing of perceptual information, (*b*) development of organizational structures that encode larger amounts of information, and (*c*) the use of verbal strategies to facilitate storage and retrieval of information. The degree to which language delay contributes to cognitive deficits and the degree to which language delays are a function of the cognitive deficits remain unclear.

Deficits in Written Language

The largest subgroup among the learning-disabled population are those children and adolescents identified as having deficits associated with learning to read and write. Children with disorders in the comprehension or formulation of written language appear to process information differently than nonlearning-disabled children. Often they fail to use effective strategies in interacting with written material and evidence deficits in their performance of reading and writing tasks.

Reading Deficits. Although most children learn to read as effortlessly as they learn to speak regardless of the method used to teach them, a small proportion of children with no clearly identifiable intellectual, physical, or social handicaps find it extremely difficult to learn to read or write. For these learning-disabled children, learning to read is a formidable task, and those who are responsible for teaching these children find the task equally difficult. However, current theoretical advances in the cognitive and linguistic sciences provide some new approaches to this problem. Insights derived from a developmental cognitive-linguistic perspective emphasize the complex, interactive nature of the reading process and provide an additional dimension for understanding the nature of reading disabilities.

This perspective assumes that there are critical age-related cognitive and linguistic characteristics that interact with reading instruction resulting in an inability to acquire specific reading skills. Key issues within such a perspective are the learner's cognitive-linguistic abilities and how these set the parameters for the child's information-processing capacities. These underlying information-processing capabilities are important for learning to read and are reflected in a student's specific reading behaviors. Because reading disability is *not* a unitary phenomenon, the actual causes of difficulties in learning to read vary. There can be various points of breakdown for different learners in the learning-to-read process. Deficits in the learner's underlying information-processing capacities relative to the skills being taught contribute to these breakdowns.

Efficient reading requires the acquisition and integration of different skills at different points in the process. The acquisition of these skills is dependent on the integrative functioning of cognitive abilities (i.e., perception, attention, and memory) and their interface with linguistic variables. Therefore, the concept of reading disability can be understood only within a developmental context that considers what learners bring to the task of learning to read and how it affects reading efficiency.

Defining the Reading Process. Reading may be broadly defined as a communication process in that it involves the ability to respond to written language. It is a process of obtaining meaning and is currently categorized not as a perceptual act, but as a language-based activity. Goodman (1973) described reading as a "psycholinguistic guessing game" in which the reader samples only a minimal amount of the visual information, relying heavily on the redundancy of language (i.e., phonology, semantics, and syntax) to predict structures. As the reader processes the subsequent language, these predictions are tested against the semantic content and are confirmed. Reading is viewed as a constructive process in which the reader's knowledge about the language and the world (i.e., past experience) interact with the textual information (Anderson, Spiro, & Montague, 1977).

In order to bridge the gap from print to meaning, the reader must engage a number of subprocesses that involve auditory and visual perceptual abilities, cognitive abilities (i.e., attention, memory, organization), language knowledge, and past experiences. Reading performance can be viewed as a product of the reader's cognitive and linguistic abilities, prior knowledge, and mastery of specific reading skills. (See Figure 11–2.)

Figure 11–2. Interactive Model of Reading Performance

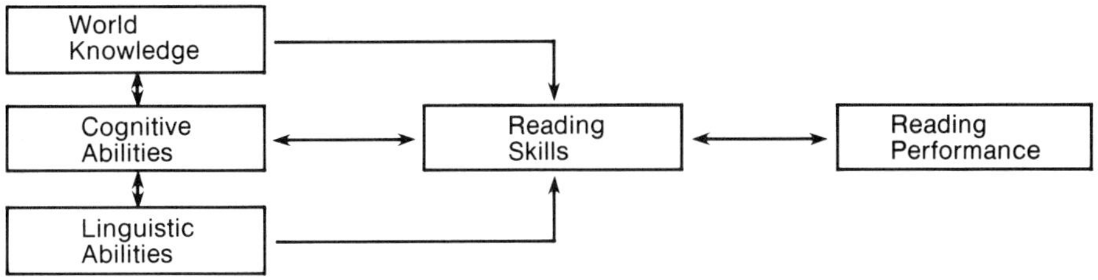

Reading performance reflects the interaction of these diverse factors, each of which contributes collectively to the reading process and, therefore, to observable reading behaviors.

Although reading may start with print and the specific skills taught in reading instruction, the level of reading efficiency demonstrated at any given point in the learning-to-read process is linked to the reader's information-processing capabilities within the different components of the model. Reading performance reflects the knowledge and competencies available to the learner and how these are activated and coordinated during the reading process.

Deficits in Verbal Processing. The possibility of verbal deficiencies in poor readers is currently receiving greater attention than it has in past years. Verbal skill deficits are reflected in various types of reading disabilities as well as other cognitive tasks (Vellutino, 1979).

A number of studies support the idea that poor readers are less adequate than normal readers in both short- and long-term memory for verbal material. However, such inadequacies appear to be associated with semantic processing deficits and are manifested in a number of linguistic deficiencies such as deficits in basic naming and labeling (Denckla & Rudel, 1976; Perfetti & Hogaboam, 1975), word retrieval problems (Ceci, 1982; Torgesen & Houck, 1980), and lexical development (Jansky & deHersh, 1972; Vellutino, 1979). Some poor readers also appear to have more difficulty than normal readers in the naming or labeling of letters and/or words (Perfetti & Lesgold, 1979; Ring, 1976).

A number of additional studies implicate other aspects of linguistic functioning in reader group differences. These studies indicate that poor readers are not as proficient as normal readers in understanding syntactically complex sentences (Brittain, 1970; Hook and Johnson, 1978; Vogel, 1975), in comprehending and using inflectional morphology (Berko, 1958; Bougere, 1969), in using syntactic constraints to assist in word identification (Samuels, Begg, & Chen, 1976; Steiner, Werner, & Cromer, 1971), and in phonological segmentation ability (Fox & Routh, 1980; Liberman, Shankweiler, Fisher, & Carter, 1974; Vellutino & Scanlon, 1979).

Because reading achievement necessitates the efficient use of all of the learner's cognitive and linguistic abilities, deficits in linguistic functioning have impact on both initial reading skill acquisition and on the later stages of the learning-to-read process.

Vellutino (1979) maintained that the apparent visual perceptual problems (i.e., word identification) encountered by beginning readers are, in fact, associated with problems in verbal mediation and/or phonological deficits. He contended that many of the errors implicated in reading disability can be understood as linguistic intrusion errors, rather than deficits in visual perception. Thus, when poor readers call a *b, d* or *was, saw,* it is not because they are processing the visual information inaccurately, it is because they have not yet learned the correct name for the letter or word. Similarly, he suggested that awareness of the phonetic structure of spoken language is important for the acquisition of word-decoding skills. Success in beginning reading, specifically in code acquisition (e.g., learning sound-symbol relationships) requires that learners have the ability to segment words at the phonemic level and to associate the separate phonemics with their counterparts in print. Poor readers appear to lack the phonological segmentation ability and, therefore, have difficulty in phonetic decoding and in developing phoneme/grapheme correspondences.

Deficits in Metacognitive and Metalinguistic Abilities. In addition to the importance of linguistic competence for the reading process, it has also been suggested that efficient reading requires a more comprehensive awareness of cognitive and linguistic functioning. Metacognition, for example, is the ability to deal abstractly with one's own thought processes in comprehension and reasoning tasks and to identify and regulate the use of appropriate strategies. Deficits in metacognitive knowledge appears to be a factor that affects the acquisition of effective reading comprehension skills among poor readers.

Research on metacognitive differences between good and poor readers indicates that poor readers are less able to evaluate task difficulty and to identify possible reading strategies (Bransford, Stein, Shelton, & Owings, 1980; Paris & Meyers, 1981). They are also characterized as overreliant on ineffective or inappropriate reading strategies. Poor readers continue to use inappropriate bottom-up strategies (word decoding strategies) that affect comprehension, or inappropriate top-down strategies (conceptual strategies based on prior knowledge) that interfere with accurate word recognition. (Pearson & Spiro, 1980). Additionally, poor readers tend not to use effective strategies for integrating word and sentence meanings, for extracting important information from the text, for drawing inferences, and for integrating background knowledge with the text (Golinkoff, 1976; Wong, 1978). Also, less skilled readers appear to be unaware of their own failures to comprehend (Markman, 1977).

It has also been suggested that reading requires a level of linguistic awareness above that required for the development and use of spoken language (Seidenberg, 1982). Many learning-disabled children appear to have deficits not solely in their verbal language systems but also in their metalinguistic awareness. For example, word segmentation ability required for the acquisition of phonic skills is a metalinguistic ability, and there are developmental differences in children's ability to analyze and differentiate the phonemes in words (Cazden, 1972). The ability to analyze words, blend word parts, and reconstruct the word requires metalinguistic skills. Also the ability to recognize the syntactic structures in written text is related to problems in reading comprehension. Learning-disabled children appear to have deficits in the ability to hold together grammatical structures and abstract meaning from larger contexts (Denner, 1970). Some disabled readers are unable to segment text into meaningful units and are, therefore, unable to attend to the focal or propositional information (Fleisher, Jenkins, & Pavey, 1979).

There are form and content differences between the language of speech and the language of text, as well as differences in the way they are used and processed (Olson, 1977). A fundamental deficit for some learning-disabled children appears to be their inability to use effective linguistic and/or cognitive strategies for the comprehension of written language.

Writing Deficits. Generally, the student with learning disabilities involving either oral language skills or reading skills will also experience difficulties in the acquisition of writing skills. Research indicates that writing skills are among the best correlates of reading, and that a strong relationship exists among reading, the receptive aspect of written language, and almost all other aspects of written language (Hammill & McNutt, 1981). Writing is a highly complex, interactive process which builds on preexisting cognitive and linguistic structures. It is the final and most formal aspect of language that has to be learned. Writing disorders can be understood only within a multiple framework encompassing knowledge of what the writer must bring to the task (i.e., underlying cognitive and linguistic abilities) and knowledge of the nature of the writing task itself.

There are two major categories of problems associated with writing disorders: (*a*) those due to deficits in underlying cognitive or linguistic processes required for writing, and (*b*) those due to the nature of the complex components inherent in writing activities and their interaction with underlying abilities. Written language facility involves a number of component skills including handwriting, spelling, punctuation, capitalization, vocabulary, syntax, and the formulation and organization of ideas. Typically, learning-disabled students have difficulty in more than one aspect of written language. Therefore, it is important to understand the development of these component skills and their relationship to proficiency in written language.

Acquisition of Written Language Skills. The abilities to read and write follow developmentally the abilities to listen and speak. Myklebust (1965, 1978) described the hierarchical process of language acquisition as developing through auditory receptive, auditory expressive, visual receptive, and visual expressive forms. He maintained that the development of abilities in the language hierarchy relies on the initial intactness of the oral language capacity. If there are significant oral language problems, then all capacities above this level will be affected. The many cognitive and linguistic abilities outlined earlier underlie basic oral language capacities. Therefore, those aspects of functioning that affect the verbal language system will also affect writing performance.

However, the ability to write requires an additional kind of analysis beyond that required for oral language. Writing is a form of representation that is further from the reality it represents than is spoken language. Vygotsky (1962) referred to writing as a "second order symbol system." Writing does not represent experience directly, but represents a previously acquired linguistic code, a system of arbitrary signs, by means of a new system. Vygotsky concluded that writing is highly abstract compared to the immediacy of spoken language. Although written language is similar to oral language in thought and imagery, its structure and mode of functioning differ.

Because of the complexity of writing, underlying processing capacities of attention and memory as well as higher levels of cognitive functioning need to be adapted and used in unique ways. For example, children must acquire the linguistic awareness that enables them to use effectively the syntactic and semantic aspects of language in writing. A writing task demands an awareness and control of linguistic processes that are different by nature and medium from speech. The conventions of writing have their own discourse rules which demand more formal use of complete syntactic conventions, such as connectives and embedded clauses, than those required for speech. There is also a demand for more cohesiveness, less redundancy, and fewer examples or illustrations.

Children need to develop metacognitive skills so that they are capable of monitoring their own production, evaluating what they are writing in light of their purpose, taking perspective into account, and using an expanded knowledge base. Finally, they need to develop a concept of text, an understanding of the way that coherence or unity is achieved in written language. Children need to acquire the concept of a "story," as well as other genres, which they will bring to the writing task. It is this concept of text structure that appears to support organization and memory during the writing activity (Applebee, 1978).

In addition to the linguistic and cognitive processes underlying writing acquisition, the task requires the ability to perform the motor act of writing and the attainment of a level of proficiency in spelling. Handwriting is a grapho-motor skill and is primarily dependent upon visual-perceptual ability, visual memory, and the eye-hand coordination. Johnson and Myklebust (1967) termed the inability to learn the appropriate motor behaviors for writing as *dysgraphia.* Severe deficits in handwriting may include the inability to maintain an appropriate pencil grasp. Less severe problems may result in handwriting that is poorly spaced, awkward, or immature. Handwriting difficulties may be only one manifestation of more generalized difficulties in the performance of motor activities (i.e., catching or throwing a ball, buttoning a coat, or following a pattern or sequence of movements).

Handwriting difficulties also may be affected by the rate of performance. In order for writing to be efficient, it must be performed at a rate appropriate for the task. Although the learning-disabled child's handwriting may appear adequate, it may have been produced slowly and with difficulty. Such problems result from a lack of automatic motor patterns for letter formation or from slowness in processing and organizing information for the writing task.

Another of the skills necessary for writing is the ability to recall the spelling of words. Cicci (1980) outlined some of the underlying abilities necessary in order for children to learn to spell words. The abilities to articulate the word correctly, recall the spoken pattern (i.e., the auditory sequence of the phonemes or syllables), and recall the visual letter sequences are necessary for learning to spell. Also, children must be able to recall the motor pattern for writing a word and to execute the plan for the motor act. Because the complex nature of the writing task requires the simultaneous use of semantic, syntactic, and graphophonic information, trying to satisfy all of these constraints at one time makes writing difficult.

Disorders in Written Language. Because the complexity of the writing task involves the integration of linguistic, cognitive, and motoric activities, writing presents a major problem for many learning-disabled students. Lerner (1981) suggested that poor facility in expressing thoughts through written language is the most prevalent disorder in the acquisition of communication skills. Students who have responded well to remediation in spoken language or reading instruction during the elementary grades often continue to have difficulties with written expressive language. In the learning-disabled population, written language disorders often persist into adolescence and adulthood (Blalock, 1981; Johnson, Blalock, & Nesbitt, 1978).

Spelling difficulties often persist in learning-disabled children even after they have learned to read. Some learning-disabled adolescents who exhibit severe spelling deficits may also show subtle oral language deficits including problems in word retrieval and in phonological segmentation ability.

Wiig and Semel (1976) reported that on writing tasks, learning-disabled students frequently make errors in word omissions, word order, incorrect verb and pronoun usage, incorrect word endings, and lack of punctuation. They also indicated that, at the syntactic level, learning-disabled children frequently produce agrammatical sentences in which elements of several transformations are combined or reversed. Learning-disabled children have been found to score significantly lower on indices of syntax and ideation when their writing samples were compared with those of nondisabled peers (Myklebust, 1973). Learning-disabled students also show significant deficits on standardized measures of spelling, grammatical correctness, capitalization and punctuation, thematic maturity, and vocabulary. In addition, their written language performance becomes more discrepant as grade-level increases (Poplin, Gray, Larsen, Banikowski, & Mehring, 1980).

Although reading and writing make different demands on underlying linguistic and cognitive capabilities, the skills needed for conveying meaning in writing are clearly interrelated with the skills necessary for extracting meaning from reading. Therefore, the reciprocal relationship inherent in reading and writing activities cannot be overemphasized. It assumes special significance in our understanding of the nature of the learning disabilities associated with written language.

ASSESSMENT OF LEARNING DISABILITIES

The measurement of a student's psychoeducational abilities and skills has historically been a major theme in the development and delivery of special education programs and services. Assessment, the collection and interpretation of relevant data, is a supporting activity for all subsequent decision-making activities. Before the need for a special education program or the instructional focus of the educational program can be determined for a student suspected of having a learning disability, a comprehensive functional assessment must be done.

Functional assessment and testing are not the same. Assessment involves far more than the administration of a group of tests. When we assess students, we have to consider the way they perform a variety of tasks in a variety of settings or contexts (e.g., the child with a short attention span for reading instruction but not for model plane building), the meaning of their performance in terms of their total functioning (e.g., the child's short attention span is directly related to the task demand—reading vs. model plane building) and explanations for the performance (e.g., the nature of the reading instructional program may be inappropriate for the child's information-processing capacities). Assessment is always an evaluative, interpretive appraisal of performance that provides information to teachers and other school-based personnel, allowing them to make effective educational decisions for children.

Comprehensive Evaluation

A single set of indicators cannot be used to decide that a child is learning disabled because there are different causes for and, therefore, different types of learning disability. Therefore, a careful clinical description of the individual child is of primary importance in making an appropriate identification. Assessment of learning-disabled children must be flexible and responsive to the individual differences exhibited by these children.

Because of the heterogeneity of the learning-disabled population, the regulations of Public Law 94–142 mandate that a comprehensive evaluation be done by a multidisciplinary team. For the assessment of children suspected of having specific learning disabilities, the regulations (Section 121a. 540) explicitly state that the team must be made up of:

- A person knowledgeable in the area of the suspected disability
- The child's classroom teacher, or if the child does not have a classroom teacher, a teacher qualified to teach the child
- At least one additional specialist such as a psychologist, a speech-language pathologist, or a remedial reading specialist, qualified to administer individual diagnostic assessments

Because of the interactive relationship between language disability and learning disability for many learning-disabled students, competent assessment requires a comprehensive evaluation which includes findings from both of these disciplines as well as other disciplines (i.e., physician, psychologist, reading specialist, regular teacher, etc.). It is very important to the overall identification of specific learning disabilities that the team's assessment approach reflect a multidimensional model, taking into account factors ranging from the purposes of assessment to a broad-based conceptualization of the nature of learning.

The Assessment Model

Assessment is undertaken to determine if special education is warranted and, if so, to determine the nature of the student's special educational needs. In order to make these decisions, a systematic approach to the organization and interpretation of evaluation data must be used. Testing information must identify meaningful patterns of functioning and provide data which is relevant for learning.

An information-processing model is one of the most fruitful approaches to understanding learning disabilities. Such a model accommodates the major concerns and problem areas in learning, including the cognitive and linguistic processes necessary for the acquisition of academic skills. Also, aspects of information-processing theory serve as the foundation for an important component of intervention which must address and integrate both the process-oriented data (e.g., cognitive, linguistic) and the content-oriented data (e.g., component skills needed for acquisition of reading, writing, etc.).

There is always a potential for bias in assessment, and it can affect both the descriptive and programmatic phases of assessment. Diverse professionals involved in the assessment process are generally influenced by the knowledge base in their respective disciplines and look for what they understand to be important aspects of learning and behavior. The adoption of a comprehensive assessment model can clarify the interrelationships among disciplines and improve current practice in the evaluation and programming of the learning-disabled student.

The translation of a comprehensive assessment model into strategies for obtaining information relevant for identification and educational planning places considerable demands upon the multidisciplinary team. It requires that team members have a strong foundation of knowledge pertaining to both the process-oriented and content-oriented aspects, and skills in translating these factors into specific assessment techniques. Team decision making requires that members have a sound knowledge base, the ability to recognize interactive patterns, and a firm understanding of how a particular testing paradigm affects the interpretation of test results. The assessment of learning disabilities, therefore, must have a sound theoretical base and the team members must be informed specialists who have kept up with current research and developments in their own and related fields.

Assessment for Identification

Until we refine our understanding of what constitutes a learning disability, the decision to classify a child as learning disabled is made on the basis of a discrepancy between expected and attained achievement and by the progressive exclusion of other causes for the learning deficits. In order to do this, the professional expertise of the multidisciplinary team is of critical importance and the basis for making the decision must be carefully documented. Assessment to determine eligibility for special education obtains objective descriptions of a child's cognitive, linguistic, and social/emotional status as well as descriptions of educational performance.

In general, formal tests, tests which are norm-referenced or standardized, are used extensively for screening and identification purposes. A child suspected of having learning disabilities should be measured in each of the domains (cognitive, linguistic, and social/emotional). Although the cognitive domain can be defined in many different ways, in practice, it almost always refers to the measurement of intelligence. The Wechsler Intelligence Scale for Children-Revised (Wechsler, 1974) is used most often and is related to and predictive of academic success. With the learning-disabled child, the intelligence test is used to establish that the child is functioning intellectually within the normal range. Data from the test can also provide information on the underlying abilities that constitute intelligence. For the learning-disabled child, extensive scatter or unevenness within the profile of cognitive abilities may provide insight into the child's information-processing abilities. The skilled clinical analysis of the data can provide information which can be useful in the development of an intervention program.

As is the case in cognitive assessment, formal measurement in the social/emotional domain is used to provide identification information and to rule out severe emotional disturbances as the primary cause of the learning deficits. A language assessment determines whether the child has difficulties in processing linguistically encoded information. Many learning-disabled children have language problems that impact directly on academic learning.

Formal measures of academic achievement are used to provide information on the difference between actual achievement and estimated potential in order to implement the identification procedures outlined in the federal rules and regulations. For the most part, the learning disabilities classification has not been operationally defined and still remains largely a matter of clinical judgment, underscoring the importance of team decision making.

Assessment for Instructional Programming

The Individualized Education Program. In order to ensure that a handicapped child receives appropriate services that are based on planned educational goals and activities determined by the child's parents and school-based personnel, an Individual Education Program (IEP) is included as a key component of Public Law 94–142. The team decision-making process described earlier is an important component of the law and is also built into the IEP process.

The specific demands of the IEP require that collected data be organized and analyzed systematically. Therefore, it is important that information be collected methodically, organized in an interpretable way, and analyzed for instructional implications. The formal tests that are administered for identification represent only the starting point in the IEP process and generally will be useful only for the most basic aspects of instructional planning. Informal assessment procedures are often the necessary bridge between formal procedures and the instructional program. Data derived from informal measures can be readily used in the construction of the IEP.

Formal measures have serious limitations in terms of generating data to explain underlying systems or in providing directly relevant intervention alternatives. Informal measures are often more descriptive and relevant to the individual, and are useful in educational planning for children with learning disabilities, where an understanding of individual differences is critical to effective intervention. Informal assessment approaches assess behavior in more natural contexts (i.e., classroom observations) and in the specific curriculum content of the classroom (e.g., criterion-referenced tests, teacher-made tests, etc.). Informal assessment which generates both qualitative and quantitative data corresponds more closely to actual behavior. The data and conclusions are specific, representative, and relevant. Informal assessment data can be directly translated into an intervention program more closely tied to meaningful goals, strategies, and activities based on the content of the regular curriculum, the context of the classroom, and the performance patterns of the child.

Quantitative and Qualitative Data. Although formal measures are used primarily to provide identification information rather than instructional programming information, both quantitative and qualitative data can result from the administration of a formal test. Quantitative data refers to the actual scores achieved on the test. Examples of quantitative data are statements such as "James scored at the 83 percentile on the Comprehension subtest of the Stanford Diagnostic Reading Test," or "Robin earned a scaled score of 12 on the Picture Completion subtest of the Webster Intelligence Scale for Children-Revised."

Qualitative information consists of (*a*) observations made while a child is being tested (e.g., child's response characteristics such as frustration tolerance, self-directive behavior, risk-taking, etc.), and (*b*) systematic analysis of the child's performance in order to understand *how* the child achieved the score (e.g., item analysis). In assessment, the nature of the child's errors is often more important than knowing the child's score. For example, James, on the measure of reading comprehension ability, may have performed best on factual questions while demonstrating a weakness in the ability to respond to questions requiring inferential reasoning. And, although Robin was able to score in the above-average range on the Picture Completion subtest of the WISC-R, some of her word choices indicated word-retrieval difficulties: she pointed to the "nostril" and said "ear," substituted "the things you pull on" for "knobs," and said, "the thing over here on the door" for "hinge," etc. When tests are used in assessment, the score earned by a child is often the *least* relevant piece of information.

Capacity Versus Strategy Deficits. In clinical assessment, a distinction should always be made between underlying abilities and performance. Performance on a task always involves the availability of four aspects of cognitive functioning: (*a*) underlying abilities (i.e., perception, attention, memory), (*b*) acquired knowledge (i.e., language skills, knowledge of the world in general based on past experience), (*c*) strategies (i.e., activities undertaken to achieve specific objectives), and (*d*) metacognition (i.e., awareness of one's own thought processes and the executive functions necessary to regulate the use of basic abilities, knowledge and strategies).

The purpose of assessment is to measure not only acquired knowledge and how it is used, but also what the child is capable of learning. A child may have the underlying abilities but not an appropriate strategy for effectively acquiring, accessing, or applying knowledge. For example, the learning-disabled child may have the underlying ability or capacity to store verbal information in short-term memory but may not have an effective verbal rehearsal or category clustering strategy for coding the information for storage and retrieval. On the other hand, word retrieval difficulties may be implicated in short-term memory deficits, in that the child may not have readily accessible high-quality verbal memory codes to represent information in short-term memory. Some learning-disabled children appear to have poorer access to a phonetic code or access to a degraded phonetic representation on memory span tasks (Shankweiler, et al., 1979). Similarly, reduced language performance does not always indicate that a child does not have adequate knowledge of the linguistic system. Knowledge of the language system may be intact, and reduced language the result of memory processing constraints or situational constraints (Ervin-Tripp, 1971; Slobin, 1971). Performance characteristics in response to specific tasks do not always clearly reflect specific underlying systems; therefore, data available from testing alone cannot always be taken as evidence of underlying ability and/or knowledge deficits.

Assessment that focuses on quantitative data deals only with the products of underlying systems (e.g., the observable responses). Such assessment is more restrictive in determining educational goals than assessment that also measures the patterns of functioning that reflect underlying systems. Patterns of performance that more fully describe the nature of the individual's difficulties are important aspects of a comprehensive assessment and guide the development of effective educational goals and strategies.

Planning Assessment for Intervention. For planning educational interventions, two levels of assessment must be considered and integrated: the content-oriented level and the process-oriented level. At the level of content, assessment must determine what academic abilities or skills the child has already learned and what aspects still remain to be learned. The second level of assessment relates to *how* academic skills are learned, the underlying cognitive or linguistic processes relevant to the acquisition of academic skills. Information obtained from such a broadened perspective may not indicate which specific areas require intervention, but it provides considerable insight into patterns of performance, the child's readiness for structured intervention in academic areas, and appropriate strategies for either intervention or compensatory techniques.

In order to integrate the content-oriented and process-oriented approaches, the assessment process must be based on identification of the component skills that underlie performance of a specific academic task (e.g., reading, writing, etc.) and the subsequent development of specific procedures to assess the prerequisite skills and underlying processes required to learn these component skills. For the assessment of specific reading disability, the reading battery should be based on knowledge of the reading acquisition process (e.g., knowledge of letter-sound correspondences, automatization of word recognition skills, comprehension skills, etc.); the cognitive battery should be based on an analysis of the cognitive and metacognitive processes relevant to learning to read (e.g., short-term verbal memory, phonemic segmentation ability, etc.); and, the language battery should be based on an analysis of the language acquisition process relevant to the acquisition of oral and reading skills (e.g., understanding sentences and paragraphs, morphophonemic processing, etc.). With this data, the team members can make relevant decisions concerning the *why, what,* and *how* of intervention. The summary of a case history included later in this chapter illustrates how members of an evaluation team can integrate assessment data to make relevant decisions about the educational needs of a language learning-disabled student.

Because a more complex picture of learning problems has emerged based on linguistic science and information-processing models of learning, assessment of the learning-disabled child requires a multifaceted approach. An effective, interactive team approach to assessment provides the initial foundation for determining the need and nature of an intervention program.

THE INTERVENTION PROGRAM

Intervention as well as assessment requires a multidimensional approach. Decisions to intervene must be made jointly, and interventions must be well planned, integrated, and carefully monitored. The specialists and regular classroom teachers who work with learning-disabled children will, to a great extent, be faced with a series of individual problems, and, the goal will be to capitalize on the strengths and minimize the limitations of the individual in the interactive learning environment. Learning disabilities are usually identified after children enter school and encounter academic failure. Intervention procedures must take into account the continuing educational demands upon the child despite cognitive and/or linguistic deficits. In addition to providing specialized instruction, the specialists working with the child, in collaboration with the regular teacher, must develop procedures that will ameliorate some of the child's problems by modifying the failure-producing aspects of the regular classroom learning environments (e.g., language of the classroom, task demands of the curriculum, etc.).

Also, it is important to maximize intervention efforts by integrating planning and implementation across disciplines. Intervention should be an integrated comprehensive set of activities involving systematic ongoing implementation and evaluation. Specialized content and procedures, including remedial techniques, should be reconceptualized to focus on intervention both within a specific discipline and across disciplines. A generic understanding of intervention planning and implementation across disciplines helps to clarify the interrelationships among disciplines, expands the range of options available, and improves current practice in the delivery of specialized instruction for the learning disabled.

The basic ideas related to intervention theory are generic and are applicable across disciplines. Some of the factors basic to all interventions include:

- *Content match*—the information, tasks, etc. must not be too disparate from the child's current knowledge base and way of understanding and learning
- *Sequence*—instruction must be sequentially ordered to correspond to the sequence of information needed by the child
- *Pace*—instruction must provide for practice, repetition, and overlearning of information that needs to be accessed automatically
- *Structure*—intervention components should be taught within and across disciplines and should correspond with the demands of the regular curriculum content
- *Motivation*—interventions need to accommodate interests, attitudes, and learning style. Activities that are reinforced will be continued, and immediate feedback supports the maintenance of attention. This attribute is intrinsic to the individual.

The Transdisciplinary Approach. Practitioners should have a comprehensive and generic understanding of intervention planning and implementation across disciplines. This understanding requires a sound grounding in the fundamentals and interrelationships of the diverse disciplines involved in the diagnostic-instructional process. Educational interventions undertaken on behalf of the learning disabled are often arbitrary and fragmented. We are only beginning to understand the developmental and behavioral characteristics of the learning disabled. Potential interventions based on linguistic science and information-processing models of learning are emerging. They strongly suggest the need for a holistic, integrated, transdisciplinary approach to educational planning. The complex interactive nature of cognitive and linguistic processes and academic learning indicates the need for a broad-based, multidimensional approach to the development of an educational program for the learning-disabled child. This approach should focus on the commonalities in intervention efforts and the interrelatedness of instructional goals and objectives across diverse disciplines.

With specific reference to the language/learning-disabled student, the interactive nature of underlying information-processing abilities and academic learning has specific implications for the development of interrelated educational goals, objectives, and activities. Integration of instruction across diverse disciplines can enhance both the compensatory and remedial aspects of instruction for the language/learning-disabled student.

Compensatory aspects of instruction can be addressed by the language specialist who can make recommendations for modifications in both the style and structure of the language of the classroom. There are aspects of language processing that are applicable to the educational management of the child whose processing abilities have not developed optimally. Instructional personnel could be guided to simplify the language of instruction by using shorter, less complex sentences, and by making longer pauses and more frequent restatements of information. Knowledge of more specific aspects of language processing is also important. Instructional personnel should be aware that formulating oral or written instructions or directions in the affirmative, whenever possible, rather than the negative will reduce language-processing difficulties. Also, because implicit negatives such as different (e.g., not the same), absent (e.g., not present), and except (e.g., not all) are processed in the same way as explicit negatives, these will be equally difficult for some children.

Similarly, the integration of remedial aspects of instruction can increase the impact of educational planning for the language learning-disabled student. An assessment model which identifies the interactive cognitive and/or linguistic correlates of reading skill acquisition at both the initial and transitional stages of reading instruction has implications for the integration of instruction. For example, at the initial stages of reading instruction, phonemic segmentation skills are critical in learning to use phonic cues (i.e., to make use of letter-sound correspondences) to help in identifying the words represented by a sequence of letters. Many learning-disabled children have trouble learning to use phonic cues because they do not recognize that words can be segmented into syllables and syllables into distinct phonemes, and that phonemic segmentation is represented graphically by the use of specific letters placed in sequence. Assessment and subsequent remedial training of phonemic segmentation skills could be jointly undertaken by both the language and learning disabilities specialists. Also, modifications in the method of teaching initial reading need to be made for the child with poor segmentation skills. An instructional procedure that places less initial emphasis on phonic skills (e.g., whole-word method, language experience approach, etc.) should be used.

Similar interrelated educational goals and activities can be identified at the transitional stage of reading acquisition. The syntactic language problems evidenced by a language learning-disabled student will also be reflected in various reading behaviors such as understanding syntactically complex sentences or in using syntactic constraints to assist in word identification. Remedial training to intensify awareness of the syntactic structure of complex sentences by manipulating clausal units would be a valid transdisciplinary activity that could be integrated into language, reading, and writing instruction. The learning-disabled child's linguistic skills and linguistic awareness can be improved by training in sentence combining and/or sentence decombining exercises (Seidenberg, 1982; Wallach & Wallach, 1976). To avoid unnecessary confusions for the language/learning-disabled student, both the language and learning disabilities specialists must integrate their efforts to maximize the impact of the intervention program.

The need to integrate intervention efforts underlies the mandate of Public Law 94–142. Educators need to assume new collaborative roles and responsibilities to meet this challenge and to fulfill the promise of meeting the special educational needs of learning-disabled students.

CASE STUDY

The following summary of a case history for Robert, a 1st-grader, illustrates how members of a multidisciplinary team identify a child as learning disabled. The screening team, comprised of professionals from diverse disciplines, meets at the time of initial referral and, based on the nature of the referral information, develops a plan to guide the assessment process. Wherever possible, they see the child jointly in order to avoid miscommunication based on different disciplinary outlooks. There is adequate articulation among the different professionals (e.g., school psychologist, learning disability specialist, language specialist, etc.) involved in the evaluation process and the final report reflects the conclusions of each team member.

Identification Information

Name: Robert G.	Birthdate: April 10, 1976
Age: 6 yrs. 6 mos.	School Placement: Windmere Elementary School
Grade: First	Date of Report: January 15, 1982

Reason for Referral

At the request of his classroom teacher and with the written consent of his parents, Robert was referred for a psychoeducational evaluation. Robert, a 1st-grader, was reported to be having difficulty in learning to read and write. The teacher reports that he exhibits written reversals, transposition of letters, and poor phonic decoding skills. She also states that Robert's difficulties appear to be associated with distractibility, confusions in directionality and sequencing, and poor ability to process auditory information. An evaluation is being done to better understand Robert's current functional ability and to assist in educational planning.

Summary of Behavioral Observations

Robert is a sturdy, well-built youngster. He appears active and alert and was not overly apprehensive during the initial testing session. Robert speaks in well-organized sentences that are logical and easy to follow, and his vocabulary appears to be within normal limits. He exhibits some articulation difficulties. Robert was able to work steadily and persistently on many of the tasks presented. However, there were also tasks on which he performed poorly or was completely unable to perform, and restlessness and increased distractibility were observable at these times.

Summary of Background Information

Birth and developmental milestones for Robert are described as "normal." Robert's health history indicates hospitalization for a myringotomy just prior to school entrance. He also experiences an allergic reaction to milk or milk products. He still has a recurrent hearing problem, and his most recent audiological examination again detected fluid in the middle ear. This may account, in part, for his articulation problems.

Summary of Assessment Procedures

Tests administered include:

1. *Wechsler Intelligence Scale for Children—Revised (WISC-R)*

Verbal IQ	115
Performance IQ	105
Full Scale IQ	112

Verbal Scaled Score	
Information	10
Similarities	15
Arithmetic	11
Vocabulary	14
Comprehension	13
(Digit Span)	(9)
Performance Scaled Score	
Picture Completion	13
Picture Arrangement	9
Block Design	9
Object Assembly	15
Coding	8

2. *Bender Visual-Motor Gestalt Test* (Initial and Recall)
3. *Human Figure Drawing*
4. *Wepman Auditory Discrimination Test*
5. *Clinical Evaluation of Language Functions* (CELF)
   Producing Model Sentences
   Producing Formulated Sentences
   Processing Relationships and Ambiguities
6. *Detroit Test of Learning Aptitude*
   Oral Commissions
7. *Key Math Diagnostic Arithmetic Test*
8. *Metropolitan Readiness Test—Level II* (Form P)
   Beginning Consonants
   Sound-Letter Correspondence
   Visual Matching
   Listening

In addition to the formal tests, Robert was asked to copy numbers, letters, and words. He also completed a trial reading lesson using a language-experience approach. He dictated a brief story and then was asked to "read" his story to the examiner. Robert also identified a word in his own story that he wanted to learn to read and write. A multisensory approach was used successfully to teach word recognition and spelling skills.

Summary of Test Results

Robert's scores on the WISC-R indicate that he is functioning intellectually in the high average range. However, there are variations in the subtest scores ranging from below average to superior.

Robert's fund of information was average, with failures on comparatively easy items and successes on more difficult ones. Verbal fluency appeared to interfere with performance on this task, and he would comment, "I know the name but I forget," or "I can't think of the name of it." At the same time, expressive vocabulary was in the superior range, and he was able to make excellent responses when he was not limited to retrieving a specific word from memory but could make semantic substitutions.

Abstract verbal reasoning (similarities) and judgment, common sense, and reality testing (comprehension) were all in the high average range. The quality of his responses indicated good ability to make abstractions and understand superordinate classification.

His ability to do in-the-head arithmetic was above average, and his lowest score was on the Digit Span subtest, which was below average. He was able to repeat up to five digits forwards, but was unable to repeat more than two digits backwards without reversing the order of presentation.

On the performance tasks, Robert's highest score (very superior on Object Assembly) reflects an ability to organize and work toward a concrete goal. His visual memory necessary for recognition of essential details, was also above average. On the remaining tasks, such as replicating designs of blocks and sequencing a series of pictures in a logical order, he scored below average. His lowest score was for the transposition of symbols within a time limit (Coding) and was in the defective range. Robert appears to have visual-motor coordination difficulties. He is also experiencing problems with more integrative visual skills, such as sequencing, directionality, and perception of spatially-defined complex stimuli (e.g., block designs). On the other hand, Robert's figure drawing was age appropriate and indicated the ability to integrate and organize the spatial details.

Robert's performance on the Bender-Gestalt, an assessment of his own response to his perceptual organization of visual information, also indicated difficulty in integration of details and organization of spatially defined stimuli. Problems with integrative skills were evidenced in his loss of angulation and difficulties in maintaining the overall structure of shapes. He has difficulty in reproducing details and in storing visual information. His visual memory for designs indicates that he was able to recall only two of the Bender designs after the initial copying task. Also, there is evidence of slowness of response to grapho-motor tasks, not only on the Coding subtest of the WISC-R, but also in his handwriting.

Robert's performance on a number of formal and informal language-processing measures showed an inconsistent response pattern similar to his intelligence test profile. Informal observation of his language skills indicated that he is able to understand everyday conversation and to express his ideas in age-appropriate syntax.

On the Wepman Auditory Discrimination Test, Robert was able to differentiate the phonemic likenesses and differences in word pairs. However, he has articulation difficulties which appear to be persistent and systematic. Further assessment is indicated in this area. On the sentence repetition subtest of the Clinical Evaluation of Language Function (CELF), Robert performed well above age expectancy (5th-grade level). However, on the sentence formulation task of the CELF, Robert performed at only the beginning 1st-grade level. He performed well above age expectancy on the sentence repetition task (5th-grade level), but at only a beginning 1st-grade level for a task requiring the formulation of sentences (e.g., "Make a sentence with the word *car*"). His performance was age-appropriate for a task tapping his understanding of logical relationships coded in language, but he had difficulty in retaining a series of oral directions in short-term memory and executing them. Robert attempted to use verbal rehearsal strategy to facilitate recall, but because his phonological reproduction and verbal fluency are faulty, rehearsal is also impaired.

Robert's performance on the Metropolitan Readiness subtests indicated slightly better performance (60 percentile) for a task requiring the matching of beginning sounds than for the other subtests administered (50 percentile). In making sound-letter correspondences, both initial consonant and consonant blend inaccuracies were noted. He was not able to match the letters *c, g, d, pl, tr, gr,* and *cl* to their phonemic counterparts in words (e.g., cat, goat, etc.). However, on the visual matching subtest, Robert was able to match all of the letter sequences accurately and only encountered difficulty with the letter-like shapes or designs. His performance on the listening subtest indicated good ability to integrate and draw inferences when information is presented orally, but poor comprehension of comparative relationships (e.g., taller, bigger, etc.).

On the Key Math Diagnostic Test, Robert scored at an overall grade equivalent of 1.5. His understanding of the number system was at a 2.5 grade level, and his numerical reasoning and ability to solve simple one-step story problems was at a 2.0 grade level. His ability to perform written, single-digit addition and subtraction computations was at a 1.6 grade level. He had difficulty with money problems (e.g., coin values), but he can recognize and apply common units of measurement (e.g., ruler, thermometer) and units of time (e.g., clock, calendar). Robert was able to write the numbers from 1 to 10, but there were still some directional confusions noted (e.g., 6, 9, and 10) that are not inappropriate for a beginning 1st-grader. Although his grapho-motor responses are slow and labored, he can copy letters and numbers accurately.

Summary of Conclusions

Robert appears to be a child of above-average intelligence with indications for better potential. He would be expected to function in academic areas at or above his grade placement. At this time, he is impeded academically by specific learning deficits in oral language, reading, and writing. His uneven performance patterns indicate that he is experiencing difficulties in those areas involving expressive language abilities (e.g., speech production, verbal fluency, and sentence formulation), auditory and visual sequential memory, spatial concepts, and visual-motor integration. He also exhibits fatigue and distractibility, especially when tasks are hard or frustrating. His arithmetic concepts and ability to do in-the-head arithmetic are excellent, but he is not doing as well as most of the other children in his grade in the acquisition of reading and writing skills. The evaluation data indicates that Robert will not acquire reading and writing skills consistent with expectations without special education and related services, and, therefore, the classification of learning disabled is indicated.

Summary of Recommendations

Robert's oral expressive language deficits are implicated in his learning difficulties and indicate the need for further assessment by the speech-language pathologist. In-depth testing of Robert's receptive and expressive language skills is recommended, including a phonological, semantic, syntactic, and pragmatic analysis of a language sample. The content of an appropriate language intervention program for Robert will depend on the results of the language assessment.

A traditional synthetic phonics approach to initial reading instruction would not be appropriate for Robert at this time. Although he uses immediate rehearsal to recreate a discrete phoneme (sound), the phonological reproduction is inaccurate, resulting in impaired or inconsistent recall of phonemes and phonemic patterns. In order to utilize his cognitive and linguistic strengths, a language-experience approach, where he dictates and then reads his own stories, could be used as an effective approach to initial reading instruction. He would also profit from a more integrative approach for the acquisition of word analysis or decoding skills for word recognition and spelling. Any method that integrates the visual-tactile and auditory aspects (e.g., Fernald technique) for teaching word recognition, particularly if based on the words found in his own stories, could be used successfully with Robert at this time.

Robert has difficulty in attending to oral directions. He attempts to use verbal rehearsal to facilitate recall, but his reproductions are inconsistent and inaccurate, and interfere with his retrieval of the auditory information. It is important, therefore, that his teachers speak clearly, use short sentences with simple syntax, and check periodically on the accuracy of his recall of the information. Robert could be asked to repeat directions to be sure that he recalls them accurately.

Robert uses a great deal of verbal mediation, that is, he talks himself through tasks. This is an excellent strategy for him and should be encouraged. For example, he could be taught to use verbal supports or associations to focus attention on relevant directional aspects of letters or numbers and thus guide his grapho-motor responses.

Handwriting skills will need to be taught in carefully sequenced incremental steps, and particular attention will need to be paid to establishing the fine-motor patterns needed for writing. Also, lengthy tasks requiring grapho-motor responses should be adjusted for Robert's current level of functioning (e.g., workbook exercises, copying from the chalkboard, etc.). He attempts to compensate cognitively for his visual-motor difficulties. He can be successful if given adequate structure and time.

As is typical of underachieving youngsters with excellent potential, Robert is beginning to experience confusion in reconciling the apparent conflict in feedback from the important adults in his life. That is, on the one hand, that he is a capable youngster; and, on the other, that he is having difficulties in learning. He is becoming extremely frustrated and unhappy because of his uneven functioning. Therefore, it is important that the educational program planned for Robert provides him with opportunities to use his cognitive and linguistic strengths and helps him to compensate for his deficit areas.

SUMMARY

That deficits in learning are a major cause of school failure is currently well accepted, and new approaches to identification and educational planning have developed based on information-processing theory. Learning disabilities derive from innate disorders that alter cognitive processes. These alterations in cognitive functioning vary in type and degree of severity and, therefore, in behavioral consequences.

An understanding of the interactive nature of language and cognition contributes to our understanding of the problems in comprehension and formulation of written language experienced by many learning-disabled children. Both reading and writing performance reflect the knowledge and the linguistic and cognitive competencies available to the learner and how these are activated and integrated during the acquisition of reading and writing skills. In addition to disorders in verbal language, a fundamental deficit for many learning-disabled children appears to be an inability to use effective cognitive strategies for the comprehension or production of written language.

Because of the heterogeneity of the learning-disabled population, the assessment process must be flexible and responsive to individual differences. Practitioners from diverse disciplines need to collaborate in decision-making activities. A multidisciplinary approach based on a comprehensive assessment model that provides for the systematic collection, organization, and analysis of assessment data needs to be adopted. The data must adequately describe the nature of an individual's difficulties and guide the development of an effective educational program. An interactive, collaborative, team approach to assessment and intervention also provides the foundation for the integration of learning experiences and educational services for children with learning disabilities.

STUDY QUESTIONS

1. Identify and discuss the major components of the information-processing model. Include in the discussion the implications for understanding the perceptual, attentional, and memory deficits of the learning-disabled student.
2. Briefly present six characteristics which may be exhibited by learning-disabled students with language deficits.
3. How does the interaction of linguistic and cognitive variables affect the acquisition of reading and writing skills?
4. Outline the research findings pertaining to cognitive and/or metacognitive deficits in relation to the learning-disabled student's acquisition of reading skills.
5. Briefly discuss several factors which may be related to writing disabilities. Discuss some writing behaviors exhibited by learning-disabled students.
6. Discuss the advantages and disadvantages of formal and informal assessment in the identification of learning-disabled students.
7. What are the important characteristics of an effective intervention program for the learning-disabled child?

BIBLIOGRAPHY

Anderson, B.F. (1975). *Cognitive psychology.* New York: Academic Press.

Anderson, R.C., Spiro, R.J., & Montague, W.E. (1977). *Schooling and the acquisition of knowledge.* Hillsdale, NJ: Lawrence Erlbaum.

Applebee, A. (1978). *The child's concept of story.* Chicago: University of Chicago Press.

Bauer, R.H. (1977). Memory processes in children with learning disabilities. *Journal of Experimental Child Psychology, 24,* 415–430.

Berko, J. (1958). The child's learning of English morphology. *Word, 14,* 150–177.

Berry, M.F. (1980). *Teaching linguistically handicapped children.* Englewood Cliffs, NJ: Prentice-Hall.

Blalock, J. (1981). Persistent problems and concerns of young adults with learning disabilities. In W. Cruickshank & A. Silvers (Eds.), *Bridges to tomorrow: The best of ACLD* (Vol. 2). Syracuse, NY: Syracuse University Press.

Bougere, M. (1969). Selected factors in oral language related to first grade reading performance. *Reading Research Quarterly, 5,* 31–58.

Bransford, J.D., Stein, B.S., Shelton, T.S., & Owings, R.A. (1980). Cognition and adaptation: The importance of learning to learn. In J. Harvey (Ed.), *Cognition, social behavior and the environment.* Hillsdale, NJ: Lawrence Erlbaum.

Brittain, M.M. (1970). Inflectional performance and early reading achievement. *Reading Research Quarterly, 6,* 34–48.

Bryan, J.H. (1981). Social behaviors of learning disabled children. In J. Gottlieb & S. Strichart (Eds.), *Developmental theory and research in learning disabilities.* Baltimore, MD: University Park Press.

Campione, J.C., & Brown, A.L. (1978). Toward a theory of intelligence. *Intelligence, 2,* 279–304.

Cazden, C.B. (1972). *Child language and education.* New York: Holt, Rinehart & Winston.

Ceci, S.J. (1982). Extracting meaning from stimuli: Automatic and purposive processing of the language-based learning disabled. *Topics in Learning and Learning Disabilities, 2,* 46–53.

Chalfont, J.C., & Scheffelin, M.A. (1969). *Central processing dysfunctions in children: A review of research.* NINDS Monograph No. 9. Bethesda,

MD: U.S. Department of Health, Education and Welfare.

Cicci, R. (1980). Written language disorders. *Bulletin of the Orton Society, 30,* 240–251.

Cruickshank, W., Bentzen, F., Razburg, F., & Tannhauser, M. (1961). *A teaching method for brain-injured and hyperactive children.* Syracuse, NY: Syracuse University Press.

Denckla, M.B., & Rudel, R. (1976). Naming of pictured objects by dyslexic and other learning-disabled children. *Brain and Language, 39,* 1–15.

Denner, F. (1970). Representational and syntactic competence of problem readers. *Child Development, 41,* 881–887.

Edwards, H.T., & Kallail, K.J. (1966). *Ability of learning disabled and regular classroom adolescents to cloze structure and content words.* Paper presented at the national convention of the American Speech and Hearing Association, Chicago.

Ervin-Tripp, S. (1971). Social backgrounds and verbal skills. In T. Moore (Ed.), *Language acquisition: Models and methods.* New York: Academic Press.

Farnham-Diggory, S. (1980). Learning disabilities: A view from cognitive science. *Journal of the American Academy of Child Psychiatry, 19,* 570–578.

Fleisher, L.S., Jenkins, J.R., & Pavy, D. (1979). Effects on poor readers' comprehension of training in rapid decoding. *Reading Research Quarterly, 15,* 30–48.

Fox, B., & Routh, D.K. (1980). Phonemic analysis and severe reading disability in children. *Journal of Psycholinguistic Research, 9,* 115–119.

Frostig, M. (1968). Education for children with hearing disabilities. In H. Myklebust (Ed.), *Progress in learning disabilities.* New York: Grune & Stratton.

Golinkoff, R.M. (1976). A comparison of reading comprehension processes in good and poor comprehenders. *Reading Research Quarterly, 11,* 623–659.

Goodman, K.S. (1973). Psycholinguistic universals in the reading process. In F. Smith (Ed.), *Psycholinguistics and reading.* New York: Holt, Rinehart, & Winston.

Hallahan, D., Gajar, A., Cohen, S., & Tarver, S. (1978). Selective attention and locus of control in learning disabled and normal children. *Journal of Learning Disabilities, 4,* 47–52.

Hallahan, D., & Reeves, R. (1980). Selective attention and distractibility. In B. Keogh (Ed.), *Advances in special education.* Greenwich, CT: JAI Press.

Hammill, D., Leiger, J., McNutt, G., & Larsen, T. (1981). A new definition of learning disabilities. *Learning Disability Quarterly, 4,* 336–342.

Hammill, D., & McNutt, B. (1981). *Correlates of reading: The consensus of thirty years of research.* Austin, TX: Pro-Ed.

Hook, P.E., & Johnson, D.J. (1978). Metalinguistic awareness and reading strategies. *Bulletin of the Orton Society, 28,* 62–78.

Jansky, J., & deHirsch, K. (1972). *Preventing reading failure: Prediction, diagnosis, intervention.* New York: Harper & Row.

Johnson, D., Blalock, J., & Nesbitt, J. (1978). Adolescents with learning disabilities: Perspectives from an educational clinic. *Learning Disability Quarterly, 1,* 24–36.

Johnson, D., & Myklebust, H. (1967). *Learning disabilities: Educational principles and practices.* New York: Grune & Stratton.

Kephart, N. (1971). *The slow learner in the classroom.* Columbus, OH: Charles E. Merrill.

Kirk, S.A. (1963). Behavioral diagnosis and remediation of learning disabilities. *Conference on Exploration into the Problems of the Perceptually Handicapped Child.* Evanston, IL: Fund for Perceptually Handicapped Children.

Kirk, S.A., & Kirk, W.P. (1972). *Psycholinguistic learning disabilities.* Urbana: University of Illinois Press.

Leonard, L.B. (1979). Language impairment in children. *Merrill-Palmer Quarterly, 25,* 205–232.

Lerner, J.W. (1981). *Learning disabilities* (3rd ed.). Boston: Houghton Mifflin.

Liberman, I.Y., Shankweiler, D., Fisher, F.W., & Carter, B. (1974). Explicit syllable and phoneme segmentation in young children. *Journal of Experimental Child Psychology, 18,* 201–212.

Markman, E.M. (1977). Realizing that you don't understand: A preliminary investigation. *Child Development, 48,* 986–992.

Mattingly, J.G. (1972). Reading, the linguistic process and linguistic awareness. In J.F. Kavanaugh & J.G. Mattingly (Eds.), *Language by ear and by eye.* Cambridge, MA: MIT Press.

Menyuk, P., & Looney, P. (1972). A problem of language disorder: Length versus structure. *Journal of Speech and Hearing Research, 15,* 264–279.

Miller, G.A., Galanter, E., & Pribam, K. (1960). *Plans and the structure of behavior.* New York: Holt, Rinehart, & Winston.

Moran, M.R., & Bryne, M.C. (1977). Mastery of verb tense markers by normal and learning disabled children. *Journal of Speech and Hearing Research, 20,* 529–542.

Myklebust, H.R. (1965). *Development and disorders of written language,* Vol. 1: The picture story language test. New York: Grune & Stratton.

Myklebust, H.R. (1973). *Development and disorders of written language,* Vol. 2: Studies of normal and exceptional children. New York: Grune & Stratton.

Myklebust, H.R. (1978). Toward a science of dyslexiology. In H. Myklebust (Ed.), *Progress in learning disabilities* (Vol. 4). New York: Grune & Stratton.

Olson, D. (1977). From utterance to text: The bias of language in speech and writing. *Harvard Educational Review, 47,* 257–281.

Orton, S.T. (1937). *Reading, writing and speech problems in children.* New York: Norton.

Paris, S.G., & Myers, M. (1981). Comprehension monitoring, memory and study strategies of good and poor readers. *Journal of Reading Behavior, 13,* 7–22.

Pearson, P.D., & Spiro, R.J. (1980). Toward a theory of reading instruction. *Topics in Language Disorders, 1,* 71–88.

Perfetti, C.A., & Hogaboam, T.W. (1975). The relationship between single word decoding and reading comprehension skill. *Journal of Educational Psychology, 67,* 461–469.

Perfetti, C.A., & Lesgold, A.M. (1979). Coding and comprehension in skilled reading and implications for reading instruction. In L.B. Resnick & P.A. Weaver (Eds.), *Theory and practice of early reading* (Vol. 1). Hillsdale, NJ: Lawrence Erlbaum.

Poplin, M., Gray, R., Larsen, S., Banikowski, A., & Mehring, T. (1980). A comparison of components of written expression abilities in learning disabled and non-learning disabled students at three grade-levels. *Learning Disability Quarterly, 3,* 46–53.

Ring, B.C. (1976). Effects of input organization on auditory short-term memory. *Journal of Learning Disabilities, 9,* 59–63.

Samuels, S.J., Begg, G., & Chen, C.C. (1976). Comparison of word recognition speed and strategies of less skilled and more highly skilled readers. *Reading Research Quarterly, 1,* 73–86.

Seidenberg, P.L. (1982). Implications of schemata theory for learning disabled readers. *Journal of Learning Disabilities, 15,* 352–355.

Shankweiler, D., Liberman, I.Y., Mark, L.S., Fowler, C.A, & Fischer, F.W. (1979). The speech code and learning to read. *Journal of Experimental Psychology, 5,* 531–545.

Slobin, D. (1971). *Psycholinguistics.* Glenview, IL: Scott, Foresman.

Steiner, R., Werner, M., & Cromer, W. (1971). Comprehension training and identification of poor and good readers. *Journal of Educational Psychology, 62,* 506–513.

Strauss, A., & L. Lehtenen, (1947). *Psychopathology and education of the brain-injured child.* New York: Grune & Stratton.

Tarver, S.G., Hallahan, D.P., Kaufman, J.M., & Ball, D.W. (1976). Verbal rehearsal and selective attention in children with learning disabilities: A developmental lag. *Journal of Experimental Child Psychology, 22,* 375–385.

Torgesen, J.K. (1977). The role of nonspecific factors in the task performance of learning disabled children: A theoretical assessment. *Journal of Learning Disabilities, 10,* 27–34.

Torgesen, J.K. (1980). The use of efficient task strategies by learning disabled children: Conceptual and educational implications. *Journal of Learning Disabilities, 13,* 364–371.

Torgesen, J.K. (1982). The study of short-term memory in learning disabled children. In K. Gadow & I. Bialer (Eds.), *Advances in learning and behavioral disabilities* (Vol. 1). Greenwich, CT: JAI Press.

Torgesen, J.K., & Houck, G. (1980). Processing deficiencies in learning disabled children who perform poorly on the digit span task. *Journal of Educational Psychology, 72,* 141–160.

U. S. Office of Education. (1977, December). *Federal Register, Part III.* Education of handicapped children: Assistance to states: Procedures for evaluating specific learning disabilities. Washington, DC: US Department of Health, Education and Welfare.

Vellutino, F.R. (1977). Alternative conceptualizations of dyslexia: Evidence in support of a verbal-deficit hypothesis. *Harvard Educational Review, 47,* 334–354.

Vellutino, F.R. (1979). *Dyslexia: Theory and research.* Cambridge, MA: MIT Press.

Vellutino, F.R., & Scanlon, D.M. (1979, April). The effect of phonemic segmentation training and response acquisition on coding ability in poor and normal readers. Paper presented at the American Education Research Association annual meeting, San Francisco.

Vogel, S.A. (1975). *Syntactic abilities in normal and dyslexic children.* Baltimore, MD: University Park Press.

Vygotsky, L.S. (1962). *Thought and language.* Cambridge, MA: MIT Press.

Wallach, M.A., & Wallach, L. (1976). *Teaching all children to read.* Chicago: University of Chicago Press.

Wechsler, D. (1974). Wechsler Intelligence Scale for Children, Revised (Manual). New York: Psychological Corporation.

Wiederholt, J.L. (1974). Historical perspectives in the education of the learning disabled. In L. Mann & D. Sabatino (Eds.). *The second review of special education.* Philadelphia: Journal of Special Education Press.

Wiig, E.H., & Semel, E.M. (1973). Comprehension of linguistic concepts requiring logical operations by learning disabled children. *Journal of Speech and Hearing Research, 16,* 627–636.

Wiig, E.H., & Semel, E.M. (1974). Logico-grammatical sentence comprehension by learning disabled adolescents. *Perceptual Motor Skills, 38,* 1331–1334.

Wiig, E.H., & Semel, E.M. (1975). Productive language abilities in learning disabled adolescents. *Journal of Learning Disabilities, 8,* 578–586.

Wiig, E.H., & Semel, E.M. (1976). *Language disabilities in children and adolescents.* Columbus, OH: Charles E. Merrill.

Wiig, E.H., & Semel, E.M. (1980). *Language assessment and intervention for the learning disabled.* Columbus, OH: Charles E. Merrill.

Wiig, E.H., Semel, E.M., & Crouse, M.A. (1973). The use of English morphology by high risk and learning disabled children. *Journal of Learning Disabilities, 6,* 457–465.

Wong, B. (1978). The effects of directive cues on the organization of memory and recall in good and poor readers. *Journal of Education Research, 72,* 32–38.

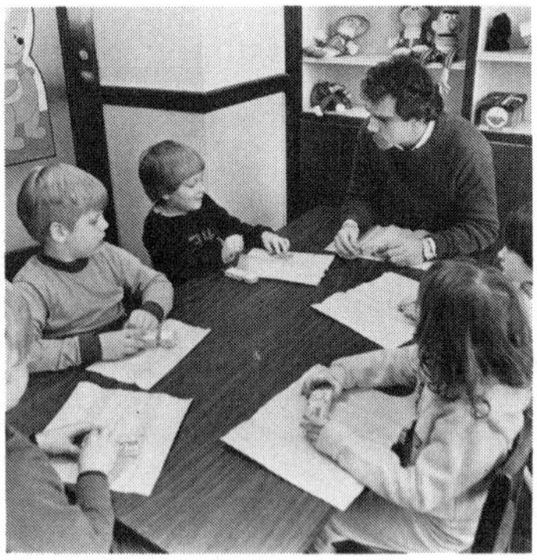

12

Language Intervention in School Settings

Language intervention services in America's schools can be considered unique because of the procedural variations necessary to make language interaction relevant. Actually, the principles of language intervention should vary little from setting to setting. It is the purpose of this chapter to provide insight into both the unique set of requirements related to the provision of services in the schools and the common set of principles for fostering language and communication development in children in any setting.

A number of forces influence the decisions that are made regarding the provision of services in schools. To be effective, speech-language pathologists working in school settings need to draw not only on their professional preparation and understanding of language disorders, but also on an understanding of the multiple levels of influence that affect service delivery. They must also be aware of possibilities for variation within school settings and be prepared to facilitate change in the system when it is needed.

In this chapter several questions are addressed. What are the special considerations for providing services in schools, the advantages and disadvantages and the levels of influence that affect it? What are the unique procedures that are a part of providing language intervention in school settings as a result of the implementation of Public Law 94–142? What are some guiding principles for planning language intervention regardless of setting? Finally, how would one go about meeting the requirements and using the principles to provide services to an individual child? The answers to these questions provide the organizational framework of this chapter.

This chapter was written by Dr. Nickola Wolf Nelson, Western Michigan University.

SPECIAL CONSIDERATIONS

The motivating principles for providing language intervention services remain the same regardless of setting. The focus should be on providing the best possible services to meet the total needs of the children within family, educational, and social contexts. Settings must be adapted to meet the needs and further the abilities of children with problems rather than squeezing children into preexisting outdated or inappropriate molds. The twice weekly therapy model that was popular when speech-language pathologists in schools worked primarily with groups of articulation-impaired children may need to be revised. The speech-language pathologist must be familiar not only with the language abilities of their students but also with the language demands associated with educational settings.

School language differs from home language in many important respects. When children begin kindergarten and as they continue through the grades, they must learn to rely on meanings that are more and more completely encoded linguistically. At home, routines were familiar and could be understood based on primarily nonverbal cues. In school, however, nonverbal context is provided less frequently as grade level increases and as instruction relies more heavily on written language activities (Nelson, 1984). Language skills provide an important key to academic success. Children who do not have a firm language foundation lag further and further behind.

The ability to read is perhaps the single most important skill children acquire in school. An awareness of the complicated interaction of speech and language skills children must bring to the task of learning to read, and reading to learn, is a critical realm of knowledge for speech-language pathologists working in school settings. Goodman (1973) has described the process of mature reading as being accomplished by cycles of *sampling* from the printed text, *predicting* meaning or forming hypotheses about what is meant based on knowledge of language and how it is structured, and then *testing* and *confirming* those hypotheses or *revising* them as needed. All these steps are accomplished almost simultaneously by mature readers. They rely on the printed text only to the extent needed to confirm that they are reading what is actually printed on the page.

Similarly, children who are learning to read use semantic and syntactic knowledge to enable them to predict what words might come next in a sentence. Sound-symbol associations, made possible by reference to well-developed phonological processing systems, enable children to check those predictions and sound out unfamiliar words. Children who have more fully developed speech and language skills, who have been read to, and who have learned to process the explicit language associated with written forms will have many advantages over language-impaired youngsters as they approach the task of learning to read. Being read to will also help children learn to use the organizational structure of stories known as story grammar (Johnston, 1982) or text-linguistics (Westby, 1982), to help them predict what kinds of events might occur next in the material they are reading and narrow the range of possibilities. Speech and language skills at sound, syllable, word, phrase, sentence, and discourse levels are all critical to the processes of using language to learn. They are the legitimate focus of language intervention activities in school settings, whether or not speech-language pathologists view their role as including the teaching of reading to children with language disorders.

Advantages and Disadvantages of School Settings

The practice of speech-language pathology and audiology in school settings offers significant advantages for working with language-impaired students in the settings in which they spend a major portion of their time. The effects of their language impairments on other areas of functioning may be readily determined, and the possibility that language intervention programming will be relevant to children's real life needs is increased. In school settings, many opportunities also arise for interacting directly with significant others in the children's lives, particularly their teachers, but also professionals from other disciplines who are concerned with providing appropriate evaluation and remediation services to handicapped children.

Historically, two primary disadvantages have been associated with the provision of language, speech, and hearing services in school settings: (*a*) the relative unavailability of parents, and (*b*) the perpetuation of delivery styles that were the mode when "speech correctionists" first initiated services in the public schools. The first of these has been addressed by Public Law 94–142, The Education for All Handicapped Children Act of 1975. Many of the requirements for implementing PL 94–142 (to be considered later in this chapter) are designed specifically to encourage the involvement of parents in all aspects of the implementation process.

Nevertheless, a problem of parent involvement unique to the school setting frequently remains. Whereas in most clinical and hospital settings, clients and their families come to the professional seeking help, in the schools, professionals are sometimes placed in the position of informing the child and family that a problem exists—or that a partial explanation for some of the problems the child has been having may be a communication disorder. Although such cases are increasingly rare as public awareness of language, speech, and hearing disorders improves, some will likely continue to arise. It is important that identification activities and services be available for all who need them, for subtle as well as obvious impairments, and for individuals who would not otherwise seek or be able to afford services. Speech-language pathologists and other professionals practicing in schools fulfill these needs.

The second disadvantage is the perpetuation of service delivery models that were frequently used when speech correction services were originally introduced into the public schools. In many districts across the United States, speech therapy was the first special education service to be offered as a part of public education. Continuing through the 1960s (and even today, in some instances), the focus was almost exclusively on the remediation of articulation, voice, and fluency problems in children who otherwise functioned largely as their age peers did in meeting academic requirements. Less was known then about normal language, language disorders, and the interaction of language skills with educational processes and other handicapping conditions. Caseloads consisted of large numbers of children (often more than 100), who were seen in groups of 5 or more, usually for articulation therapy. Clinicians traveled among as many as seven or more schools. Hence, the term *itinerant therapy* continues to be associated with the type of service delivery model in which children are pulled out of the classroom to be worked with in small groups two or three times per week for approximately one-half hour each.

As the knowledge base has grown, understanding of communicative disorders and the best ways to remediate them has expanded to include a variety of possibilities.

Professionals in most districts now recognize the responsibility to provide a continuum of services for children with all types of communicative disorders of all degrees of severity. The interaction of language disorders with overall educational performance is increasingly appreciated, and speech-language pathologists now have the skills to work with other educational specialists in remediating language disorders. These disorders include not only those associated with speaking and listening, but also with reading, writing, and thinking as well.

Comprehensive appropriate programming for language-impaired youngsters, many of whom have multiple handicaps, requires time and flexibility. In order to obtain both, many speech-language pathologists have learned to work together with school administrators, boards of education, and legislators to ensure that regulations encourage, rather than reduce, the likelihood that appropriate services will be provided. For example, revised views of the number of students that can be reasonably served by any one speech-language pathologist have led the American Speech-Language-Hearing Association (ASHA) to recommend maximum caseload sizes from around 25 to 40 students, or even lower when serving severely or multiply involved youngsters (ASHA, 1984). Teacher certification requirements and program descriptions have also been revised in some states to allow speech-language pathologists to (*a*) function as classroom teachers in self-contained classrooms for severely language/learning-disabled students, (*b*) provide public school-operated programs for speech and language-impaired preschoolers, or (*c*) serve as resource room teachers at middle and high school levels with students scheduled to see them as a regular (special education) course offering.

Levels of Influence

The provision of services in school settings is generally influenced by regulatory controls arising from three or four levels. First, local districts, often referred to as Local Education Agencies (LEAs), have direct responsibility for providing appropriate educational programs for all children, whether they are handicapped or not. Second, intermediate (between local and state educational agencies) or countywide districts provide a consolidation of services and coordinate communication between state and local agencies, although not all states have intermediate districts. Third, state departments of education (regulated by state boards of education and/or legislatures) determine the policies of states regarding provision of regular and special education services. They write state plans (with public input) to describe such policies and procedures. These are underwritten and approved by the United States Department of Education Office of Special Education Programs, which is charged with seeing that PL 94–142 is implemented to provide "free appropriate public education" to all handicapped children. In general, the rules and regulations established at each of these levels have been written to protect the rights of handicapped children and their parents. When professionals determine that particular regulations hamper rather than facilitate this process, it is their responsibility to facilitate needed change.

The information presented in this chapter relative to legal requirements for provision of special education programs to language-impaired children is based on the Rules and Regulations for Implementing Public Law 94–142, The Education for All Handicapped Children Act, that were published in the August 23, 1977 *Federal Register*. Although efforts were made early in the 1980s to deregulate implementation of the law, most advocacy groups agreed that the majority of its provisions are not excessive and that the regulations meet the purpose of the law to ensure appropriate educational opportunity for all students. Time-consuming requirements that have little direct positive effect on children frequently can be traced to overinterpretation at state, intermediate, or local levels. Generally speaking, regulations and policies arising from these levels are easier to change if a need to do so becomes apparent as they are implemented. Testimony from individuals and groups led to the proposed rule changes being withdrawn by the Reagan administration in 1983, and no new changes are planned. However, it is possible that changes could be suggested in the future, and professionals should make an effort to keep themselves informed.

PROCEDURES

Procedural considerations for providing programs for language-impaired children in the schools relate to identification, parent notification, evaluation, placement decisions, individual education plan (I.E.P.) meetings, I.E.P. content and review, and reevaluation. Official regulations change. The broad procedures outlined here are generally appropriate in any area of the United States and comply with PL 94–142. For a detailed understanding of procedures in any particular district, the professional is referred to the special education office of that district. Copies of state, intermediate (if any), and local policy statements should be available there. A flowchart outlining general procedures discussed here is presented as Figure 12–1.

Identification

Educators have a responsibility to identify all and only the handicapped children in a district as needing special education. The need to identify *all* children has led to a variety of "Child Find" projects identifying preschool handicapped children. Because the federal legislation has been in effect for several years, most previously unserved school-age children have been identified. However, states vary in age levels of handicapped children served as a part of public education depending on statutes within the states. Some states' public education systems serve handicapped children from birth, and many provide special education programs for children who are 3 years of age and above. Child Find teams often employ speech-language pathologists, and occasionally audiologists, as team members. In fact, the original impetus for referring children with many kinds of handicapping conditions is often delay or abnormality in the early stages of learning to talk. Preschool children who are not developing normally might be referred by physicians, community health agencies, family courts, early detection centers, parents, or school personnel.

School-age speech- and language-impaired children must also be identified. The traditional method of identifying elementary-age children with communicative disorders has been to screen whole grades of students to identify which children should become a part of the caseload. This activity was usually conducted in the fall, and each year placement decisions were made anew. Such a practice is no longer followed routinely for many reasons, primarily because children must be considered individually. They must be given individualized comprehensive multidisciplinary evaluations, and they

Figure 12–1

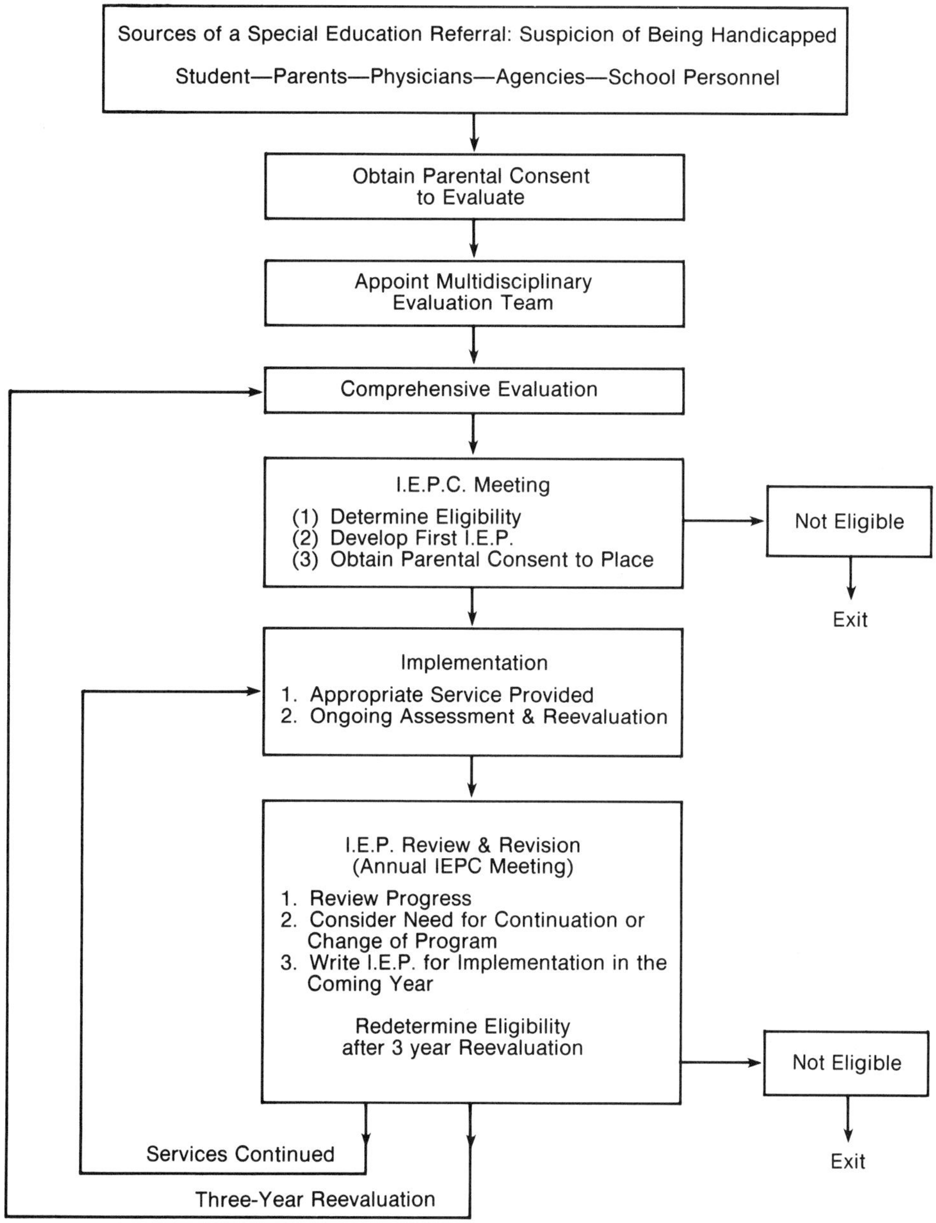

Note. From *Program Suggestions for Speech and Language Services* (p. 2) by the Michigan Department of Education, 1982. Reprinted by permission.

must be provided services as outlined in I.E.P.s. The I.E.P.s are reviewed and revised at least annually until it is determined, again at an I.E.P. meeting, that the student no longer needs the program.

The need for several people to be involved in determining a child to be handicapped, or no longer handicapped, makes group screening and unilateral decision making inappropriate. A further requirement of PL 94–142, and one that has been controversial and difficult to interpret, has been that a child's handicap must "affect educational performance" in order to qualify for special education and related services under the law. Oral/aural communication is an essential component of educational performance and much of learning is accomplished using language as a tool for organizing and transmitting thought. Language and speech skills are such an integral part of all other activities, both in and out of school, that they are often taken for granted.

Classroom teachers have the best opportunity to observe students' performance using language in a variety of ways. They can become the best resource available for identifying language-impaired school-age children. Although they may need guidance in knowing which aspects of communicative behavior to observe, they often become effective members of multidisciplinary evaluation teams, not as administrators of formal assessment devices, but as contributors of valuable information about ways in which the child's apparent communication disorder is expressed in real life situations. After they are made aware that language disorders may be subtle but significant, and may or may not involve obvious speech impairments, many teachers become sensitive observers of children's communication skills. They are then able to assist in identifying children who are experiencing a variety of difficulties with classroom routine and who may have communicative disorders.

Although teacher referral is generally considered to be a more valid and appropriate means of identifying potentially speech- and language-impaired children at the school-age level than whole-grade screening, screening may still be used in some districts, particularly for children who are just entering kindergarten. This process sometimes is used to help teachers learn to identify children with language problems. If the screening procedures are comprehensive, they can ensure that children with language disorders are provided early intervention that may lessen later problems of educational performance. However, children may no longer be placed in special education programs, including speech and language intervention, on the basis of screening results alone. A nonbiased comprehensive multidisciplinary evaluation must be provided to ensure that *only* children who have true speech and language impairments are placed in special programs. Children who score below norms not because they are speech and language impaired, but because they have language experiences that do not match those measured by most evaluation tools must not be labeled as handicapped. On the other hand, children from diverse cultural communities who have true language disorders must be identifiable. Speech-language pathologists may be required to use specialized techniques, to become bilingual themselves, or to use interpreters in evaluating children who come from different cultural backgrounds and linguistic communities and who are suspected of being speech and language impaired.

In addition to previously unidentified preschool and school-age children, students with multiple handicaps require attention in the identification phase of special programming. Children with a variety of handicapping conditions may exhibit language disorders as well. For example, communicative disorders are often integrally related to such other conditions as learning disabilities, mental retardation, autism, and hearing impairment. Recent changes, many of which are associated with the implementation of PL 94–142, have led to children with more severe handicaps being served in regular education settings in some districts. In other districts, children in some of the above categories are served in special schools operated by local or intermediate districts which are sometimes called *center programs,* and some children are still placed in residential state schools (e.g., for the deaf or blind) or state "hospitals" for the severely mentally or multiply impaired.

A debate is currently being waged over the relative benefits of providing service in these various settings. Although most educators view the swing of the pendulum away from automatic institutionalization of severely handicapped infants as extremely positive, there is less agreement about the relative merits of using center programs to provide special facilities and services. There is also some disagreement about using intensive mainstreaming within regular education to provide opportunities for handicapped and nonhandicapped children to have daily contact with each other. Some educators are concerned that children who are more completely mainstreamed may receive less attention to their individual needs and fewer opportunities to excel. Speech-language pathologists may provide services within any of these settings and must adapt programs to the characteristics of the various settings. If appropriate settings do not exist within a school system, it is important for the speech-language pathologist to provide input to increase the likelihood that they will be made available.

Different philosophies also exist regarding the role of speech-language pathologists in serving populations with multiple impairments. For example, some parents and professionals hold the view that all handicapped children who do not score at chronological age level on standardized language evaluation tools need direct speech and language intervention services several times per week. It is indeed possible that increases in a child's speech and language skills may result in concomitant improvements in other areas of development. However, many children whose language skills are commensurate with other areas of development can benefit most from a comprehensive classroom program with language included as an integral part of the curriculum. Having a speech-language pathologist serve as classroom consultant is often the most appropriate way of meeting the needs of such students. A process that can be used for making this type of decision is described later in this chapter.

At the other end of the spectrum from overrecommendation of speech and language services is underrecommendation for children who clearly need speech and language intervention. Speech-language pathologists may not be included as members of some children's multidisciplinary evaluation teams (sometimes called *Committees of the Handicapped*) even when a major aspect of the child's disability is speech and language impairment. The attitude that speech and language programs are *related* but not *necessary* services may be symptomatic of a need to demonstrate the value of effective speech and language programming. When children who need evaluations of their communication skills do not receive them as part of their original multidisciplinary diagnoses, it becomes more complicated to add services later on. Providing parents and teachers with information about the types of communicative problems likely to be encountered by all kinds of children will reduce this problem. Prior chapters in this book can help prepare the professional to provide others with a balanced picture of etiologic and symptomatic views of language disorders.

Parent Notification

Signed informed parental consent is required at two points under PL 94–142. The first is prior to conducting a preplacement evaluation, and the second is prior to initial placement of a handicapped child in a program providing special education and related services.

The procedure for obtaining parental consent requires that parents receive information about their rights under the law as well as information about what activities are planned. Generally, use of a form that has broad descriptions of language, speech, and hearing evaluations printed on it satisfies this need prior to the preplacement evaluation. Parents sign and return one copy of the form and keep the other one that includes a description of the evaluation process and their rights under PL 94–142 and the Family Rights and Privacy Act. If placement in a special education program is recommended after comprehensive evaluation, the first I.E.P. meeting, at which parents are important participants, provides an opportunity to explain the recommended placement. Thereafter, any time the educational agency proposes to make changes in the child's identification as speech and language impaired or in the I.E.P., parents must be provided with written notification of what is being planned.

Whether parental consent is being sought for initial evaluation or placement, or parents are being notified about potential changes in their child's program, several regulations apply to the notification process. Information must be presented in such a way as to be understandable by parents, including the use of translators when parents do not speak English. Parents must also understand that their consent is voluntary and may be retracted later. They also should be informed of their rights to request a review of their child's I.E.P. more frequently than at the required one-year intervals if they have concerns about its appropriateness. Parents are also informed of their rights under the Family Rights and Privacy Act to have access to their children's school records. Their permission must be given before information in those records is shared with anyone outside the school district.

Evaluation

Once parental permission is obtained, evaluation of children suspected of being language impaired has two major purposes: (*a*) determination of eligibility for placement in a program as speech and language impaired, and (*b*) identification of specific intervention needs, if so indicated. These two areas of concern are considered separately in the following sections, but they overlap in actual practice.

Determining Eligibility. The determination of eligibility is guided by state rules and regulations that are generally more specific than those in the federal document. Rules often exist for each of the categories in which children may be eligible for special education services. Although efforts are currently being mounted in some areas to reduce the labeling that accompanies a categorical approach to special education, teacher certification and program reimbursement often depend upon the use of such categories, and the categorical approach is unlikely to be abandoned. Definitions for determining language disorders vary, but most specify that a child must show language deficits in one or more of the systems of language—phonology, morphology, syntax, semantics, or pragmatics.

In addition, requirements regarding the evaluation process may be specified. As a minimum, the federal regulations for implementing PL 94–142 specify that a full and individual evaluation must be conducted with more than one procedure, and that each procedure must be validated for the purpose for which it is used. Procedures must also be selected and administered so as not to be racially or culturally discriminatory. A child must be evaluated in all areas related to the suspected disability (as previously discussed in this chapter in the section on identification), and the evaluation must be conducted by a multidisciplinary team, which might include the regular education classroom teacher for some children. Other professionals frequently serving on evaluation teams for language-impaired children besides speech-language pathologists and audiologists are special education teachers, particularly learning disability specialists, psychologists, occupational therapists, and others knowledgeable about the child or the suspected handicapping condition.

The speech and language evaluation must also be comprehensive. The principles of evaluation discussed in chapter 6 are as appropriate in school settings as any other. Often the quantitative requirements of language evaluation are met by using a broad comprehensive language assessment instrument comprising a number of subtests and followed by specific evaluation in areas suspected to be relatively more intact or disordered. Many language-disordered children show uneven profiles of relative strengths and weaknesses. Identifying these areas is an important function of the evaluation process. It leads to accomplishment of the second, more qualitative goal of assessment, determining individualized intervention needs.

Determining Intervention Needs. It is important that descriptions of language-disordered children be specific enough to allow recommendations regarding focus of intervention. I.E.P.s may then be written prior to placement, as required. I.E.P.s include goals and short-term objectives in addition to specific details about program implementation. The assessment must provide sufficient information to enable the I.E.P. committee to write appropriate initial objectives at the time of the preplacement I.E.P. meeting. Some examples may make this process clearer.

Consider the child whose evaluation makes it apparent that he needs further development in the area of conceptual vocabulary. A preliminary survey of specific vocabulary might lead to spatial and temporal words being targeted in the child's I.E.P. Another child's language sample indicates that beyond having difficulty with the syntactic rules of language, she needs specific work on past tense morphemes and auxiliary verb structures. In yet another example, it may be determined that a child has difficulty with the pragmatic rules for using language and would benefit most from attention to conversational turn-taking skills and staying on topic. Although I.E.P.s are often written with little detail beyond a specification of the broad areas needing remediation, using the initial evaluation to identify specific targets of intervention lessens the time needed to get started with intervention activities themselves when the program actually begins.

The process of arriving at the most appropriate areas for intervention depends on utilization of the six guiding principles listed later in this chapter. These guidelines include interaction during the evaluation process with others who know the child well. Information gathered from parents and teachers can be used to validate areas identified with formal and informal measures as being disordered, and it can also be used to help decide which tests to use. Observing the child in the classroom can also be an important part of the evaluation, and it may be required in some states. If the child is suspected of being learning disabled or mentally retarded, psychological and educational evaluations are often mandatory as well.

Children who are physically and/or mentally impaired may present particularly complicated evaluation needs. Separating relative influences of different aspects of the handicap is often difficult. One method for approaching the evaluation process for such children has been devised by Nelson, Silbar, and Lockwood (1981). It involves the use of more formal evaluation procedures and/or informal observation to judge a child's relative abilities in each of the four areas: *cognitive bases, receptive language, expressive language,* and *social interaction and play.* The appendix presents a Reference Chart of developmental events in each of these realms. A Summary Chart with condensation of the information on the Reference Chart into a single-page format appears as Figure 12–2. A child's diagnostic profile may be sketched on the Summary Chart by shading in complete or partial boxes to illustrate the child's relative abilities and difficulties. Examples of this procedure appear in Figure 12–3. Then the decision-making charts of Figures 12–4 and 12–5 may be used to determine what kinds of programming might be appropriately selected.

For example, as illustrated in Figure 12–3a, a physically handicapped child may be able to show cognitive development up through Piaget's sensorimotor stage V by using novel means to seek familiar ends if given access to the means. The evaluator must be careful because physical impairment may be easily mistaken for lack of cognitive support for communication. However, many speech-language pathologists providing services in school programs are becoming increasingly sophisticated about using a variety of augmentative communication systems. For example, especially young or handicapped children might be taught to activate electronic toys or other devices using any of a variety of switches. In this way, they can be given the means to demonstrate the acquisition of concepts of cause and effect, using means to achieve desired ends, and the intentional uses of communication.

The child whose behavior is profiled in Figure 12–3a might have demonstrated late intentional *cognitive bases* of language by grasping at a ring that could be used to draw a favorite toy closer or by vocalizing with increased intensity when a snack was removed prematurely. For the severely physically handicapped child, sustained gaze might be the only means available to indicate cognitive potential at this level. This same child might be able to use sustained and focused eye gaze (eye pointing) to identify words out of context at the same level in the column on the Reference and Summary Charts representing *receptive language.* However, *expressive language* constrained by the physical impairment may be limited to reflexive vocalizations (except for the nonverbal expressive communication skills already described). In the area of *social interaction and play,* the child might be able to show behaviors at the third developmental stage on the Reference Chart by reacting to the emotions of others or by gazing at desired objects. The profile for such a child would lead to the decision outlined in the third or fourth column of the Placement and Decision Chart depicted in Figure 12–4. That is, this child appears ready to enter the stage of representational thought, showing cognition at the level of late intentional thought (substage 5), a discrepancy between cognition and

SUMMARY CHART

Name: ______________ BD: ______________ Speech-Language Clinician: ______________

Date: ______________ Classroom Teacher: ______________

COGNITIVE BASES	RECEPTIVE LANGUAGE	EXPRESSIVE LANGUAGE	SOCIAL INTERACTION & PLAY
Preintentional (Birth to 8 months) *Sensorimotor I, II, III* ____ Infant moves from being purely reflexive to showing the initial beginnings of goal-oriented behavior ____ Developing object permanence	____ Startles to sound ____ Turns to sound ____ Reacts to human voice ____ Responds to tone of voice	____ Cry ____ Reflexive Vocalizations	____ Engages in interaction ____ Maintains interaction ____ Initiates interaction ____ Indicates preference for familiar people and objects
Early intentional (8 to 12 months) *Sensorimotor IV* ____ Uses familiar means to achieve novel ends	____ No word comprehension yet ____ Imitates on-going action ____ Looks where parent looks	____ Differentiated cries ____ Syllabic babbling	____ Plays nursery games ____ Plays with toys
Late Intentional (12 to 18 months) *Sensorimotor V* ____ Invention of new means to achieve familiar ends	____ Responds appropriately to single words in context	____ Hi/bye routines ____ First words ____ Words used as 'performatives' (to manipulate environment)	____ Solitary or onlooker play ____ Hugs doll, pulls toy
Representational (18 to 24 months) *Thought* *Sensorimotor VI* ____ Begins symbolic thinking	____ Understands words without context (points to pictures) ____ Follows 2-word commands	____ Novel one-word utterances ____ Asks "What's that?" ____ Onset of 2-word utterances	____ Parallel play
Early Preoperations (2 to 3½ yrs.) ____ Thought is preconceptual ____ Inference is sometimes but not always correct	____ Begins to understand Wh-questions ____ Answers yes/no questions	____ Two-word utterances ____ Basic sentences develop ____ Morphological markers develop	____ Symbolic play
Late Preoperations (3½ to 7 yrs.) ____ Beginning of intuitive thought ____ Problem solves by trial & error (not always correct)	____ Points to pictures representing sentences ____ Uses word order to understand agent-object relationships	____ Uses compound and complex sentences ____ Uses language to relate experiences ____ Talks about remote experiences ____ Adequate voice, articulation, fluency	____ Plays in small groups
Concrete Operations (7 to 12 yrs.) ____ Classifies on 2 characteristics	____ Understands conditional causal sentences	____ More clauses per sentence ____ Uses language to converse, persuade, tease	____ Genuine cooperative play

Instructions:

1. Place a check mark beside characteristics demonstrated (reference chart or other evaluation tools may be used as necessary)
2. Shade in areas which describe functioning (areas may be partially shaded)
3. Refer to program decision chart

Recommendations:

Nelson, Silbar, Lockwood, 1981.

Figure 12–3a
SUMMARY CHART

Name: ______ BD: ______ Speech-Language Clinician: ______

Date: ______ Classroom Teacher: ______

COGNITIVE BASES	RECEPTIVE LANGUAGE	EXPRESSIVE LANGUAGE	SOCIAL INTERACTION & PLAY
Preintentional (Birth to 8 months) *Sensorimotor I, II, III* ____ Infant moves from being purely reflexive to showing the initial beginnings of goal-oriented behavior ____ Developing object permanence	____ Startles to sound ____ Turns to sound ____ Reacts to human voice ____ Responds to tone of voice	____ Cry ____ Reflexive Vocalizations	____ Engages in interaction ____ Maintains interaction ____ Initiates interaction ____ Indicates preference for familiar people and objects
Early intentional (8 to 12 months) *Sensorimotor IV* ____ Uses familiar means to achieve novel ends	____ No word comprehension yet ____ Imitates on-going action ____ Looks where parent looks	____ Differentiated cries ____ Syllabic babbling	____ Plays nursery games ____ Plays with toys
Late Intentional (12 to 18 months) *Sensorimotor V* ____ Invention of new means to achieve familiar ends	____ Responds appropriately to single words in context	____ Hi/bye routines ____ First words ____ Words used as 'performatives' (to manipulate environment)	____ Solitary or onlooker play ____ Hugs doll, pulls toy
Representational (18 to 24 months) *Thought* *Sensorimotor VI* ____ Begins symbolic thinking	____ Understands words without context (points to pictures) ____ Follows 2-word commands	____ Novel one-word utterances ____ Asks "What's that?" ____ Onset of 2-word utterances	____ Parallel play
Early Preoperations (2 to 3½ yrs.) ____ Thought is preconceptual ____ Inference is sometimes but not always correct	____ Begins to understand Wh-questions ____ Answers yes/no questions	____ Two-word utterances ____ Basic sentences develop ____ Morphological markers develop	____ Symbolic play
Late Preoperations (3½ to 7 yrs.) ____ Beginning of intuitive thought ____ Problem solves by trial & error (not always correct)	____ Points to pictures representing sentences ____ Uses word order to understand agent-object relationships	____ Uses compound and complex sentences ____ Uses language to relate experiences ____ Talks about remote experiences ____ Adequate voice, articulation, fluency	____ Plays in small groups
Concrete Operations (7 to 12 yrs.) ____ Classifies on 2 characteristics	____ Understands conditional causal sentences	____ More clauses per sentence ____ Uses language to converse, persuade, tease	____ Genuine cooperative play

Instructions:
1. Place a check mark beside characteristics demonstrated (reference chart or other evaluation tools may be used as necessary)
2. Shade in areas which describe functioning (areas may be partially shaded)
3. Refer to program decision chart

Recommendations:

Nelson, Silbar, Lockwood, 1981.

Figure 12–3b
SUMMARY CHART

Name: ______________________ BD: ______________________ Speech-Language Clinician: ______________________

Date: ______________________ Classroom Teacher: ______________________

COGNITIVE BASES	RECEPTIVE LANGUAGE	EXPRESSIVE LANGUAGE	SOCIAL INTERACTION & PLAY
Preintentional (Birth to 8 months) *Sensorimotor I, II, III* ____ Infant moves from being purely reflexive to showing the initial beginnings of goal-oriented behavior ____ Developing object permanence	____ Startles to sound ____ Turns to sound ____ Reacts to human voice ____ Responds to tone of voice	____ Cry ____ Reflexive Vocalizations	____ Engages in interaction ____ Maintains interaction ____ Initiates interaction ____ Indicates preference for familiar people and objects
Early intentional (8 to 12 months) *Sensorimotor IV* ____ Uses familiar means to achieve novel ends	____ No word comprehension yet ____ Imitates on-going action ____ Looks where parent looks	____ Differentiated cries ____ Syllabic babbling	____ Plays nursery games ____ Plays with toys
Late Intentional (12 to 18 months) *Sensorimotor V* ____ Invention of new means to achieve familiar ends	____ Responds appropriately to single words in context	____ Hi/bye routines ____ First words ____ Words used as 'performatives' (to manipulate environment)	____ Solitary or onlooker play ____ Hugs doll, pulls toy
Representational (18 to 24 months) *Thought* *Sensorimotor VI* ____ Begins symbolic thinking	____ Understands words without context (points to pictures) ____ Follows 2-word commands	____ Novel one-word utterances ____ Asks "What's that?" ____ Onset of 2-word utterances	____ Parallel play
Early Preoperations (2 to 3½ yrs.) ____ Thought is preconceptual ____ Inference is sometimes but not always correct	____ Begins to understand Wh-questions ____ Answers yes/no questions	____ Two-word utterances ____ Basic sentences develop ____ Morphological markers develop	____ Symbolic play
Late Preoperations (3½ to 7 yrs.) ____ Beginning of intuitive thought ____ Problem solves by trial & error (not always correct)	____ Points to pictures representing sentences ____ Uses word order to understand agent-object relationships	____ Uses compound and complex sentences ____ Uses language to relate experiences ____ Talks about remote experiences ____ Adequate voice, articulation, fluency	____ Plays in small groups
Concrete Operations (7 to 12 yrs.) ____ Classifies on 2 characteristics	____ Understands conditional causal sentences	____ More clauses per sentence ____ Uses language to converse, persuade, tease	____ Genuine cooperative play

Instructions:
1. Place a check mark beside characteristics demonstrated (reference chart or other evaluation tools may be used as necessary)
2. Shade in areas which describe functioning (areas may be partially shaded)
3. Refer to program decision chart

Recommendations:

Nelson, Silbar, Lockwood, 1981.

expressive language (even though receptive language is at least as high as cognition), and social interaction at a level slightly lower than language skills. A prescriptive/ integrative intervention approach might be recommended, including the development of an individualized program to be implemented in the classroom following demonstration by the speech-language pathologist. Services could be implemented directly by the speech-language pathologist as well. Further recommendations about mode of communication might be made using the Augmentative Communication decision chart in Figure 12–5, because this child also exhibits the behaviors described in the input box on the decision chart for selecting augmentative systems.

The child exemplified by the profile on the Summary Chart in Figure 12–3b presents a different set of abilities and needs. This child indicates behaviors at consistent levels across realms, has only partially developed the skills of the first level, and does not yet exhibit cognitive bases for developing more sophisticated communication skills. Such a child fits the description of Column 2 in the Decision Making Chart of Figure 12–4. The recommendations for this child would involve consultation by a speech-language pathologist regarding prelinguistic communication objectives to be implemented by the classroom teacher and caretakers at school and at home.

The decision regarding types of service delivery to recommend and specific areas and methods of intervention should be guided by evaluation results. No one type of service delivery is right for all children. In addition to the delivery models described in this chapter, others may be designed to fit particular needs of individual children and capabilities of districts. Part of the federal legislation for handicapped children, however, is that placement decisions must be based on the needs of children and not on the availability of programs. Actual decisions regarding placement are finalized at initial I.E.P. meetings, during which parental permission is obtained for the initial placement in a special education program.

Placement Decisions and Planning

In the schools, a continuum of service delivery systems should be available for meeting the variety of needs evidenced by language-disordered children. Some of these systems have been illustrated in Figure 12–4. Children who are severely impaired and who demonstrate behavioral characteristics typical of prelinguistic stages of development may benefit most from having consultant services provided by a speech-language pathologist. Consultant services may be provided as part of home programs or to classroom teachers and aides, or both. In either case, the consultation generally focuses on assisting those who provide primary care for the child to "tune in" to primitive communication attempts and to encourage the development of the cognitive underpinnings of language. Home programs might also provide appropriate means of delivering language intervention services to handicapped infants and preschoolers who are too young for classroom placement and would be served best by their own parents or other caretakers at home.

Children with language disorders accompanying other handicapping conditions may also benefit from close interaction between speech-language pathologists and classroom teachers. For example, as discussed in chapter 9, the communicative disorders experienced by autistic children are an integral part of the syndrome of autism. Such children need a program in which more than 30 minutes two times per week are

Figure 12–4

Placement and Program Decision Chart

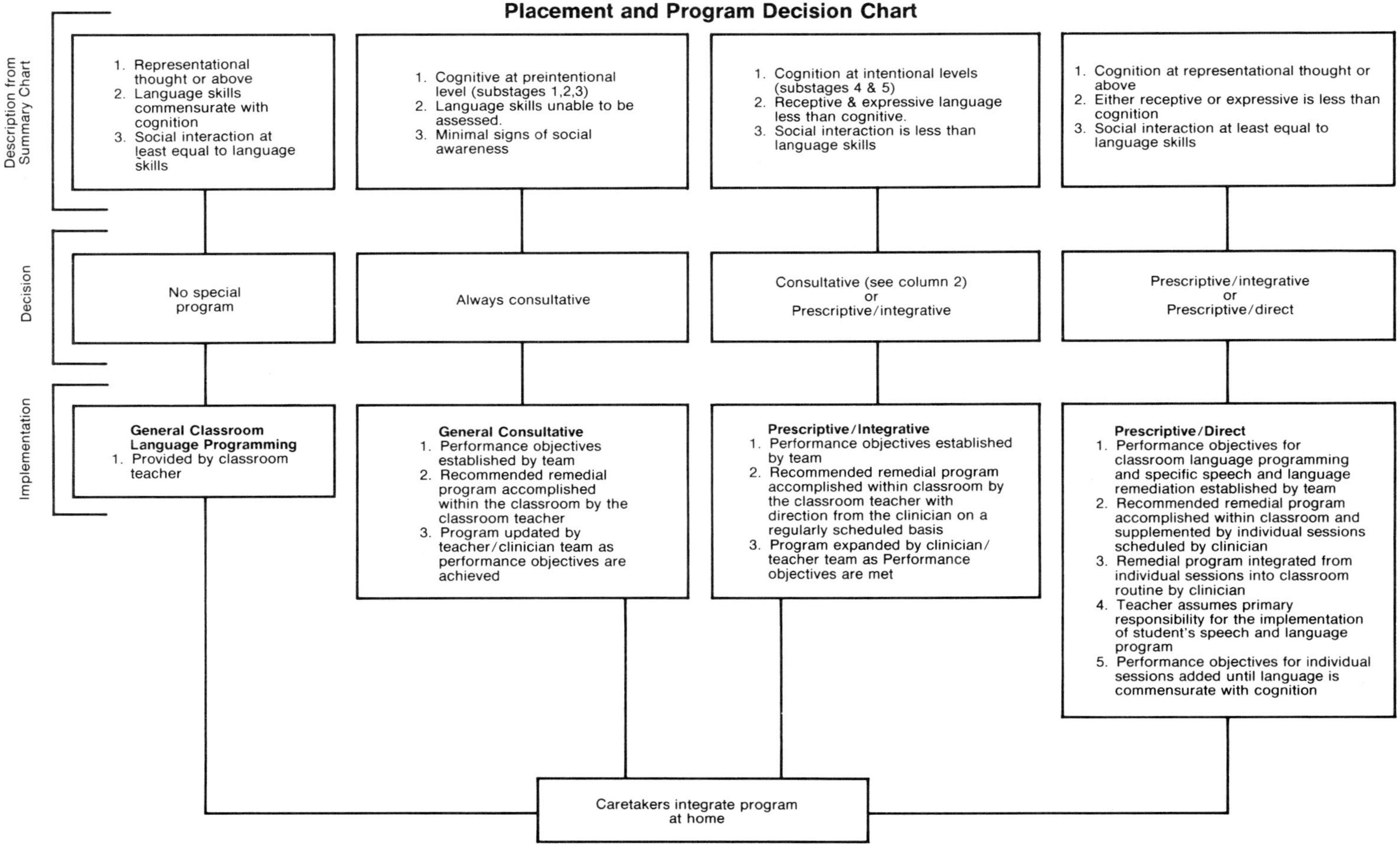

Figure 12-5

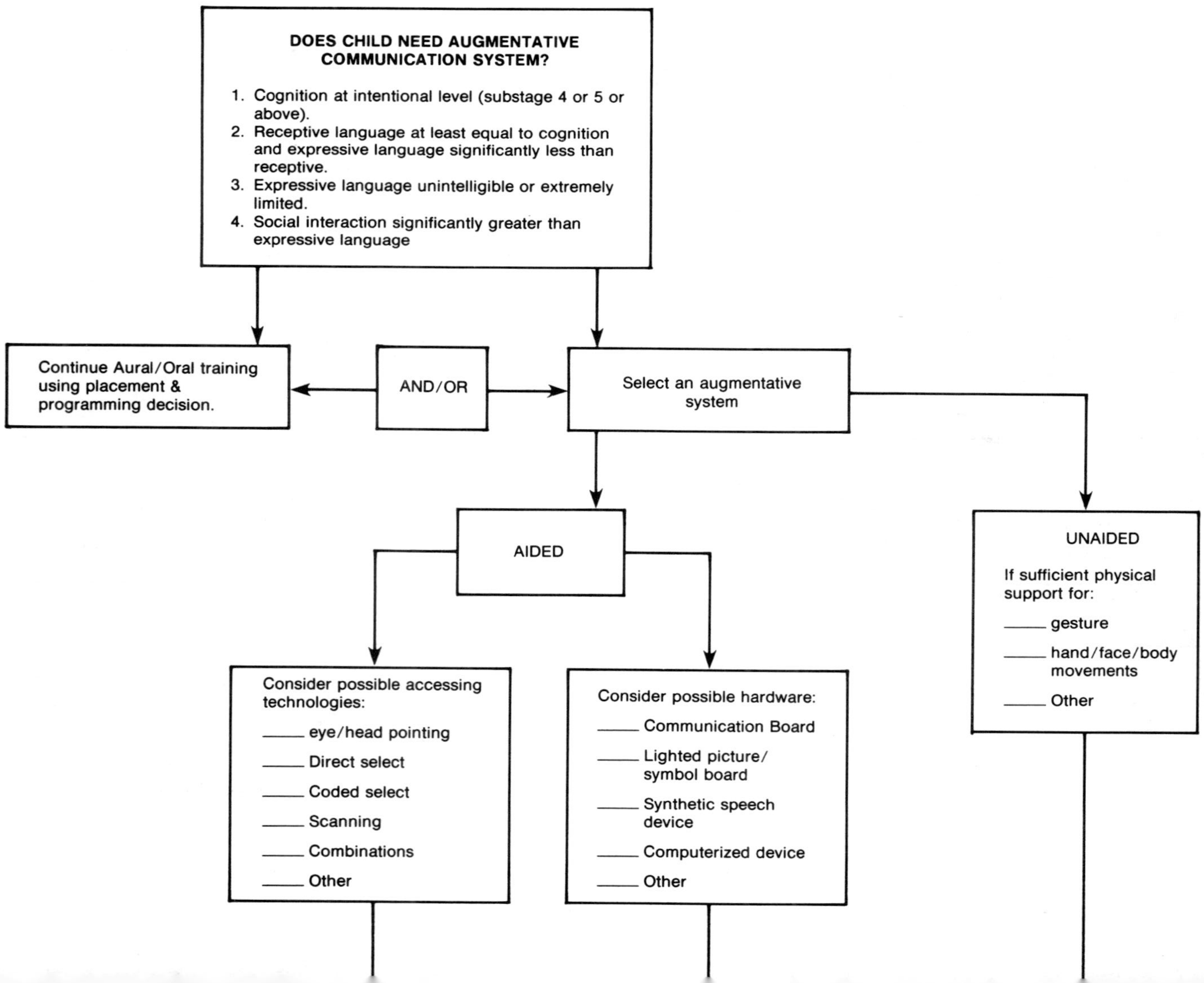
DOES CHILD NEED AUGMENTATIVE COMMUNICATION SYSTEM?
1. Cognition at intentional level (substage 4 or 5 or above).
2. Receptive language at least equal to cognition and expressive language significantly less than receptive.
3. Expressive language unintelligible or extremely limited.
4. Social interaction significantly greater than expressive language
Continue Aural/Oral training using placement & programming decision.
AND/OR
Select an augmentative system
AIDED
UNAIDED
If sufficient physical support for:
____ gesture
____ hand/face/body movements
____ Other
Consider possible accessing technologies:
____ eye/head pointing
____ Direct select
____ Coded select
____ Scanning
____ Combinations
____ Other
Consider possible hardware:
____ Communication Board
____ Lighted picture/symbol board
____ Synthetic speech device
____ Computerized device
____ Other

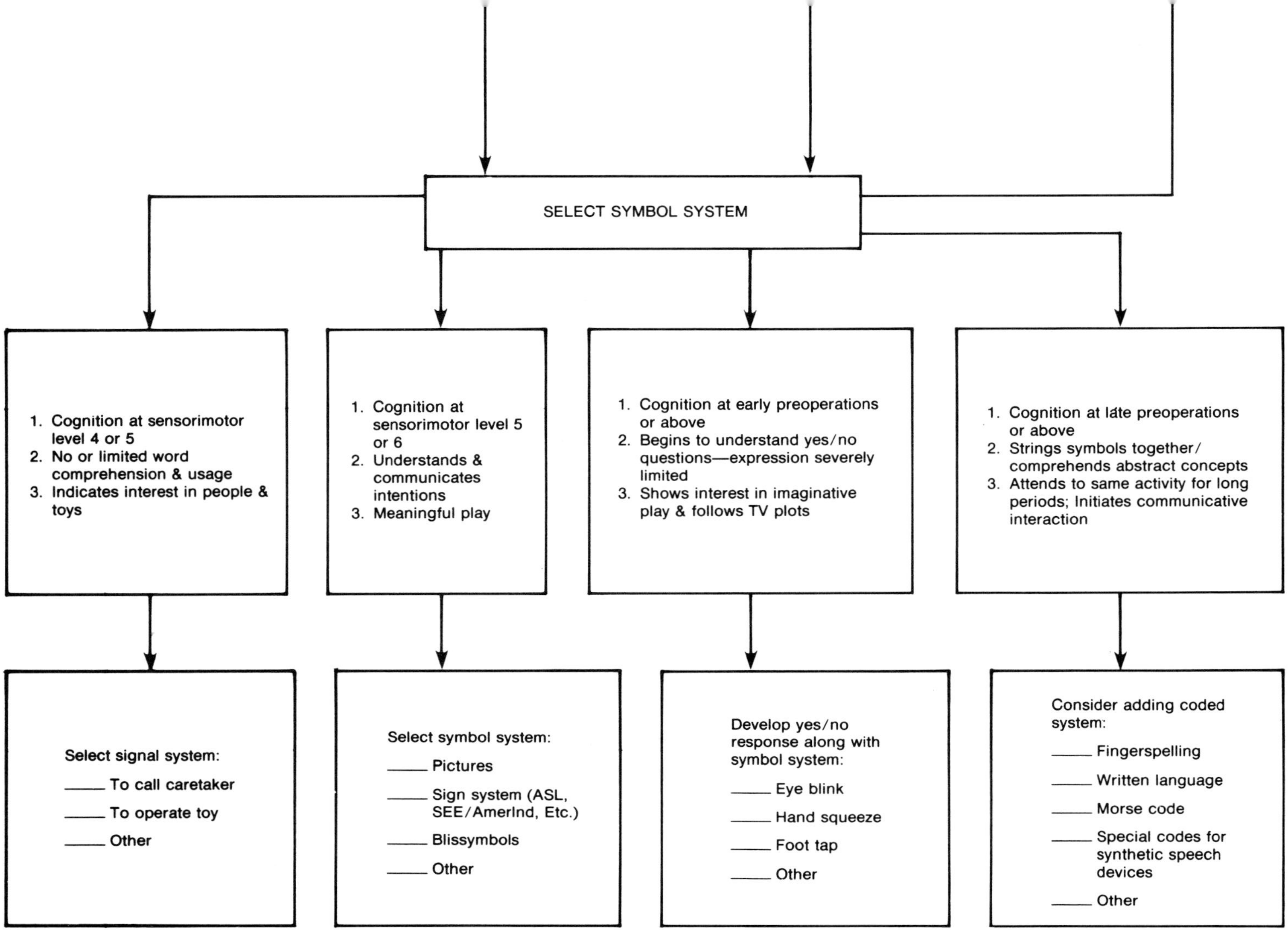

Nelson, Silbar, Lockwood, 1981

devoted to meeting their needs for communication intervention. Team teaching is one way of meeting these needs. Using classroom contexts, teachers and speech-language pathologists can work together to provide comprehensive programs. Manual communication systems or microcomputer-based learning experiences may provide initial access to language for some autistic children. Meaningful, but structured, communication experiences can be devised and repeated in classroom contexts many more times than if the speech-language pathologist removes the child to an isolated setting down the hall.

In some instances, speech-language pathologists themselves serve as classroom teachers. This is most frequently the case when language-learning disabilities are determined to be the primary impairments of a group of preschool or school-age children. Advantages of self-contained or resource room programs are that language may be encouraged in its most relevant and communicative forms. Language intervention generally proceeds best in meaningful contexts, and it requires intensive contact with more severely involved children to be most effective. Speech-language pathologists serving as classroom teachers can provide these kinds of language intervention services. However, when speech-language pathologists assume the role of classroom teachers, they also accept responsibility for meeting the students' total developmental and educational needs. For example, preschoolers need activities designed for encouraging the development of gross and fine motor and cognitive skills as well as structured and natural language intervention activities. School-age youngsters would require attention to academics and preparation to deal with the regular classroom curriculum in addition to specialized instruction in spoken and written language.

A less intensive service delivery model should also be available for mild to moderate language-impaired children. Many language-disordered children in the schools can handle regular educational experiences if language intervention is provided early enough and with enough intensity to allow them to acquire the psycholinguistic foundations for much of later learning. These children may best be served by attending special speech and language sessions several times per week. This approach might be recommended either for children who spend some time in a resource room with another special education teacher, or for children who receive no other special education services. Such a delivery model would be more appropriate than self-contained classrooms for children who could make optimal progress with less intensive service. This is an important part of meeting the requirement of PL 94–142 that children be served in the "least restrictive environment" (L.R.E.) possible. Provision of services two or three times per week individually or in small groups is often referred to as *itinerant* or *traditional therapy.*

Although children are most often pulled from regular classroom activities for these sessions, the speech-language pathologist sometimes enters the classroom or consults with the regular teacher, who may implement a portion of the program. A caution here is that the symptoms of attention deficit and distractibility that often accompany language disorders may contraindicate provision of language intervention activities in the classroom at the same time other activities are taking place. The separate room with quiet surroundings may provide the best context for learning new language forms for some children. Quiet rooms are not always easy to obtain. As many school districts are consolidating buildings, speech-language pathologists may find themselves needing to persuade principals and school boards that sharing a spare room with the reading teacher with only a visual barrier, and not an acoustic one, between them, is not an appropriate setting for meeting the needs of language-impaired children.

The program should not stop with carefully controlled protective contexts for encouraging the acquisition of new language forms. If new forms are to be used for new functions, conscious plans will need to be drawn by the speech-language pathologist, the child's parents, and teachers for requiring use of the new forms in a variety of contexts. It is also possible to set up relatively naturalistic contexts with one or two children in settings outside the classroom. For example, younger children might be engaged in a snack preparation or art activity designed to increase the likelihood that targeted language content, syntactic and morphological structures, or communicative functions would be produced. For older students, activities might include conversational interactions, role playing of social situations, replicating classroom activities, and other opportunities to use new skills. Less structured activities also give the speech-language pathologist a chance to probe newly acquired behaviors in situations that are more like those of real life in order to judge whether they are sufficiently automatic to be maintained outside the relatively protective environment of the therapy room.

I.E.P. Meetings

Decisions regarding the selection of a particular type of program for a particular child are not made unilaterally. They are made on the basis of a multidisciplinary evaluation by an I.E.P. committee. Regulations exist for specifying the kinds of individuals who must be present at the I.E.P. meeting. These include:

1. *A representative of the public agency, other than the child's teacher, who is qualified to provide, or supervise the provision of special education.* This person may be the special education coordinator for the district, the building principal, or another speech-language pathologist or special education teacher.
2. *The child's teacher.* This person may be the speech-language pathologist; however, in some states, if the child is in a regular education classroom, the child's regular education teacher must attend the I.E.P. meeting.
3. *One or both of the child's parents.* The regulations for implementing PL 94–142 are specific about the steps a public agency (school system) must take to ensure that parents are afforded the opportunity to participate in their child's I.E.P. meeting. These include notifying parents of the meeting early enough; scheduling the meeting at a mutually agreed upon time and place; taking care that parents are fully informed about the purpose of the meeting and who will be there; and, providing special assistance to help them understand the proceedings if necessary. Meetings may be held without parents if school districts can show that, though repeated attempts were made, they were unable to convince the child's parents to attend the meeting. Although requirements related to obtaining parental participation in the planning process may become one of the most time-consuming aspects of provision of language intervention services in school settings, the expectations are no more than would generally be a part of service provision in any other environment. Quite apart from meeting legal requirements, they are also important in meeting the

principles outlined in this chapter as forming a basis for effective language intervention programs.

4. *The child, where appropriate.* Modifying communicative behaviors entails the shaping of skills that are largely automatic, though never trivial nor simple. Although the conscious participation of the individuals being served is not required to accomplish this, their active and self-motivated involvement greatly increases the likelihood of success. When the child can be appropriately included in the goal-setting phases of program planning, goal-directed learning may be enhanced. Children who are old enough to understand that they have more problems in some areas than many of their peers also have a right to have these difficulties explained to them in an understandable fashion. If left to draw their own conclusions, they too often conclude that they are too dumb, or otherwise inferior, to be good in school. Providing children with some simple language to explain their problems and the special services they and others receive may be one of the more important initial or ongoing functions of the communication specialist.
5. *Other individuals.* The child's parents or the educational agency may request other individuals to attend the I.E.P. meeting if they wish. If the agency chooses to do so, the parents must be informed regarding who will be there. At the first I.E.P. meeting, it is required that someone who is capable of explaining the evaluation procedures and results be present. If the I.E.P. meeting is scheduled for a child who has some other primary impairment accompanied by a language disorder, the speech-language pathologist who performed the evaluation should make every effort to be at the meeting. In this way, not only the language evaluation per se can be explained, but it may be more possible to sort out the confounding effects of language, cognition, and cultural and environmental factors, as required by the regulations of PL 94–142.

I.E.P. Content and Review

The format for writing I.E.P.s varies widely from district to district across the United States. Most districts have designed their own forms, and the same form is used regardless of handicapping condition. Some forms feed easily into computerized information-processing systems. Others are processed with a number of manual steps to meet accountability needs. Regardless, each I.E.P. must include information in five areas:

1. *A statement of the child's present levels of education performance* is generally written to record the highlights of the comprehensive multidisciplinary evaluation. It may be entered on the form prior to the I.E.P. meeting, or it may be recorded while the results are being explained at the meeting. For the language-impaired child who is functioning primarily at grade level, anecdotal evidence that the child can handle the regular curriculum except for the noted areas of special difficulty is sufficient. Formal test scores of academic achievement are not necessary. For the learning-disabled or mentally retarded child, psychological and educational assessments are frequently conducted as part of the preplacement evaluation. A summary statement of the results of these assessments is then included in describing present levels of education performance.

The degree of detail in the statement regarding levels of education performance varies depending on the philosophy of the district. If greater detail is included in order to provide baseline or criterion referenced data, the information may be used as a point of comparison for the evaluation plan, which serves as component number five in the specifications for I.E.P. content. The statements should not become too narrow, however. The main purpose of this part of the I.E.P. is to provide an accurate sketch of the total child at a particular point in development. With this in mind, a microscopic look at some of the critical aspects related to the disability is appropriate, but not at the expense of a macroscopic view of the child as a whole person.

2. *A statement of annual goals, including short-term instructional objectives* provides a time frame for the process. The challenge facing individuals who come together at I.E.P. meetings is to establish goals that are broad enough to be significant (avoiding triviality), yet specific enough to be manageable (avoiding lack of clarity). The goals and short-term objectives will be revised within at least one year.

The leveling between goals and short-term objectives built into the regulations for PL 94–142 also assists with the decision-making process. Using both formal and informal evaluation results, individuals at the I.E.P. meeting can work together at the goal-setting level to identify broad areas of focus. The principles outlined earlier in this chapter can be used to underlie the selection of goal areas to meet any of a variety of criteria. For example, the selection may be based on: (*a*) areas that are next in developmental sequence and appear to be ripe for change, (*b*) areas that are particularly impaired, (*c*) areas that show potential for rapid development to act as catalysts for other delayed processes, or (*d*) areas that have a particular significance for the child and others who are close to him or her.

Each educational specialist who will be working with the child establishes goals for his area. For the speech-language pathologist, two or three goals are usually needed to define a meaningful program. For example, "to improve communication skill," may focus the group on the need to be concerned about communication in general, but including language intervention as a specific service to be provided to the child probably accomplishes as much. It is a more efficient use of I.E.P. space to indicate as annual goals that the child needs to demonstrate: (*a*) expanded use of conceptual vocabulary, (*b*) expressive syntax of greater length and complexity than the baseline sample, and (*c*) spontaneous use of language for a greater number of communicative functions and in a wider variety of situations than exhibited in the preplacement inventory. One may decide to select more than three goals, depending on the time available to implement the plan. Keeping in mind the need to integrate behaviors in the realms of content, form, and use may help make goal setting more manageable.

Short-term objectives are more precise and define further the areas of focus selected as annual goals. They are sufficiently detailed to determine whether a program is working to move a child closer to appropriate targets. The targets may be chronologically normal skills for some children, or more functional, independent living skills for others. The targets (goals) will be based on macroscopic views of what is important for the individual child. The short-term objectives offer a relatively more microscopic view of how to meet the goals that have been selected to move the child toward eventual targets.

At least two short-term objectives are usually provided under each of the established goals, and may be viewed as measurement points in moving the child toward the goal. They are most useful if written as operational definitions of observable, quantifiable behaviors. Writing objectives behaviorally does not necessitate that behavior modification techniques be used to implement them. For example, although the precision of behavior modification techniques may help a mentally retarded child acquire such skill as naming objects, more naturalistic approaches are usually most effective in developing creative spontaneous language functions. Objectives may be written for more structured or more naturalistic activities by operationally defining the desired skill as an observable, quantifiable behavior. For example:

Goal One: The child will acquire new skill in object naming.

Objective 1. The child will point to pictures representing at least three sets of five objects as they are named by the speech-language pathologist (50% tangible reinforcement, 100% social reinforcement; two consecutive sessions with no errors).

Objective 2. When presented varied examples of objects and pictured objects, the child will name them in response to the question "What is this?" asked by the classroom teacher (social reinforcement only; at least 15 new names used on two occasions with a week's interval between).

Goal Two: The child will demonstrate spontaneous use of new communicative functions.

Objective 1. The child will ask questions when presented with an interactive language experience which leaves important information unknown (child given bowl of ice cream with no spoon). Criterion: four spontaneous verbal questions with rising intonation (any syntactic maturity) in five required contexts over two situations.

Objective 2. The child will initiate appropriate communication exchanges with a variety of adults at least two times during 5-minute interactions without being prompted (at least five situations with three different adults).

The short-term objectives in these examples are all written to include three kinds of information: (*a*) a statement of what the *child will do,* (*b*) under what *conditions,* and (*c*) *how well.* Each of these objective components provides important information about the design of the child's individualized language intervention program.

The *do statement* is the behavioral one. It is written in terms of the child's behavior, not the speech-language pathologist's. The focus is on establishing behaviors that demonstrate that a child is moving closer to desired targets in selected areas. If written in terms of what the speech-language pathologist or teacher will do, the child-oriented focus is diminished. It is also important to write the "do" statement in terms of behavior that is observable and measurable. In the examples given, such behaviors as pointing, naming, and verbal question asking are observable and their occurrence can be documented. If these behaviors had been written as understanding or discriminating skills, the nonobservable hidden quality of those processes would have made it impossible to determine that the desired event had occurred. When the speech-language pathologist determines that skills such as understanding and discriminating are important to encourage, the behaviors that can demonstrate such events must be defined.

The *conditions* portion of the short-term objective indicates the type of approach and environmental contexts that are predicted to be the most effective for helping the child acquire the new behavior. Conditions statements can specify content for a number of different variables. Among these, kinds and complexity of stimuli may be described, along with the degree of structure or spontaneity to be provided or expected in the communicative exchanges. Also important are the environmental contexts and people with whom the new behavior is to be demonstrated. The short-term objectives that are written into I.E.P.s are intended to provide measurement points and not to outline the entire intervention program. In fact, it may be desirable in some cases to leave them slightly more open-ended than those in the examples to allow some flexibility as the program is implemented. Some states do require more specific, step-by-step programs to be written to supplement the I.E.P. If so, additional time after the initial I.E.P. meeting is usually allowed before this requirement must be met. An example of an objective sequence designed for this purpose (Nelson, 1979) appears as Figure 12–6.

The third component of a well-written short-term objective is a specification of *criteria* for determining when the objective has been met. Criteria are integrally tied to descriptions of conditions. Being able to demonstrate a new behavior spontaneously without any modeling by the speech-language pathologist may be an important part of the criteria for determining that an objective has been met. Criteria may also include specification of how complete, how frequent, or how rapid correct responses must be. For example, the speech-language pathologist must decide how many occurrences of a new behavior must be observed on how many occasions in order to be confident that the current objective has been met and the child is ready to move on to a higher level.

Percentages (e.g., 80–90% correct) are often used to specify criteria for meeting objectives. However, percentages have little meaning unless a time frame or number of trials is specified as a basis for computing them. Otherwise, 80% may mean 4 out of 5 possible occurrences, or it may mean 40 out of 50 possible occurrences. The speech-language pathologist must decide whether the differences between these are significant in a particular instance and which is most appropriate for determining the acquisition of a particular skill. Those criteria are written into the short-term objectives on a child's I.E.P.

Putting all of these components together—what the child will do, under what conditions, and how well—meaningful short-term objectives can be written to move children closer to the longer-term goals that have been set for them. By writing at least two short-term objectives under each goal, movement toward the goal can be measured at least at two points during the year that each I.E.P. is in effect.

3. *A statement of the specific special education and related services to be provided to the child, and the extent to which the child will be able to participate in regular education programs* describes the placement of the child in a particular program and the amount of time the child will spend in the program relative to the amount of time to be spent in regular education. The type of delivery model recommended for a particular child is recorded. If the district offers a continuum of service delivery possibilities, the child's needs can be considered foremost in selecting the style of program to be adopted. Possibilities may include consultation, intermittent therapy, resource room placement, or placement in a specially designed self-contained classroom program. Regardless of the type of program recommended, a specification of the time to be spent in the program is required. Possible examples are, "one hour per week," "one hour per day," or "full time except for art, music, and gym with regular education

Figure 12-6. Language: Semantic Acquisition of Conceptual Vocabulary

Date: ____________

STUDENT: ____________ AGE: ____ SCHOOL: ____________ GRADE/LEVEL: ________ SPEECH-LANGUAGE CLINICIAN: ____________

GOAL: The student will spontaneously and appropriately use the vocabulary being formally taught and will begin to acquire new vocabulary from the natural environment more rapidly.

DIAGNOSTIC: Cognitive ____________ MLU ________ PPVT ________ TACL ________
Affective ____________ Other Language Measures ____________
Speech ____________
Audiological ____________ Other: ____________

LONG-RANGE OBJECTIVE: The student will verbally label (older student will define) at least five previously untrained stimuli (objects/object relationships/pictures/actions/verbal descriptions) representing the category indicated (two consecutive sessions with no prompting).

SHORT-TERM OBJECTIVES	Category: ____ Vocabulary: ____		Category: ____ Vocabulary: ____		Category: ____ Vocabulary: ____		COMMENTS TECHNIQUES EVALUATION
THE STUDENT WILL:	Date In.	Date Accom.	Date In.	Date Accom.	Date In.	Date Accom.	
1. point to objects/pictures or perform an action, following concrete demonstration earlier in session, to represent target vocabulary items named by clinician (two consecutive sessions; 4 of 5 trials correct each item; minimal prompting).							
2. point to previously untrained objects/pictures or perform an action to represent concrete and obvious demonstration target vocabulary items named by clinician (two consecutive sessions; 4 of 5 trials correct each item; no prompting).							
3. label objects/object relationships/pictures/actions representing the target vocabulary, following demonstration earlier in session, in response to clinician's verbal question or fill-in task (two consecutive sessions; 4 of 5 trials correct each item; mixed presentation; minimal prompting).							
4. demonstrate ability to discriminate less obvious examples representing the target vocabulary by pointing or performing an action (two consecutive sessions; two trials correct each item; mixed presentation; no prompting).							

classes." Parents are often particularly concerned with this part of the I.E.P., because it is the component that assures that their children will receive the services they need to benefit from education.

4. *The projected dates for initiation of services and the anticipated duration of services* are determined. The federal regulations specify that an I.E.P. meeting must be held within 30 calendar days of the determination that a child needs special education and related services. States have differing rules for meeting the placement decision and first I.E.P. requirements. Some districts combine these two functions in the same meeting. Other requirements may be established by states for timelines between the initial I.E.P. meeting and the initiation of services. However, it is a federal requirement that an I.E.P. must be in effect before special education and related services are provided to a child. If the evaluation has included a qualitative analysis as well as a quantitative one, it will have been possible to write meaningful objectives to be included in this first I.E.P. Although details of programming method and style may need to be added later after the speech-language pathologist has worked with the child for a short time, areas of language development needing focus will have been identified as a part of the evaluation. Most districts require that children begin to receive the services outlined in their I.E.P.s within a few days after the initial I.E.P. meeting.

Within one year, another I.E.P. meeting must be convened to revise the I.E.P. and to consider whether the child still needs the special education and related services outlined in the plan. This one year interval is usually used to define the "anticipated duration of services" required in this component of the I.E.P. Although some states interpret this as meaning the establishment of a prognosis for the child's need for special education over a number of years, it is more often viewed as a requirement to enter a date on the I.E.P. form indicating that the I.E.P. will be reviewed and revised before a year has passed. Different management schemes are used by different districts for spreading I.E.P. annual review meetings throughout the year. An I.E.P. must be implemented all the time it is in effect. Children must begin receiving speech and language intervention services when school begins in the fall if an I.E.P. is in effect for them from the prior school year.

5. *Appropriate objective criteria and evaluation procedures and schedules for determining whether the short-term instructional objectives are being achieved* occur at least annually. If short-term instructional objectives have been written so that they are measurable, this requirement will have been partially met. Criterion statements form an integral part of short-term objectives. In addition, pre- and posttest formats may have been adopted for determining progress. Formal tests may, of course, be selected for this purpose, and they may be identified by name or generically (e.g., "a standardized vocabulary test will be administered") as part of the evaluation plan on the I.E.P. form.

Another procedure for pre- and posttesting language-disordered children, and one that may yield more usable information, is to institute a plan for gathering periodic spontaneous language samples. Different kinds of observations may be made on these language samples depending on the goals selected for intervention. Multiple observations may be made on the same language sample, making this an efficient process. Rich information about aspects of language a child knows and can use makes it a valid process. For example, the same 15-minute sample may yield information on the number of obligatory contexts in which a child used selected bound morphemes or failed to use them, as well as the number of false starts, filled pauses, or other hesitation phenomena that signal word selection delays or problems. Mean length of utterance in words and/or morphemes may also be computed. Then, 6 months later another 15-minute sample may be gathered using similar conditions, after which it can be transcribed and analyzed for the same variables. If written coded transcriptions are saved, an ongoing record of changes will be available.

Although the time needed for such activities has been limited in the past, and it remains so where inappropriately large caseloads are allowed, the technology is available to make such procedures possible for any school-based speech-language pathologist. As microcomputers become standard clinical tools, it will be possible to transcribe language samples directly onto computer discs, and to store a series of language samples on the same child. Then, a variety of comparative measurements can be made in a matter of seconds (Miller & Chapman, 1983).

Reevaluation

The final requirement of PL 94–142 to be considered in this discussion of language intervention in school settings is that of reevaluation. In order to be certain that children continue to receive the most appropriate education possible, it is necessary to step back occasionally and take another comprehensive look at the child's abilities and needs. An implicit goal for most children is to assist them to function as much like their normally developing age peers as possible. However, it is easy to get lost in the day-to-day details of meeting behavioral objectives. To ensure that professionals maintain a broad perspective as well as a detailed one, a requirement has been established that a comprehensive reevaluation must be conducted at least once every 3 years. This comprehensive reevaluation must meet all of the requirements of the preplacement evaluation. However, instead of obtaining parental permission prior to testing, the district must notify parents in writing that their child is undergoing a reevaluation that may result in a change in the identification of their child as handicapped. Following the comprehensive reevaluation, another meeting, which may coincide with the regularly scheduled annual review process, is scheduled to explain the results of the evaluation and to make further plans (see Figure 12–1).

GUIDING PRINCIPLES

Although it is important to be aware of regulatory influences when providing services to school-age children, guiding principles should arise more directly from what is known about language-disordered children and effective ways of serving them. Six interrelated principles are useful in guiding the development of programs for language-disordered children wherever they are served.

Individualization

Language intervention should be individualized using the diagnostic profiles of children. The group of children with language disorders is a heterogeneous one. Some have relatively more difficulty with the *content* of language—the semantic system including the lexicon (vocabulary) and the ideas that language represents. Some have more difficulty with the *form* of language—its syntax and morphological systems including rules and strategies for speaking and for processing auditory sequential input or for understanding and producing written language. Some have more difficulty with the *use* of language—the pragmatic system including a variety of communicative functions and strategies for selecting alternative ways of expressing oneself related to the contexts and purposes of events. Programs should recognize these relative differences and provide activities designed to meet individual needs.

Integration of Content, Form, and Use

Language intervention should lead to integration among the linguistic components of content, form, and use, even though children may have relatively greater difficulty with one component than another. One of the problems traditionally faced by speech-language pathologists has been planning activities that will encourage the *use* of newly acquired content and form categories in spontaneous communication events. The second principle of intervention suggests that program design should involve conscious plans to encourage such integration. Furthermore, activities for doing so should be built into all phases of intervention and not just the final ones.

A relatively new insight is also that for some children language *use* must be the primary area of focus. Language *use* involves skill in performing a variety of functions with language—for example, to request action, to request information, to give information, to demand, to command, to entertain, to be polite, or to use and interpret indirect forms. Children who have difficulty with the uses of language, whether at the preschool or secondary level, need to have some objectives for learning those skills included as a part of their I.E.P.s. Acquiring competence with various language uses may involve learning additional rules in the area of language form as well.

Form and function often advance, not simultaneously, but in stepwise progression. Slobin (1971) explained that new functions are first served by old forms and new forms first serve old functions. In other words, a clinician should not expect a child to be able to combine new forms and new functions in the same activity. New forms require multiple practice opportunities before they can be used for functions that carry a significant communicative load in many language-impaired children.

Combination of Structured and Natural Activities

Language intervention should offer a combination of structured and natural activities. Most children learn language, especially auditory/oral language, with relatively little effort. They are able to induce its regularities and organize its systems internally by forming hypotheses based on a mixture of linguistic input from their own and others' conversations. Parents and other adults do simplify their linguistic input to young children learning language (Broen, 1972; Snow, 1977). However, the limited evidence on parent input to language-disordered children suggests that it may be less well matched to the children's communicative needs than language addressed to younger normal children usually is (Lasky & Klopp, 1982). Children who are having difficulty learning language may need greater structuring of language input to make its regularities more apparent. In most cases, what is needed is amplification and replication of the aspects of language that have been selected for special focus. Greater structuring of the environment might be required to encourage the most rapid progress. Greater structuring of the environment can also provide occasions for such old functions as imitative and modeled responses that enable some language-disordered children to concentrate on using forms that have previously been omitted when their attention was consumed by more complex content and use concerns.

In keeping with the preceding principle regarding the integration of the systems of content, form, and use, a language intervention plan must also include more naturalistic activities for keeping language relevant and communicative. Language interaction opportunities work best for developing aspects of language use, and language content is generally acquired through direct experiences with the objects and relationships it represents. Combined with more structured activities to develop the form of a language-disordered child's communication repertoire, naturalistic activities provide the experiences for integrating the systems of content, form, and use and allowing them to be stabilized.

Involvement of Others

Language intervention should involve others in the environment. Language is not learned in isolation, but in meaningful contexts in communication with others. Regular and special education teachers are important assets in all stages of the language intervention process. A speech-language pathologist may act as a consultant, giving specific suggestions about how to include the forms and content which have been the target of special language intervention activities into the daily routine of the classroom. Using the content of the classroom for language intervention activities offers an alternative approach for utilization of this same integrative principle. Perhaps the most important steps to be taken involve leading teachers to recognize that language is not something that can be relegated to an hour or half-hour of the daily schedule, but is an integral part of all other activities.

Parents are also essential partners in the language intervention process. Ongoing communication avenues need to be established to keep parents involved in all stages of the program. This involvement ranges from participation in formal meetings to regular feedback and suggestions about ways parents can use natural opportunities to facilitate acquisition of targeted language skills and general communicative ability.

Practice in Context

Language intervention should emphasize opportunity for the practice of language in forms and contexts that are as intact as possible. Specific processing abilities, such as memory span for related or unrelated syllables, or discrimination of individual phonemes, and other auditory and visual perceptual skills are often impaired in association with disordered language development. It is tempting to focus on such "splinter skills" in remediation on the assumption that their improvement may be prerequisite to further language acquisition. However, the evidence for the success of this type of approach has been disappointing (Bloom & Lahey, 1978; Hammill & Larsen, 1974). It is unclear whether such isolated symptoms are involved more as causes or as effects of language disorders. There is as much evidence that effective language users apply language skill to assist in solving perceptual tasks as vice versa (Smith, 1973, 1975).

These findings imply that if the goal is to improve reading skill, students should read rather than perform activities thought to underlie reading. Similarly, if the goal is to improve syntactic structure, students should practice using the targeted syntactic structures rather than recalling or discriminating unrelated items. The uniqueness of intervention should involve the careful selection of stimulus materials and practice activities rather than breaking skills down to levels of underlying processes.

Developmental Validity

Language intervention should follow normal developmental stages unless clear justification exists for doing otherwise. One of the most obviously valid bases for sequencing the steps in language intervention is the information on normal developmental stages. Earlier developing forms, content, and uses of language can be expected to be learned more easily by children who are having difficulty learning language just as they are by younger children learning language normally. However, one of the findings of researchers who have attempted to differentiate language disorders from language delay has been that development in language-disordered children may be uneven across realms (Leonard, 1972). Some language-disordered children seem to have difficulty using earlier developing forms during the same stages when they have acquired partial control of skills usually mastered later in normal development.

In some instances, these later developing skills may be used to support development in areas in which a child is experiencing difficulty. For example, children who have developed a sizable vocabulary may use that vocabulary to help identify words as they read a paragraph. However, if other decoding skills are not developed at a commensurate level, the stronger skills may actually interfere with the application of the weaker ones. The only reason to discourage children from using the comprehension strategy for reading would be if they were using it to the *exclusion* of any other approach, and making semantic substitution errors as a result. Then, the best intervention plan might involve two types of activities. In one activity, they would be given practice in making sound-symbol associations and using those skills to identify nonsense or real words for which no contextual cues were available. At some other time in the day, in another activity, experience stories might be used to encourage a comprehension-based reading approach even though some words might be misidentified. As skills developed, a third activity could be introduced to lead children to focus alternatively on form and content in order to arrive at accurate meanings.

Although children may demonstrate uneven development *across* the realms of content and form, similar problems may occur *within* one of the realms of content, form, or use. For example, a child who is using complex sentence forms may show restriction of earlier developing forms when doing so. Muma (1973) has called these *co-occurring restricted structures,* in that when a sentence requires the application of two or more rules that are at a child's developing level of competence, the increased complexity of the task may lead to at least one of the rules being restricted. Lee (1974) commented on the increased likelihood of language-impaired children to show "grammatical overload." Program planning for children who show such characteristics might involve careful sequencing of activities designed to elicit the earlier developing morphemes in sentences and situations with graduated increments of complexity, until finally requiring simultaneous use of the earlier and later developing forms.

In a final example, violation of normal developmental sequences might be justified in some instances when more than one modality is involved. In normal development, the acquisition of listening and speaking skills is generally thought to precede learning to read and write. However, for some children, later developing skills may be used to help them acquire earlier ones that are deficient or disordered (Nelson, 1981). Consider the child who demonstrates multiple articulation and speech-sound discrimination problems. Such a child may be helped to hear and say the sequence of sounds in syllables, and syllables in words, by learning to associate written symbols with acoustic and motokinesthetic input. The association method, which was originally developed by McGinnis (1963), and has since been adapted by Monsees (1972), offers such an approach. In this approach, children are given multiple opportunities to make sound-symbol associations in controlled environments. Intensive experiences in reading and writing first sounds, and later words and sentences, give children skills in hearing and saying language structures they would otherwise be unable to process.

These six guiding principles are not unique to language intervention in school settings. They are a part of good clinical practice in any setting. The regulatory requirements of PL 94–142 are particularly tied to school services, but they should be used to help facilitate, not interfere with, the implementation of these six guiding principles. The integration of principles and procedures is illustrated by the following case example, drawn from the author's professional experiences in the school setting.

CASE STUDY

The case report presented here was written for the annual review of a 4-year 11-month-old child I shall call Alison. Alison had been placed for 5 months in a new self-contained classroom program for learning- and language-impaired preschool children operated by Berrien County Intermediate School District in Michigan. An unusual amount of formalized pre- and posttesting was completed for this child in a short period of time as part of an evaluation plan to determine whether the classroom itself, which was experimental at the time, should be continued. This case provides an example not only of procedures undertaken for an individual child, but also exemplifies part of the procedures undertaken within a school district to extend the continuum of services to speech- and language-impaired students.

Background

Alison was seen by the speech-language consultant after she refused to speak out loud on her first two diagnostic visits to the preschool diagnostic team. When she continued to refuse to talk on the third visit, her parents were requested to tape record a sample of Alison's spontaneous speech for the examiners to use to observe her communicative skills.

It was found that Alison's speech consisted of short sentences with many omitted function words, syllables, and phonemes. Poor word boundaries added to the unintelligibility of Alison's speech and made it sound almost jargonic at times. The earlier developmental history included reports of a difficult birth, a number of health problems including a severe burn, and long hospital stays.

Program Objectives and Progress

In the Speech and Language Preschool Classroom, Alison was provided learning opportunities with varying degrees of structure to work toward the following performance objectives. Results after 5 months in the program are reported for each objective.

1. *Phonology*
   a. Alison will produce the target phonemes from at least five "semantically potent words" (Hillard & Goepfert, 1979) spontaneously, each in at least two nondrill

words in conversation with the teacher. Accomplished as of June, 1982 for the target phonemes /w/, /j/, /tʃ/, /ou/, /ai/, /t/, and /n/.

b. Alison will show improvement on a standard articulation test beyond that which could be attributed to normal development. Accomplished as of May, 1982 (see summary of test results below).

2. *Morphology and Syntax*
   a. Alison will converse with an adult using complete sentences (where required) with an increased mean length of utterance beyond that which would be expected due to normal development. Accomplished as of July, 1982. Alison made 4 months gain in 3 months time on Lee's (1974) Developmental Sentence Scoring and moved from Level III to IV on Tyack and Gottsleben's (1977) Word-Morpheme Index.
3. *Semantics and Cognition*
   a. Alison will correctly point to objects illustrating at least five new concept words on posttest as compared to pretest with the locally designed Berrien County Intermediate School District (BCISD) vocabulary assessment instrument. Accomplished as of July, 1982. Alison responded correctly on only 75% of conceptual vocabulary items during pretesting, but she was correct on all 92 items (100%) on the posttest. Alison does continue to show some problems in answering complex questions with responses in the appropriate semantic category. Rather than answering questions directly, she frequently changes the topic.
4. *Pragmatics*
   a. Alison will communicate verbally (in an audible voice) with at least two newly introduced adults. Accomplished as of May, 1982, when Alison had helped deliver milk money to the school secretary and had talked to the school psychologist, who had come to visit the classroom.
   b. Alison will refuse to respond to no more than two direct questions in a 10-minute conversation with the teacher. Accomplished as of June, 1982.

Formal Test Results

Test Name	*Pretest Scores (March, 1982 age 4 yrs. 6 mos.) Raw Score*	*Age Score*	*% Correct*	*Posttest Scores (July, 1982 age 4 yrs. 11 mos.) Raw Score*	*Age Score*	*% Correct*
Carrow Test of Auditory Comprehension of Language	70	4;8		74	5;3	
Sequenced Inventory of Communication Development	rec:85/102 exp:103/125	3;4 3;0	83 82	92/102 112/125	3;4 3;8	90 90
Goldman-Fristoe Test of Articulation	40/61		67	50/61		82
Developmental Sentence Score (DSS)	4.06	2;8		5.25	3;2	
Mean Length of Utterance (in morphemes)	3.39	3;8		4.54	4;0	
Tyack and Gottsleben Word-Morpheme Index	3.45	Level III		4.40	Level IV	
Berrlen County Intermediate School District Test of Conceptual Vocabulary	69/92		75	92/92		100

Summary

Alison has made excellent progress during the 5 months she has been enrolled in the program. Raw scores for all of the measurement areas showed noticeable increases, and age scores for a number of the tests showed increases greater than the number of months Alison has been in the program. Her expressive language scores, measured as mean length of utterance in morphemes, Developmental Sentence Score, and Word-Morpheme Index, all showed an increase of greater than one unit. As Alison's sentences become longer and more complex, it is expected that those in her environment will experience a period of increased difficulty in understanding her until such time as her word boundaries and phonological productions become clearer. This possibility should be interpreted to her parents.

Recommendations

1. *Placement*

At the time of the team meeting, July 18, 1982, it was the consensus of the professionals involved that Alison should remain in the Language Preschool for one year, given her parents' permission. Although the option to attend kindergarten in the fall was available, the team made this recommendation because (*a*) Alison's birthday (August 18, 1977) is late, (*b*) she spent so many early months ill and hospitalized, (*c*) she continued to have expressive language skills at least one year below her chronological age, and (*d*) she was making good progress in the program. Following one more year in the special program, it is felt that Alison will probably be ready for regular kindergarten with intermittent speech and language intervention services.

2. *Further speech and language intervention should be directed toward*

a. Diagnostic teaching to determine the extent to which Alison has difficulty comprehending complex sentences.

b. Improving the clarity of Alison's individual words while working within her existing sentence length.

c. Increasing the use of subject noun phrases which tend to be omitted or transposed (e.g., "and be bad that too, everybody!"). The Fokes Sentence Builder might be useful in this area (Fokes, n.d.).

d. Eliminating the immature phonological processes of cluster reduction and syllable deletion. The Semantically Potent Word Approach (Hillard & Goepfert, 1979) should be used with emphasis on words which will help her eliminate the previous processes. This approach has been used successfully in the past to help Alison reduce the phonological omissions of initial and final consonants.

SUMMARY

This chapter provides a comprehensive, though abbreviated, view of the provision of language intervention in the schools. It ends as it began, with primary emphasis on the provision of meaningful language-learning opportunities designed to meet the needs of individual children, and with a secondary emphasis on the use of federal and state regulations to do so. When greater emphasis is placed on compliance with regulations, service to children becomes incidental, and needs for individualized education may not be met.

To be effective, speech-language pathologists in schools are encouraged to become involved with children's educational experiences at all levels. This involvement includes becoming more knowledgeable about local, state, and federal regulations and the political process for changing them in instances in which they are counterproductive to providing appropriate services. Membership in professional associations provides a mechanism for staying informed and for facilitating awareness of the needs of speech- and language-impaired children.

Perhaps the most consistent characteristic of the practice of speech-language pathology in school settings is the breadth of knowledge it demands of the professional. Rarely can one afford to become a specialist in any one area. Language-impaired children in schools may have voice problems, experience fluency difficulties, be motorically unable to learn intelligible speech, be severely delayed in all areas, fail to exhibit social awareness of others, be awkward in asking for assistance from teachers and peers—among countless other possibilities. A solid knowledge of communicative behaviors, a sensitivity and flexibility in working with people, and an ability to establish and work toward goals are perhaps the most critical skills a speech-language pathologist can bring to a position in a school setting.

A number of problems associated with the provision of services in school settings remain to be solved. Among these are needs to increase the precision of determining which students qualify for language intervention programs; to expand the continuum of service delivery models in all areas of the country, both rural and urban; to clarify the role of the speech-language pathologist in evaluating and serving severely and multiply handicapped individuals; to foster awareness of the professional skills of speech-language pathologists and audiologists; and, to ensure that regulations, including those relating to caseload size, will allow professional skills to be practiced. Meeting these needs, along with the need to enhance basic understanding of language and communication disorders and ways to remediate them is the challenge of the coming years.

STUDY QUESTIONS

1. In what ways is language intervention in school settings unique, and in what ways should it be similar to the provision of services in other settings?
2. List the sequential steps for placing a child in a special education program and for planning, implementing, and reviewing an I.E.P.
3. What are some guiding principles for planning language intervention regardless of setting, and how might the school setting be used to plan intervention activities using these principles?
4. What are the levels of regulatory influence on the provision of programs in school settings, and what should the role of the speech-language pathologist be in attempting to ensure that the regulatory influences are facilitative?
5. Formulate two well-written short-term objectives for each of the goal areas that have been identified for the following two children:
   A. A mentally retarded 7-year-old who needs to develop:
      1. Use of plural and possessive morphological endings
      2. Comprehension and production of constructions with three or more components (e.g., agent + action + object, and agent + action + location).

B. A 6th-grade language/learning-impaired student who needs to develop:
   1. Ability to comprehend and produce complex sentence forms (e.g., with the conjunctions *since, while, if . . . then, because,* and *except*)
   2. Ability to organize ideas and present them orally or in writing
   3. Ability to recognize and use abstract and multiple word meanings associated with other academic areas.

BIBLIOGRAPHY

ASHA. (1984). Committee on language, speech, and hearing services in the schools. Guidelines for caseload size for speech-language services in the schools. *Asha, 26,* 53–58.

Bloom, L., & Lahey, M. (1978). *Language development and language disorders.* New York: Wiley.

Broen, P. (1972). The verbal environment of the language learning child. *Monograph 17.* Washington, DC: The American Speech and Hearing Association.

Carrow, E. (1973). *Test for auditory comprehension of language.* Austin, TX: Learning Concepts.

Fokes, J. (no date). *Fokes sentence builder.* Boston, MA: Teaching Resources.

Goldman, R., & Fristoe, M. (1970). *The Goldman-Fristoe test of articulation.* Circle Pines, MN: American Guidance Service.

Goodman, K.S. (1973). Psycholinguistic universals in the reading process. In F. Smith (Ed.), *Psycholinguistics and reading* (pp. 21–27). New York: Holt, Rinehart, & Winston.

Hammill, D., & Larsen, S. (1974). The effectiveness of psycholinguistic training. *Exceptional Children, 40,* 5–13.

Hedrick, D., Prather, E., & Tobin, A. (1975). *Sequenced inventory of communication development.* Seattle, WA: University of Washington Press.

Hillard, S.W., & Goepfert, L.P. (1979). Articulation training: A new perspective. *Language, Speech and Hearing Services in Schools, 10,* 145–151.

Johnston, J.R. (1982). Narratives: A new look at communication problems in older language-disordered children. *Language, Speech and Hearing Services in Schools, 13,* 144–155.

Lasky, E.Z., & Klopp, K. (1982). Parent-child interactions in normal and language-disordered children. *Journal of Speech and Hearing Disorders, 47,* 7–18.

Lee, L.L. (1974). *Developmental sentence analysis.* Evanston, IL: Northwestern University Press.

Leonard, L. (1972). What is deviant language? *Journal of Speech and Hearing Disorders, 37,* 427–447.

McGinnis, M. (1963). *Aphasic children.* Washington, DC: Alexander Graham Bell Association.

Miller, J.F., & Chapman, R.S. (1983). Systematic Analysis of Language Transcripts (SALT). Software and users' manual. Madison: University of Wisconsin.

Monsees, E.K. (1972). *Structured language for children with special language learning problems.* Washington, DC: Children's Hospital of District of Columbia.

Muma, J. (1973). Language assessment: The co-occurring and restricted structure procedure. *Acta Symbolica, 4:* 12–29.

Nelson, N.W. (1979). *Planning individualized speech and language intervention programs.* Tucson, AZ: Communication Skill Builders.

Nelson, N.W. (1981). An eclectic model of language intervention for disorders of listening, speaking, reading and writing. *Topics in Language Disorders, 1:* 1–24.

Nelson, N.W. (1984). Beyond information processing: The language of teachers and textbooks. In G. Wallach & K. Butler (Eds.), *Language learn-*

ing disabilities in children (pp. 154–178). Baltimore, MD: Williams & Wilkins.

Nelson, N.W., Silbar, J.C., & Lockwood, E.L. (1981, November). *The Michigan decision-making strategy for determining appropriate communicative services for physically and/or mentally handicapped children.* Paper presented at the annual conference of the American Speech-Language-Hearing Association, Los Angeles, CA.

Public Law 94–142. (1977, August). Implementation of Part B of the Education of the Handicapped Act. *Federal Register.*

Slobin, D.I. (1971). *Psycholinguistics.* Danville, IL: Scott, Foresman.

Smith, F. (1973). *Psycholinguistics and reading.* New York: Holt, Rinehart & Winston.

Smith, F. (1975). *Comprehension and learning.* New York: Holt, Rinehart & Winston.

Snow, C. (1977). The development of conversation between mothers and babies. *Journal of Child Language, 4,* 1–22.

Tyack, D., & Gottsleben, R. (1977). *Language sampling, analysis and training: A handbook for teachers and clinicians* (2nd ed.) Palo Alto, CA: Consulting Psychologists Press.

Westby, C. E. (1982). Cognitive and linguistic aspects of children's narrative development. *Communicative Disorders, 7,* 1–16.

REFERENCE CHART

FOR MAKING DECISIONS ABOUT SPEECH AND LANGUAGE PROGRAMMING FOR SEVERELY PHYSICALLY AND/OR MENTALLY HANDICAPPED CHILDREN

COGNITIVE BASES	RECEPTIVE LANGUAGE
Preintentional (Birth to 8 months) *Sensorimotor stages I, II, III* ☐ Little evidence of goal oriented actions at beginning of period ☐ Assimilates new objects into reflex exercises ☐ Explores objects by mouthing or banging ☐ By end of period infant moves from being purely reflexive to showing the initial beginnings of goal oriented behavior ☐ Gradually develops object permanence ☐ Early: eyes focus on empty space where object was when it is dropped; fails to look under scarf for object ☐ Later: eyes follow object as it is moved; looks under scarf for hidden object	*Precursors* ☐ Startles to noise ☐ Orients to sound source ☐ Looks at person who calls name
Early Intentional (8 to 12 months) *Sensorimotor IV* ☐ Uses familiar means to achieve novel ends (tries to repeat or prolong an effect he/she has discovered) ☐ Imitates ongoing actions already in repertoire (e.g., pattycake, kiss mommy, peekaboo) ☐ Object permanence now established (looks for object previously seen) ☐ Looks at pictures in a book with adult ☐ Stares to gain information ☐ Reacts in anticipation prior to familiar event	*Precursors* (strategies used prior to actual linguistic comprehension) ☐ Looks at objects that mother looks at ☐ Acts on objects noticed ☐ Imitates ongoing action or sound if it is already within repertoire ☐ Laughs at familiar interaction sequences ☐ Inhibits action in response to "no" ☐ Responds to "bye-bye" ☐ Follows caretaker's gaze to common objects when labelled
Late Intentional (12 to 18 months) *Sensorimotor V* ☐ Uses novel means to achieve familiar ends (e.g. communicative gestures and stereotyped vocalization used to achieve adult attention, particular object, object's removal) ☐ Figures out ways to overcome some obstacles (opens door, reaches high objects)	*Lexical comprehension* ☐ Understands one word in some sentences when referents are present ☐ Points to objects in response to "Show me___." (e.g. body parts) *Nonverbal comprehension strategies* used to respond to commands: ☐ Attend to object mentioned ☐ Give evidence of notice ☐ Do what is usually done in a situation
Representational Thought (18–24 months) *Sensorimotor VI* ☐ Begins to replace sensorimotor grouping of previous stages with internalized problem solving using images, memories, and symbols to represent actions and objects	*Lexical comprehension* ☐ Understanding of words when referent is not present ☐ Understanding of action verbs out of routine context; carries out two-word commands, but often fails to understand three lexical elements ☐ Understanding of routine forms of questions for agent, object, locative, and action *Nonverbal comprehension strategies* used to respond to commands: ☐ Locate the objects mentioned ☐ Give evidence of notice ☐ Do what you usually do: objects into containers, conventional use ☐ Act on the objects in the way mentioned ☐ Child as agent

Note: Columns and boxes of Reference Chart correspond to those of the Summary Chart in Figures 12-2, 12-3a, and 12-3b.

REFERENCE CHART

FOR MAKING DECISIONS ABOUT SPEECH AND LANGUAGE PROGRAMMING
FOR SEVERELY PHYSICALLY AND/OR MENTALLY HANDICAPPED CHILDREN (Continued)

COGNITIVE BASES	RECEPTIVE LANGUAGE
Early Preoperations (2 to 3½ yrs) ☐ Arranges objects in patterns but not in categories ☐ Initiates drawing of verticle line (by 30 mo) ☐ Imitates drawing of horizontal line and circle (by 36 mos) ☐ Matches identical objects ☐ Draws 2 or more lines imitating a cross (by 3½ yrs) ☐ Copies short line of beads by matching individual items but fails to put them in correct order, getting only adjacent pairs correct ☐ Matches similar objects ☐ Ability to represent one thing by another increases speed and range of thinking, particularly as language develops, but thinking remains tied closely to actions ☐ Thought is preconceptual; inferences sometimes but not always correct	*Lexical comprehension* ☐ Accepts or rejects, confirms or denies in response to yes/no questions ☐ 2½ yrs. ☐ What for object ☐ What-do for action ☐ Where for location (place) ☐ 3 yrs. ☐ Whose for possessor ☐ Who for person ☐ Why for cause or reason ☐ How many for number ☐ Understanding of gender contrasts in third person pronouns ☐ 2–3 yrs–*Comprehension strategies* ☐ Does what is usually done ☐ Probable location strategy for in, on, under, beside ☐ Probable event strategy for simple active reversible sentences ☐ Supplies missing information (2 years) ☐ Supply explanation (3 years) ☐ Infers most probable speech act in context ☐ Sequence for understanding Wh-questions
Late preoperations (3½ to 7 yrs) ☐ Applies systematic trial and error problem solving strategies to classification and seriation tasks ☐ Sorts set of blocks varying in size, shape, and color into 2 piles on basis of single attribute (50% can do by age 3½) ☐ Places seven blocks varying in height in order and places 3 missing blocks in sequences (50% can do by age 4½) ☐ Begins differentiating open and closed shapes in drawings, and squares may have corners (by age 4½) ☐ Develop concepts of time and space ☐ Identifies one of three pictures not in the same category ☐ Matches pictures that "go together" ☐ Draws person with 2 parts ☐ Copies square (by age 4½) ☐ Cuts and pastes—may finish project next day ☐ Copies triangle (by age 5) ☐ Draws person with body, arms, legs, feet, nose, and eyes	*Lexical comprehension* ☐ Understands contrasts for topological locatives (in, on, under, beside) ☐ Answers how questions with manner or instrument responses ("What do we eat with") ☐ Comprehension of word order as cues to understand agent-object in active sentences (word order strategy) ☐ Responds to two-stage action commands
Concrete Operations (7 to 12 years) ☐ Formation of series and classes takes place mentally; physical actions are internalized as mental actions or 'operations' ☐ Classifies in two ways at once (e.g., can sort by both color and shape in matrix) ☐ Still solves problems primarily through trial and error rather than establishing general rules and testing hypotheses ☐ Able to correct misconceptions through discussion	☐ Understanding of conditional conjunctions *if* and *when* (usual rather than logical sense) ☐ Probable relation of events strategy for causal conjunctions ☐ Understanding of causal conjunctions *because* and *so* (8 years) ☐ Understanding of contractive conjunctions *but* and *although* as though they mean *and* (8 years) ☐ Contrastive conjunctions *but* and *although* (10 years)

REFERENCE CHART

FOR MAKING DECISIONS ABOUT SPEECH AND LANGUAGE PROGRAMMING
FOR SEVERELY PHYSICALLY AND/OR MENTALLY HANDICAPPED CHILDREN (Continued)

EXPRESSIVE LANGUAGE	SOCIAL INTERACTION & PLAY
Precursors ☐ Undifferentiated cry ☐ Reflexive vocalizations and comfort sounds	☐ Stares at large masses ☐ Grasps object placed in hand ☐ Makes eye contact briefly ☐ Quiets when picked up ☐ Actively seeks sound source ☐ Looks intently and shakes toy in hand ☐ Smiles at mirror image, familiar faces ☐ Sobers at sight of strangers ☐ Increases activity at sight of toy, familiar caretaker ☐ Works for toy out of reach ☐ Returns to activity after interruption
Precursors ☐ Differentiated cries ☐ Syllabic babbling ☐ Communication games ☐ Intentional action	☐ Responds to facial expressions ☐ Frequently cries when parent leaves room ☐ Drinks from cup, feeds self crackers ☐ Imitates arm movements for games like peekaboo, pattycake ☐ Squeezes toy to make it squeak ☐ Drops toys and watches them fall ☐ Puts small objects in and out of container ☐ Stacks rings on peg ☐ Holds crayon, imitates scribbling ☐ Cooperates in dressing ☐ Kisses, waves, holds out hands
First words ☐ Performatives (gesture accompanies vocalization or word) ☐ Hi/bye routines ☐ Comment ☐ Request object or attention ☐ Reject ☐ Communicates immediate needs by pulling or pointing	☐ Reacts to emotions of others ☐ Solitary or onlooker play, self play ☐ Scribbles spontaneously with crayon ☐ Points to objects he/she wants and claims certain objects as own ☐ Imitates sweeping, hair combing ☐ Hugs doll, pulls toy
Transition to two word combination ☐ New semantic roles ☐ Early: action-object relations; agent, action, object, recurrence, disappearance ☐ Later: object-object relations; location, possession, nonexistence ☐ Asks a "What's that" question ☐ Answers some routine questions ☐ Rapid acquisition of vocabulary ☐ Successive one-word utterances ☐ Increased frequency of talking ☐ Onset of two-word utterances (MLU 1.5)	☐ Parallel play (near others but not with them) ☐ Talks to self while playing ☐ Little social give and take—hugs, pushes, pulls, snatches, grabs, but pays little attention to what others say or do ☐ Relates action to object or another person—washes, feeds doll in addition to self ☐ Listens to short story ☐ Demonstrates pleasure in make believe games (e.g. 2 sticks to represent "airplane")
Typ *Age* Brown's *Stage* *New Development* — MLU *(morph)* 2 ☐ I Basic semantic relations — 1.75 ☐ Agent-action ☐ Existence ☐ Action-object ☐ Recurrence ☐ Agent-object ☐ Nonexistence ☐ Possessive ☐ Rejection ☐ Entity-locative ☐ Denial ☐ Action-locative ☐ Attributive ☐ II Grammatical inflections — 2.25 ☐ Some articles, plurals, possessives ☐ -ing on verbs ☐ What doing? questions 2½ ☐ III Differention of sentence — 2.75 ☐ Modalities ☐ Possession ☐ Number (noun plural) ☐ Locative containment and support (in, on) ☐ Temporary duration (ing)	☐ Parallel play predominates (24 mos) ☐ Dramatization, imagination and symbolic play (make believe and pretend) ☐ Takes turns ☐ Watches cartoons on TV ☐ Associative group play begins (3½ yrs) ☐ Organizes doll furniture accurately and plays imaginatively ☐ Builds bridge from model

REFERENCE CHART

FOR MAKING DECISIONS ABOUT SPEECH AND LANGUAGE PROGRAMMING
FOR SEVERELY PHYSICALLY AND/OR MENTALLY HANDICAPPED CHILDREN (Continued)

EXPRESSIVE LANGUAGE	SOCIAL INTERACTION & PLAY
Typ Brown's MLU *Age Stage New Development (morph)* 3 □ IV Sentence embedding 3.50 □ Immediate future (gonna) □ Regular past -ed □ Inflects verb *be* (am, was, are)	
Brown's Stage V (by approx. 3½ years) □ Sentence Conjoining □ Regular past -ed 3.75 □ Third pers. singular *Event relations* (sequence of emergence from 3½ to 7 years) □ And (coordinate and temporal) □ Because, so (causal) □ But (contrastive) □ When (conditional) □ While (simultaneity) □ After □ Before □ Past time (-ed) □ Possibility (might) *Syntactic rule emergence from 4 to 6 years* □ N + cont + cop + PN/PA/loc (He's sick) □ There expleture (There is a table) □ Pos + N + V (Jim's dog bites) □ Adj + N + V (The big truck rolled) □ N + N + V (Joe and Jim race cars) □ Reflexive (He sees himself) □ S becomes S (He went because he wanted to) □ S + V + indirect + N (He gave her a book) □ When S + S (When I go to town, I will buy an ice cream cone) □ Obligatory & emphatic do (He does not feel good. He does feel good) □ Noninversion of aux/modal (Where daddy is?) □ Aux/modal + aux modal (How can he can look? Is that's a rocket?) □ Continued use of double negation. Some problems in the truth value of negatives. □ Continued regularization of regular forms. *Syntactic rule emergence from 6 to 7 years* □ Passive transform (The boy was hit by the girl) □ If transformation (If it rains, we won't go) □ N + V + particle (I like eating) □ S/V concord (He likes candy) □ Pronominalization (John knew he would win the race. He knew John would win the race) □ Inversion of aux/modal + main V (When's going to be the party?) □ Noninversion of aux/modal (Where she's going?)	□ Increased dramatization in play □ Suggests turns, but often bossy □ Plays in group of 2 to 3 children □ Shows off □ Friendships stronger □ Plays in groups of 2 to 5 □ Able to play games by rules (by age 6) □ Spends hours at one activity □ Demands more realism in play (age 7)
Marks of maturity in language □ Longer sentences □ More clauses per sentence—8th graders use 150% more than 4th graders □ Use of adverbial clauses (He was sleeping when I walked in the door) □ Use of adjective clauses (The man with the broken foot limped along the highway) □ Nominals (Flying airplanes is fun) □ Sentence complements (They elected Jim president) □ Infinitive complements (He told Jim to feed the dog) □ Reduction of mazes and tangles (characteristic of younger children who begin a sentence which does not fulfill a communication unit and eventually drop it as if it is beyond them.) □ Uses language to converse, persuade, tease	□ Genuine cooperation with others replaces isolated play or play 'in the company of others' □ Reduction in imaginary play but development of theatrical entertainment □ Makes accurate replicas and working models □ Enjoys categorizing collections of various sorts

References

Beard, R.M. *An Outline of Piaget's Developmental Psychology for Students and Teachers.* New York: Basic Books, 1969.

Brandt, A., Berlin, C., Cunningham, R., Gisier, P., and Radke, A. *The Classroom Language Inventory.* Wayne, MI: Wayne County Intermediate School District, 1979. Contact: E.L. Lockwood, WCISD, 33500 Van Born Road, Wayne, MI 48184.

Chapman, R.S. and Miller, J.F. Analyzing language and communication in the child. In *Nonspeech Language and Communication* (Ed. by R.L. Shiefelbusch) Baltimore: University Park Press, 1980.

Fokes, J. Developmental periods and stages. (unpublished paper) Athens, OH: Ohio U., 1977.

Gard, A., Gilman, L. and Groman, J. *Speech and Language Development Chart.* Salt Lake City, UT: Word Making Productions, 1980.

McLean, J.E. and Snyder-McLean, L.K. *A Transactional Approach to Early Language Training.* Columbus, OH: Charles E. Merrill Publishing Co., 1978.

Nelson, N.W. *Planning Individualized Speech and Language Intervention Programs.* Tucson, AZ: Communication Skill Builders, Inc., 1979.

Project Perform: TMI/SMI Instructional System. Developed by Ingham Intermediate School District (Project Director, Audrey Gowman) 1979. Contact: Audrey Gowman, Project Director, 625 Hagedorn Road, Ingham Developmental Center, Mason, Michigan 48854 (517) 676-3409.

Yoder, D. Communicative competence. (Unpublished papers.) Madison, WI: U. Wisconsin-Madison, 1978, 1980.

Author Index

Subject Index

About the Authors

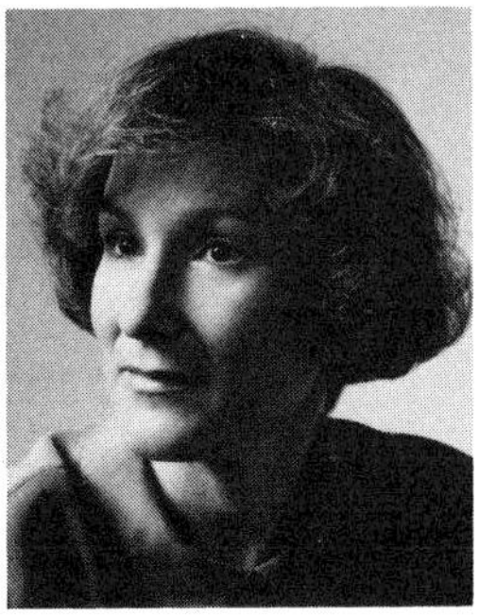

Deena K. Bernstein received her Ph. D. from the Department of Speech and Hearing Science of the City University of New York. She is a professor in the Department of Speech and Theater of the Herbert H. Lehman College of the institution. Her professional writings appear in both national and regional journals, and she lectures extensively throughout the United States and abroad. She is active in professional organizations, state and national committee work, continuing education, and teacher training.

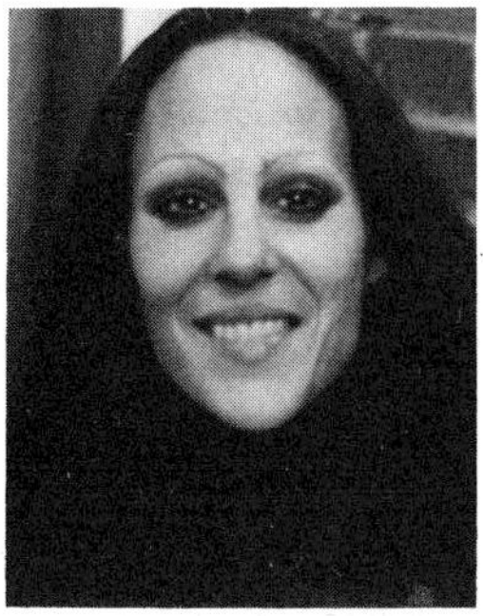

Ellenmorris Tiegerman is an associate professor at Adelphi University and Director of the Speech and Hearing Center and the Preschool Language Program. She received her doctorate in the Department of Speech and Language Pathology from the City University of New York. She has written several books and journal articles reflecting her interest in language acquisition of language-disordered and autistic children. She has made many presentations throughout the United States and is an active member of several professional organizations.

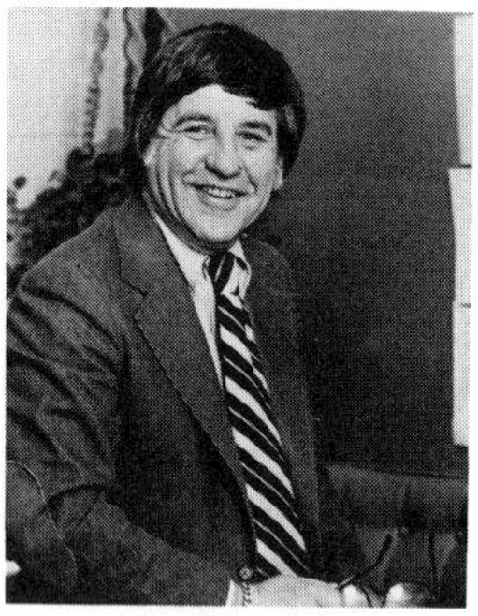

James E. McLean is a senior scientist with the Bureau of Child Research at the University of Kansas and is Director of the Parsons Research Center. His research and publications have focused on language acquisition and intervention strategies and phonological learning. He received his doctorate from the University of Kansas.

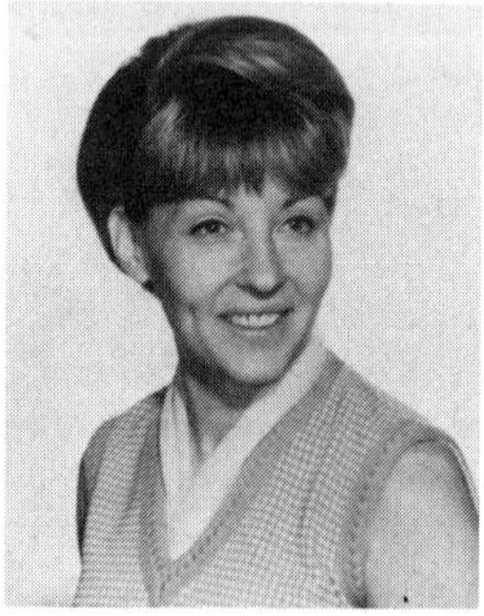

Pearl L. Seidenberg is an associate professor at the C.W. Post Campus of Long Island University. She received her Ed. D. from Yeshiva University. She has published many papers and articles and has presented many seminars on exceptional children, learning disabilities, and public policy.

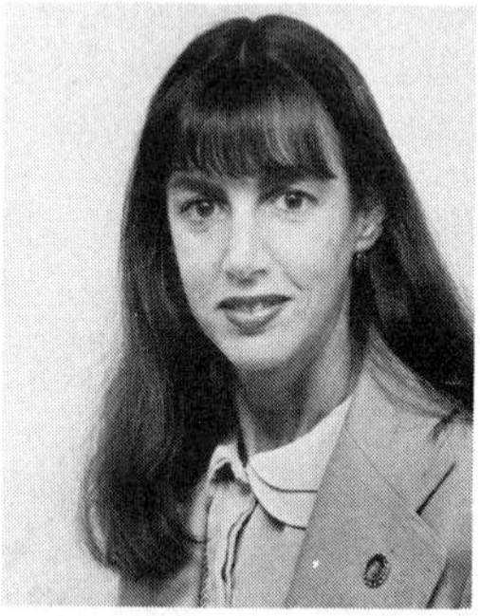

Joan Braverman-Callahan received her Ph. D. in Speech Pathology and Audiology from Adelphi University where she is currently an assistant professor in the Department of Speech Arts and Communicative Disorders. She is Coordinator of Deaf Education and the Mobile Hearing Unit and Supervisor of Adult Speechreading and Auditory Training at that institution. She is also a consultant to the New York City Board of Education. She is presently engaged in the application of computer literacy to deaf education programs.

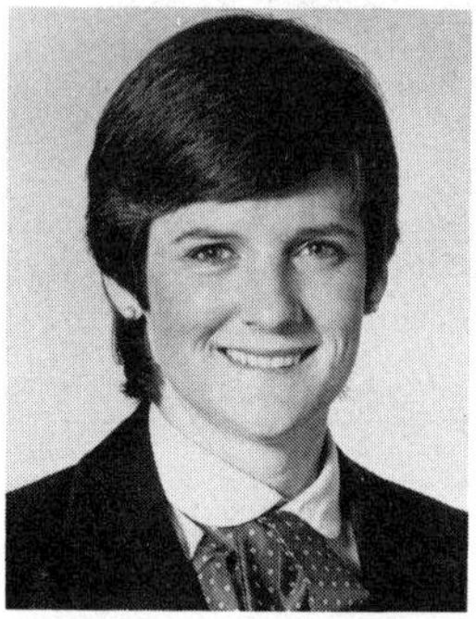

Nickola Wolf Nelson is an associate professor of Speech Pathology and Audiology at Western Michigan University. She received her doctorate from Wichita University. She is the author of *Planning Individualized Speech and Language Intervention Programs,* as well as several book chapters and journal articles. She has lectured throughout the United States and Canada.

Christine K. Radziewicz is an instructor in the Department of Speech Arts and Communicative Disorders at Adelphi University where she is pursuing her Ph. D. She is currently involved in the use of videotapes in training the parents of hearing-impaired children.

Sharon L. James is an associate professor of Communicative Disorders at Syracuse University. She received her graduate degrees from the University of Wisconsin. She is an associate editor of the *Journal of Speech and Hearing Research* and an active writer and lecturer.

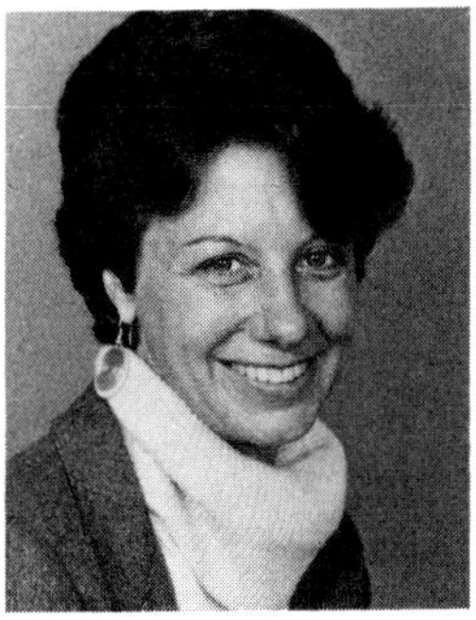

Robert E. Owens, Jr. is an associate professor and the graduate program director in the Department of Speech Pathology and Audiology at the State University of New York at Geneseo. He has published several articles, has made many presentations at professional conferences and workshops, and is the author of *Language Development: An Introduction,* published by Charles E. Merrill. He received his doctorate from the Ohio State University.

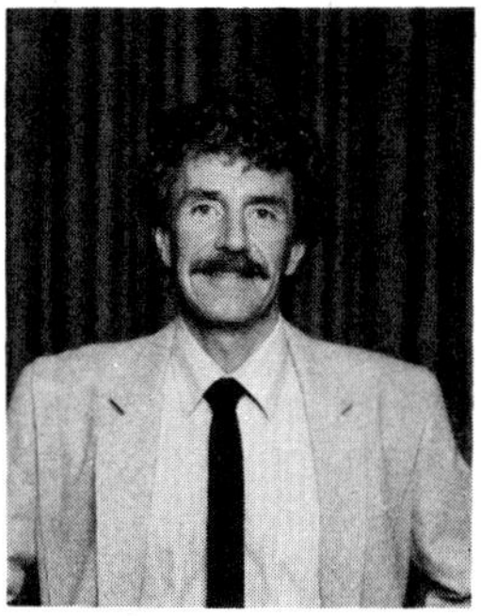